PHYSICAL ACTIVITY
AND
MENTAL HEALTH

PHYSICAL ACTIVITY
AND
MENTAL HEALTH

Angela Clow, PhD

Sarah Edmunds, PhD

University of Westminster

• EDITORS •

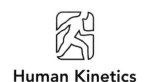

Human Kinetics

Library of Congress Cataloging-in-Publication Data

Physical activity and mental health / Angela Clow, Sarah Edmunds, editors.
      p. ; cm.
  Includes bibliographical references and index.
  ISBN 978-1-4504-3433-1 (print) -- ISBN 1-4504-3433-9 (print)
  I. Clow, Angela. II. Edmunds, Sarah, PhD.
  [DNLM: 1. Exercise--psychology. 2. Exercise Therapy--psychology. 3. Mental Disorders--prevention & control. 4. Mental Disorders--therapy. 5. Mental Health. QT 255]
  RM725
  615.8'2--dc23
                                        2013006538
ISBN-10: 1-4504-3433-9 (print)
ISBN-13: 978-1-4504-3433-1 (print)

The web addresses cited in this text were current as of June 2013, unless otherwise noted.

Acquisitions Editor: Myles Schrag; **Developmental Editors:** Judy Parks and Melissa Zavala; **Assistant Editors:** Casey Gentis, Jan Feeney, and Tyler Wolpert; **Copyeditor:** Amanda Eastin-Allen; **Indexer:** Alisha Jeddeloh; **Permissions Manager:** Dalene Reeder; **Graphic Designer:** Fred Starbird; **Graphic Artist:** Kathleen Boudreau-Fuoss; **Cover Designer:** Dawn Sills; **Photo Asset Manager:** Laura Fitch; **Visual Production Assistant:** Joyce Brumfield; **Photo Production Manager:** Jason Allen; **Art Manager:** Kelly Hendren; **Associate Art Manager:** Alan L. Wilborn; **Illustrations:** © Human Kinetics, unless otherwise noted; **Printer:** Victor Graphics

Printed in the United States of America   10 9 8 7 6 5 4 3 2 1

The paper in this book is certified under a sustainable forestry program.

Human Kinetics
Website: www.HumanKinetics.com

United States: Human Kinetics
P.O. Box 5076
Champaign, IL 61825-5076
800-747-4457
e-mail: humank@hkusa.com

Canada: Human Kinetics
475 Devonshire Road Unit 100
Windsor, ON N8Y 2L5
800-465-7301 (in Canada only)
e-mail: info@hkcanada.com

Europe: Human Kinetics
107 Bradford Road
Stanningley
Leeds LS28 6AT, United Kingdom
+44 (0) 113 255 5665
e-mail: hk@hkeurope.com

Australia: Human Kinetics
57A Price Avenue
Lower Mitcham, South Australia 5062
08 8372 0999
e-mail: info@hkaustralia.com

New Zealand: Human Kinetics
P.O. Box 80
Torrens Park, South Australia 5062
0800 222 062
e-mail: info@hknewzealand.com

E5769

Contents

8 Impact of Physical Activity on Mental Health in Long-Term Conditions 141

Sarah Edmunds, PhD • Angela Clow, PhD

Part III   Physical Activity and Mental Health Conditions .. 163

9 Depression and Anxiety 165

Amanda Daley, PhD

10 Dementia and Alzheimer's Disease 185

Juan Tortosa Martinez, PhD

Preface

Physical activity is an untapped resource for promoting well-being and mental health. Despite evidence of the power of physical activity across a spectrum of mental and physical health problems, the majority of adults do not meet accepted minimum recommendations for physical activity. The case must be made more strongly for why practitioners should promote physical activity to patients and clients and they need to be provided with practical strategies to help them do so.

This specialist text for students and practitioners provides theoretical frameworks linking physical activity with well-being and mental health, thus providing an evidence base from which to inform practice across a range of populations and conditions. It is particularly relevant to students in physical activity- and health-related courses at both undergraduate and graduate levels as well as researchers in these areas. The text is also a valuable resource that supports the development of evidence-based practice for health professionals and those working in the fitness industry. It provides practitioners with a better understanding of the theory and mechanisms by which physical activity leads to improved well-being and mental health, thus enabling them to refine their practice for the benefit of their patients and clients.

The text integrates theoretical and applied approaches with practical tips on training programmes, measurement strategies and methodological considerations. This provides students with an overview of the current evidence linking physical activity with well-being and mental health and provides insight into how this information can be applied in the real world. The text also highlights gaps in the evidence base so that researchers can target their resources to resolve key outstanding issues in the area.

The text is not limited to exploring the role of physical activity in recovery from mental ill health. It also examines the role of physical activity in promoting flourishing across the life span and across socioeconomic status and explores the role of physical activity and exercise in improving quality of life and recovery in people with a range of mental and physical health conditions. It also touches on the negative impacts of excessive exercise, considers the methodological challenges of research in this area and suggests directions for future research.

How This Text Is Organised

Although the text presents a coherent overview of the relationship between physical activity and mental health, each chapter can be read individually. Part I explores the brain systems that are affected by physical activity and how these systems affect mental well-being. This part also describes international guidelines for physical activity and exercise and identifies the challenges of accurately measuring physical activity that underlie much of the debate about the details of the relationship between physical activity and mental health.

Part II provides an innovative look at the factors—namely socioeconomic status, self-esteem, aging and long-term health conditions—that can affect how physical activity and mental health interact. Part II also raises the issue of excessive physical activity and provides guidance on identifying and supporting people who are at risk.

Part III considers the role of physical activity in mental health conditions and reviews how physical activity can attenuate progression of Alzheimer's disease, depression, schizophrenia and addictive behaviours. Each chapter includes practical suggestions for

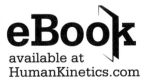
eBook available at HumanKinetics.com

introducing physical activity regimens to these clinical populations. Part III also examines exercise dependence and its relationship with eating disorders and body dysmorphia. The text concludes with an overview of previous chapters and suggestions for moving research and practice forward.

Special Features of This Text

Each chapter in the text opens with a chapter outline and an editors' introduction that provide a quick overview of the structure of the chapter and the content within. Each chapter includes a "Key Concepts" feature that covers core concepts and definitions. Sidebars, which accent topics and central information from the text, are found in each chapter. "Evidence to Practice" boxes at the end of each chapter review current knowledge and theory with a focus on practical application, and chapter summaries wrap up the text. Each chapter pulls leading research from the field. You may further explore these sources in the references section.

Introduction to Physical Activity and Mental Health

The opening section of this text provides contextual information that informs the more focussed chapters in parts II and III. Part I explores the new science of well-being and how it is related to ill-being and mental health conditions, providing context to the study of the interactions between mental health and physical activity. Although well-being and mental health are determined by diverse biological, psychosocial and environmental factors, they can be modified by external events and behaviours such as physical activity. The processes by which physical activity can modify well-being and mental health in humans are complex and include physical movement as well as elements that frequently occur alongside physical activity (e.g., social interaction, fresh air and exposure to green spaces). Chapter 1 explores the current thinking of how physical activity can improve overall brain function and buffer the negative effects of stress. These actions are thought to be a main avenue by which physical activity can promote mental well-being.

Although accumulating evidence supports the value of physical activity for improving both physical and mental health, sedentary lifestyles prevail. This situation has informed evolving national physical activity guidelines, which provide a population-based approach to promoting physical activity. Chapter 2 discusses the history of the development of physical activity guidelines and their application and use in surveillance, practice and policy. Guidelines provide a focus for policymakers and practitioners when implementing physical activity promotion in individuals, communities and whole populations. Chapter 2 also discusses how existing physical activity guidelines could be better used for mental health promotion and treatment of mental health conditions.

Chapter 3 explores the difficult issue of measuring physical activity, particularly in the context of mental health settings. This chapter discusses why self-report measures are often chosen over objective measures and the consequent limitations of the evidence base. The chapter also offers practical advice about using noninvasive and low-cost measures to support self-report measures. The key message is to strike a balance between feasibility (ease and cost) and validity (complexity and expense) in order to find an appropriate middle ground between scientific rigour and practicality.

Relationship Between Physical Activity and Mental Health

Angela Clow, PhD
University of Westminster, London, United Kingdom

Sarah Edmunds, PhD
University of Westminster, London, United Kingdom

Chapter Outline

1. Science of Well-Being
2. Relationship Between Well-Being and Mental Health
3. Physical Activity as a Complex Behaviour
4. Biological Foundations of Effects of Physical Activity on Mental Health
5. Summary
6. References

Editors' Introduction

The aims of this text are to highlight and explain the impact of physical activity on well-being and mental health and to make useful recommendations for practice and future research addressing public health and clinical imperatives. The purpose of this chapter is to introduce the terms and explain the putative pathways that underpin the documented associations between physical activity, well-being and mental health.

Adult well-being and mental health are determined by many diverse biological, psychosocial and environmental factors, many of which are impossible for individuals to modify. For example, genetic makeup, prenatal environment, parental behaviour and early life experiences all affect the development of psychological resources, temperament and vulnerabilities. However, levels of well-being are not predetermined entirely by influences outside of one's control. Pharmacological therapies such as antidepressants, antipsychotics and anxiolytics can be prescribed to treat mental health disorders. These powerful neuroactive drugs have improved quality of life for millions of people, and the development of these agents has been a major spur to understanding the biological underpinnings of mental health conditions. However, use of these drugs can often induce negative side effects, and long-term use may be disadvantageous. Recent studies have shown that individuals can learn to play a more active part in their well-being and mental health regardless of the cards they have been dealt. For example, individuals can learn to be more resilient, happier and less distressed by employing thinking strategies that minimise the negative impact of their underlying vulnerabilities (e.g., susceptibility towards depression). In other words, one can make the most of one's resources and actively attenuate negative cascades of self-destructive thought patterns. Talking to supportive friends and family can sometimes enhance resilience and promote mental well-being. People are increasingly referred to the talking therapies (e.g., cognitive behavioural therapy, which is discussed later in the text). More recently, researchers have realised the potential of physical activity to promote population well-being and alleviate some of the symptoms of serious mental health conditions. Physical activity is a self-directed behaviour that is shown to confer multiple physical and mental health benefits and few negative side effects, especially if the level of activity matches the fitness status of the participant. Physical activity has been shown to affect

KEY CONCEPTS

- Multiple and diverse biological, psychosocial and environmental factors determine well-being and mental health.
- Well-being has two domains: hedonic and eudemonic. High levels of well-being can provide resilience to mental-health conditions.
- External events or behaviours such as physical activity can modify well-being.
- A population-level increase in physical activity would increase the percentage of the population that is flourishing and reduce the prevalence of languishing and serious mental health conditions.
- The processes by which physical activity can modulate well-being and mental health in humans are likely complex and include physical movement as well as elements such as social interaction, fresh air and exposure to green spaces.

- Physical activity benefits overall brain health by reducing peripheral risk factors such as inflammation, diabetes, hypertension and cardiovascular disease and by increasing blood flow and associated delivery of nutrients and energy.
- The hippocampus in the brain is particularly sensitive to effects of physical activity and is proposed as an underlying common element in different mental health conditions.
- Physical activity enhances the activity of the nerve growth factor brain-derived neurotropic factor, which is important for neural growth and protects against damage.
- Physical activity can promote mental well-being by buffering the negative effects of psychological stress on hippocampal function.

cardiovascular health and body composition as well as the complex brain systems implicated in well-being and mental health. As such, one should not underestimate the potential of physical activity to positively affect the quality of life of millions of people.

At this early stage it is appropriate to define the key terms *physical activity* and *exercise*. Physical activity encompasses all types of bodily movement. Exercise is a subcategory of physical activity and consists of planned, structured and repetitive body movement undertaken to promote and maintain components of physical fitness; as such, physical activity does not always involve exercise. Pursuits such as walking and gardening, which one may undertake without the specific purpose of exercise, can be important elements of physical activity. See chapter 3 for further discussion of these issues.

1 Science of Well-Being

The science of well-being is relatively new. Therefore, a good place to start is to explain why it is an important issue in this text. Until recently, researchers and practitioners have focussed on alleviating poor mental health both at the population level (e.g., stress) and in a clinical setting (i.e., specific debilitating mental health conditions such as depression, schizophrenia and dementia). It was assumed that well-being occupied one end of a unidimensional continuum and that mental health conditions (i.e., ill-being) occupied the other. Under this assumption, measuring and reducing ill-being were, by default, measuring and promoting well-being. Consequently, promoting well-being was not on the agenda, either for public health professionals seeking to address population-level health issues or in clinical settings.

However, research has shown that the assumption of a unidimensional continuum is inaccurate and that some degree of dissociation exists between well-being and ill-being. One may have low levels of ill-being (e.g., stress or depression) but not have high levels of well-being (e.g., happiness and meaning in life). Similarly, one may have high levels of ill-being but coexisting high levels of well-being. Once researchers started to tease apart these relationships it became apparent that well-being, independent of ill-being, is a powerful predictor of all-cause morbidity and mortality (see Huppert, 2009, for a review). Figure 1.1 illustrates

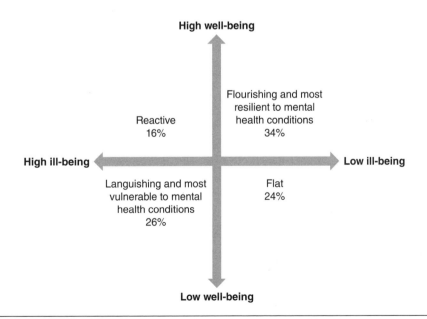

Figure 1.1 Dimensions of well-being and ill-being and typical percentages of healthy population in each segment. This shows the percentage of healthy community-dwelling adults who typically fall into each quadrant.

Data percentages from Evans et al., 2007.

the interactions between well-being and ill-being and the types of functioning associated with each combination. For example, full flourishing is enabled when high well-being coincides with low ill-being; studies show that this is characteristic of an estimated 34% of the population. The individuals in this quadrant are most resilient to experiencing mental health conditions. In contrast, coexisting low well-being and high ill-being are associated with languishing and vulnerability to future mental health conditions. Perhaps most surprising is that studies suggest that an estimated 24% of the global population has low well-being and low ill-being. The individuals in this quadrant, who are described as being "flat" or not fulfilling their potential, are still vulnerable to poor health outcomes despite low levels of ill-being (Evans et al., 2007; Huppert et al., 2009).

These findings provided impetus for the new science of well-being, which focusses on the positive rather than the negative. However, it became increasingly apparent that well-being, like ill-being, is a complex construct. People continue to debate about precise definitions and components of well-being and how it should be measured. However, broad consensus exists that well-being comprises two main domains: hedonic (i.e., subjective) well-being and eudemonic (i.e., psychological) well-being. Hedonia

is associated with the emotional aspects of well-being (e.g., moods and feelings) and includes both positive and pleasant emotions such as joy, elation and affection and negative emotions such as guilt, anger and shame. Eudemonia is more closely associated with the cognitive evaluation of one's life as a whole. Researchers believe that six domains of eudemonic well-being exist: purpose in life, environmental mastery, self-acceptance, personal growth, autonomy and positive relationships (Ryff & Singer, 2008). These eudemonic domains are thought to be relatively independent of each other and can be present to a greater or lesser extent. Hedonic and eudemonic well-being interact with one another, and—notwithstanding the nonmodifiable component of well-being referred to at the beginning of this section—external events and behaviours can influence eudemonia (see figure 1.2). This modifiable aspect of well-being makes it an important target for intervention (e.g., with physical activity).

2 Relationship Between Well-Being and Mental Health

Because well-being is modifiable it has become an important focus for researchers, policy makers and practitioners alike. An important argument in favor of promoting well-being is that, with

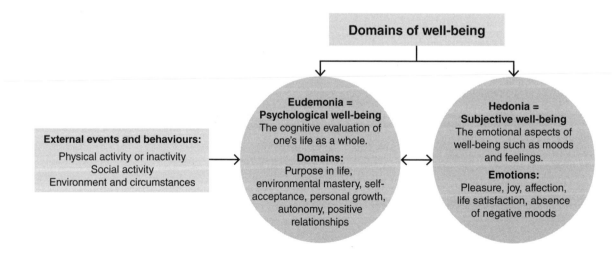

Figure 1.2 The interacting components of well-being (WB) and their susceptibility to modification by behaviours (e.g., physical activity) and external factors (e.g., social and physical circumstances).

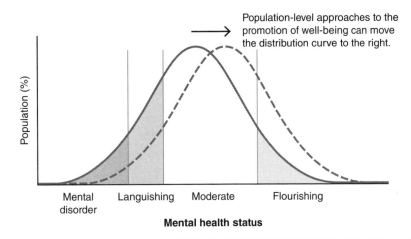

Figure 1.3 The population distribution of mental health status showing the impact of adopting a population-level approach to promoting psychological well-being. Such a population-level approach can shift the curve to the right. However, the cutoff points for mental health disorder, languishing and flourishing remain the same, meaning that fewer people manifest with disorder and languishing and more flourish.

time, shifts in the average prevalence of subclinical health deficits within the population as a whole affect the prevalence of severe health conditions (Rose, 1992). This theory has been applied to the understanding of well-being within the population such that increases in the average level of well-being within a population will ultimately reduce the prevalence of mental health conditions (Huppert, 2009), as illustrated in figure 1.3.

This normal distribution indicates that the majority of the population has moderate levels of mental health and that a relatively small percentage is fully flourishing. At the opposite end of the spectrum, a minority have incapacitating mental health conditions and others are languishing and are at risk of more serious conditions over time. The theory proposed by Rose (1992) states that public health initiatives that target the majority of the population can, with time, shift the curve to the right, thus reducing the prevalence of health disorders and increasing the percentage of individuals who are flourishing (see figure 1.3). The implication of this theory (developed and expounded by Huppert, 2009) is that well-being and mental health compose a continuum and that, with time, promoting well-being at a population level can confer resilience and reduce the risk of deteriorating psychological resources.

This concept is very significant because it means that population-level approaches can have major impacts across the spectrum of mental health status and can play a role in the prevention, treatment and management of mental health disorder. Not all interventions are suitable for population-level approaches. For example, providing everyone with a drug to improve well-being would be inadvisable. However, physical activity is an intervention that is appropriate for large-scale implementation. For these reasons, this text examines the role of physical activity in promoting population-level well-being (e.g., in relation to socioeconomic status and aging) and in specific mental health conditions.

3 Physical Activity as a Complex Behaviour

The processes by which physical activity modulate well-being and mental health in humans are complex. For example, it can be difficult to determine the precise "active ingredient" or precise element of the behavior that confers benefit in a physical activity behaviour or intervention. Physical activity is a complex behaviour that is often associated with other potentially beneficial elements such as social interaction, fresh air and exposure to green spaces. In addition, determining the direction of causality in studies linking better physical activity, increased well-being and mental health is challenging because people with greater psychological resources are likely to take part in more physical activity. It is difficult to determine whether physical activity promotes better well-being or vice versa. In human populations, this is a complex area of study and requires a systems approach and an understanding of the potential for multiple and complex interactions (see figure 1.4).

A promising conclusion to draw from examining the interactions shown in figure 1.4 is that promoting physical activity sets in motion a sustainable cycle of enhanced psychological resources. Increased physical activity improves well-being and enhances resilience to mental ill health, which in turn increases the motivation to take part in physical activity as well as associated social and behavioural factors. This systems approach also acknowledges the role of social and environmental factors in promoting physical activity and provides more targets for intervention, many of which are addressed in this text.

A more direct approach to examining the physiological impact of physical activity on brain function is used in animal (most often rodent) studies that employ wheel running as a form of physical activity. Much of the evidence

presented in the following section is derived from such work. It is interesting to note from these studies that voluntary wheel running is more beneficial for brain systems than is forced wheel running. These relatively simple behavoural intervention studies may be more complex than imagined.

4   Biological Foundations of Effects of Physical Activity on Mental Health

The observation that physical activity affects well-being and mental health implies that physical activity must affect brain function, either directly or indirectly. Evidence shows that mental health conditions (e.g., schizophrenia, depression, addiction, Alzheimer's disease) and low well-being (e.g., chronic stress) are associated with perturbations in brain function. Therefore, one may deduce that these perturbations must be attenuated in order to produce benefit.

The disturbances in brain function associated with poor mental health can be brought about by myriad and interacting factors. For example, genetic makeup, prenatal environment, parental behaviour and early life experiences all contribute to the process of brain development and maturation. Unfavorable prenatal and early life environments can lead to biological and psychological vulnerability that predisposes an individual to mental health problems such as depression, schizophrenia and addiction in later life. Alternatively, negative life events that occur in later life, such as exposure to chronic stress, can lead to downstream neurotoxic effects on brain function and secondary mental health problems. The vulnerability and neurotoxicity hypotheses of mental health are currently the focus of much interest. The causes and biological correlates of mental health disorders are complex and not yet fully understood. However, a life course approach is beginning to shed greater light on sensitive developmental periods that affect the structure and function of the brain, leading to effects that persist throughout life (Lupien et al., 2009).

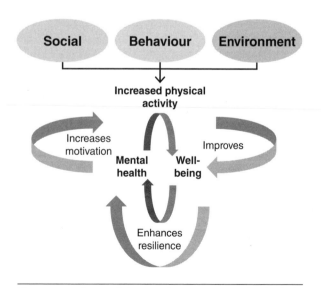

Figure 1.4 Some of the complex systems involved in linking physical activity with well-being and mental health.

It is clear that complex neuronal circuits are involved in mental health conditions and that, like ripples in a pond, disturbance in one part of the brain can have an array of effects elsewhere. The neurotransmitters dopamine, norepinephrine, serotonin and acetylcholine are implicated to a greater or lesser extent, depending on the condition. Research has demonstrated that physical activity affects levels of these neurotransmitters. In the investigation of links between physical activity and mental health, focus has recently shifted from the role of specific neurotransmitter pathways to the function of interacting systems in a particular region of the brain. The region of the brain that has been most studied in this resp ect is the hippocampus. Evidence suggests that the hippocampus is a key mediator in the links between physical activity, well-being and mental health.

4.1 Hippocampus

The hippocampus is part of the Papez's circuit or limbic system, which is known to influence emotional and cognitive regulation. The hippocampus, a subcortical structure that lies in the medial temporal lobes, is surrounded by the entorhinal, parahippocampal and perirhinal cortices (Bird & Burgess, 2008). Its size, central location and networks allow it to connect to several subcortical and cortical structures, including the anterior thalamic nuclei, the mammillary bodies, the septal nuclei of the basal forebrain, the retrosplenial cortex and the parahippocampal cortex (see figure 1.5). This central and networked location enables the hippocampus to influence surrounding structures.

The hippocampus is involved in learning, cognition, anxiety, regulation of the hypothalamic–pituitary–adrenal (HPA) axis and other vegetative functions, which are altered in individuals with mood disorders. The hippocampus also has important connections to the amygdala and prefrontal cortex that may further cause emotional and cognitive deficits.

Physical activity benefits overall brain health by reducing peripheral risk factors such as inflammation, diabetes, hypertension and cardiovascular disease (which converge to cause brain dysfunction and neurodegeneration) and by increasing blood flow and associated delivery of nutrients and energy (Cotman et al., 2007). However, the hippocampus appears to be most sensitive to the effects of physical activity. For example, in a study of rats, 3 weeks of exercise led to both increases and decreases in the expression of a number of genes in the hippocampus (Tong,

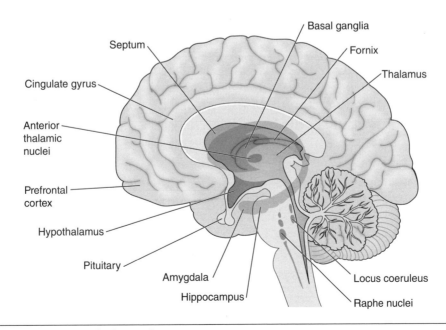

Figure 1.5   The hippocampus in the human brain.

2001). Many of these genes are involved in synaptic function and neuroplasticity (i.e., the capacity of the brain to adapt, learn and recover from damage). The remarkable findings that physical activity regulates the expression of so many genes in the hippocampus contribute to the evidence that physical activity modulates mental health mainly through attenuating disturbances in the structure and function of the hippocampus in particular.

4.2 Brain-Derived Neurotrophic Factor

A key first step in understanding the links between physical activity and brain function came in the mid-1990s. Rodent studies showed that voluntary wheel running increased the production of brain growth factors, especially in the hippocampus (Neeper et al., 1995). These nerve growth (or neurotrophic) factors support the differentiation, growth and survival of many neuronal subtypes, thus conferring a widespread positive effect on brain function. A single mechanism (e.g., increased levels of growth factor) can have multiple effects on different brain pathways and thus confer extensive and nonspecific benefit. Brain-derived neurotrophic factor (BDNF) is the growth factor that has been most studied in

this respect. The varied actions of BDNF together promote neural growth, protect from damage and enhance function (see "Actions of Brain-Derived Neurotrophic Factor").

Unlike typical neurotransmitters (e.g., dopamine and acetylcholine), the growth factor BDNF is transported in both directions in neurons to affect synaptic structure and function as described in "Actions of Brain-Derived Neurotrophic Factor." Levels of BDNF increase when the BDNF gene is activated to generate its precursor, messenger ribonucleic acid. Crucially, BDNF gene activation is activity dependent: The more active the neuron, the more BDNF is manufactured (i.e., a feed-forward positive-feedback loop). Physical activity increases firing in the neurons and, consequently, increases levels of BDNF. This process appears to be mediated via pathways from the medial septum that involve a combination of neurotransmitter systems.

Studies have examined the effect of 7 days of voluntary wheel running on levels of BDNF in the rat brain hippocampus. In rodents, running has been shown to increase levels of BDNF messenger ribonucleic acid in the lumbar spinal cord, cerebellum and cerebral cortex but not in other regions such as the striatum. Research has shown that although other growth factors, including nerve growth factor and fibroblast growth factor,

---

Actions of Brain-Derived Neurotrophic Factor

Brain-derived neurotrophic factor (BDNF) promotes neural growth and protects from damage:

- BDNF promotes the neural differentiation, neurite extension and survival of a variety of neuronal populations in culture, including hippocampal, cortical, striatal, septal and cerebellar neurons.
- Intraventricular BDNF infusion protects the hippocampus and cerebral cortex from ischemic damage.

BDNF can enhance brain function:

- BDNF stimulates synapse formation.
- BDNF enhances synaptic transmission by modulating neurotransmitter release and postsynaptic actions.
- BDNF promotes long-term potentiation (i.e., sensitisation of specific synaptic pathways) and associated learning.

Adapted from Cotman et al. 2002.

are induced in the hippocampus in response to exercise, upregulation of these growth factors is transient and less robust than that of BDNF. These animal studies suggest that BDNF is the best candidate for mediating the long-term benefits of exercise on the brain (Cotman et al., 2007; Lazarov, et al., 2010). Further work exploring these pathways and their significance in the adult human brain is under way.

4.3 Hippocampal Neurogenesis

Neurogenesis is the process by which neural stem cells proliferate and give rise to neural progenitor cells that eventually differentiate into new neurons and glia. Neurogenesis occurs most actively during prenatal brain development. The hippocampus is one of only two areas of the brain in which neurogenesis is known to take place in adulthood. (The other is the subventricular zone, or the lining of the lateral ventricles.) Neurogenesis in the adult brain is increasingly acknowledged to be of functional significance in maintaining optimal brain function and repairing damage (van Praag et al., 2002; Zhao, Deng & Gage, 2008). The brain's capacity for neurogenesis declines with age; this is thought to contribute to age-related decline in function. However, neurotrophins, like BDNF, are potent stimulants of neurogenesis (Cotman et al., 2007).

Enhanced hippocampal neurogenesis is one of the most reproducible effects of exercise in the rodent brain and is thought to be a key mechanism mediating exercise-related improvements in well-being, mental health and cognitive function (Cotman et al., 2007). Exercise stimulates neurogenesis in both young and old animals and, via properties of exercise-induced growth factors, promotes survival of these new cells. The threshold of excitability of the new neurons, which become functionally integrated into the hippocampal architecture, is lower than that of the original mature cells. This feature makes these new neurons well suited to mediate exercise-stimulated enhanced brain function.

It is well known that exercise increases peripheral levels of pituitary-derived plasma β-endorphin. This increase has been associated with the runners' high that occurs immediately after exercise. This association is unlikely because peripheral β-endorphin is unable to cross the blood–brain barrier to access the brain to induce the feelings of euphoria associated with runners high. The fact remains, however, that opioids such as β-endorphin are able to modulate the process of hippocampal neurogenesis in the adult brain. Because exercise also increases brain β-endorphin levels, it is possible that b endorphin may contribute to the observed effects of exercise on hippocampal neurogenesis (as well as contribute to the runner's high along with other putative mediators such as endogenous cannabinoids; Raichlen et al., 2012).

For maximal benefit, neurogenesis must be accompanied by the process of angiogenesis, which is the growth of new blood vessels to supply the new tissue with adequate nutrients and energy. New neurons also require an increased number of microglia, which are their support cells. Exercise leads to widespread growth of blood vessels in the hippocampus and other areas of the brain (e.g., the cerebral cortex and cerebellum) and to more microglia (Cotman et al., 2007; Ekstrand, Hellsten & Tingström, 2008). Researchers believe that these processes, which are synergistic with neurogenesis, are the primary way physical activity can affect well-being and mental health.

4.4 HPA Stress-Response System

Hippocampal neurogenesis can be enhanced by a range of environmental factors. For example, research has shown that environmental enrichment is a positive modulator of adult neurogenesis (Kempermann, Kuhn & Gage, 1997). On the other hand, negative environmental stimuli such as chronic psychosocial stress can actively inhibit neurogenesis.

Response to psychosocial stress involves finely tuned and integrated systems and is adaptive for survival in situations of short-term stress. When activated, the HPA axis secretes powerful glucocorticoid hormones. Neurons in the hypothalamus of the brain release corticotrophin-releasing hormone and arginine vasopressin. These messengers trigger the subsequent secretion of adrenocorticotropic hormone from the pituitary gland, leading to the production of glucocorticoids by the adrenal cortex. The hippocampus is inhibitory in regulating the HPA axis, whereas the amygdala is stimulatory (see figure 1.6). However, stress that is severe and sustained (i.e., chronic stress) can lead to dysregulation of these systems, which can damage mental and physical health.

The HPA axis is regulated by a sensitive system of negative feedback via the glucocorticoid receptor and the mineralocorticoid receptor. These receptors are located at different sites in the axis (see figure 1.6) but especially populate the hippocampus. One negative consequence of chronic stress is changed sensitivity of these receptors, which leads to aberrant patterns of secretion of glucocorticoids (cortisol in humans and corticosterone in rodents) into circulation. This has given rise to the glucocorticoid cascade hypothesis, which suggests that a relationship

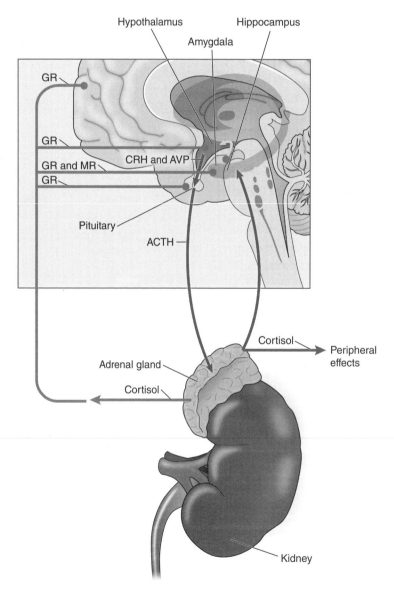

Figure 1.6   The hypothalamic–pituitary–adrenal (HPA) stress-response system and the pivotal role of the hippocampus in inhibiting its function. Glucocorticoid receptors (GR) and mineralocorticoid receptors (MR) regulate feedback and are sensitive to neurotoxicity. ACTH = adrenocorticotropic hormone; AVP = arginine vasopressin; CRH = corticotrophin-releasing hormone.

exists between cumulative exposure to high glucocorticoid levels and hippocampal atrophy (McEwen & Milner, 2007). Prolonged exposure to glucocorticoids reduces the ability of neurons to resist insults, thus increasing the rate at which neurons are damaged by other toxic challenges or ordinary attrition. In addition, high levels of glucocorticoids inhibit hippocampal neurogenesis (Lupien et al., 2009). However, physical activity can attenuate the negative impact of stress or glucocorticoid administration on neurogenesis and angiogenesis in the hippocampus and thus buffer the negative effects of psychological stress on hippocampal function (Chang et al., 2008; Cotman et al., 2007; Ekstrand, Hellsten & Tingström, 2008; Yau, Lau & So, 2011).

In addition, chronic stress has a complex array of negative effects on peripheral risk factors for brain dysfunction and neurodegeneration such as inflammation, diabetes, hypertension and cardio-vascular disease. Stress exacerbates these conditions and increases the risk of reduced well-being and mental health. Physical activity can reverse the prevalence of these physical risk factors for mental health conditions. Evidence of the effects of physical activity on peripheral stress-response systems (e.g., HPA axis response) is complicated by the wide array of physical activity and stress-ors investigated. However, evidence increasingly shows the beneficial effects of physical activity on the ability to cope with both psychological and exercise stress in both humans and animals. More research is needed to fully clarify these relationships (Tortosa-Martínez & Clow, 2012). Figure 1.7 illustrates the complex interactions between chronic psychosocial stress, physical

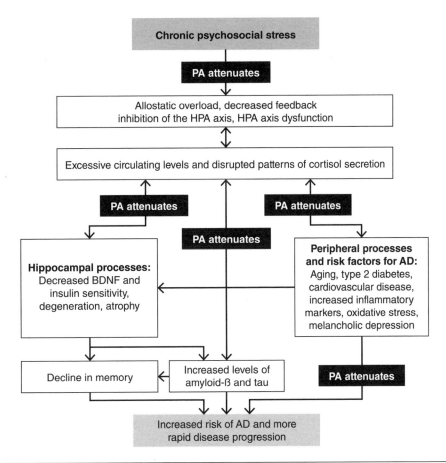

Figure 1.7 Links between stress, physical activity and dementia. Arrows indicate putative pathways. AD = Alzheimer's disease; BDNF = brain-derived neurotrophic factor; HPA = hypothalamic–pituitary–adrenal; PA = physical activity (located where it has been shown to attenuate that pathway). Amyloid-β and tau are pathological signs of Alzheimer's disease.

EVIDENCE TO PRACTICE

- Promoting physical activity is an ideal population-level strategy for increasing the prevalence of flourishing and reducing languishing and severe mental health conditions.
- Promoting physical activity is an excellent strategy for increasing mental health

in specific populations with a range of mental health conditions.

- When evaluating the impact of a physical activity intervention, one must consider the enhancement of well-being and not focus solely on changes in ill-being.

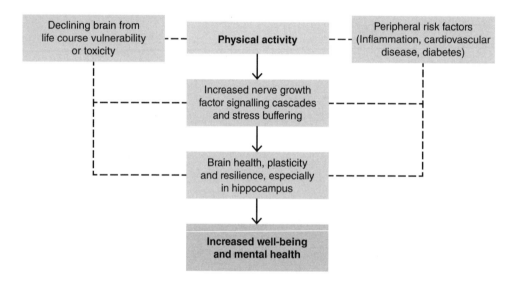

Figure 1.8   Interacting factors linking physical activity and increased well-being and mental health. Solid lines indicate facilitatory pathways and dotted lines indicate inhibitory pathways. CV = cardiovascular.

activity, peripheral risk factors and development of dementia and Alzheimer's disease. In addition, physical activity can reduce the prevalence of peripheral risk factors for deteriorating brain function such as inflammation, cardiovascular disease and diabetes (see figure 1.8).

5   Summary

Physical activity can positively affect a diverse range of mental health conditions (e.g., schizophrenia, Alzheimer's disease and depression) and well-being. The varied effects of physical activity have led to speculation that physical activity activates a common underlying pathway that is shared by all these conditions. The hippocampus, which is strategically located and highly networked in the brain, may be a common link

between physical activity and mental health. Furthermore, the hippocampus is exceptionally sensitive to the effects of physical activity. Physical activity initiates a signaling cascade involving gene activation, nerve growth factor synthesis and associated neurogenesis and angiogenesis in this region of the brain. These cascades help buffer the negative effects of excess stress-related secretion of glucocorticoids and promote neuroplacticity and brain health, which positively affects well-being and mental health. Peripheral risk factors for deteriorating brain function such as inflammation, cardiovascular disease and diabetes are also reduced by engaging in physical activity.

Although more research is needed to expand understanding of these processes and replicate the results from animal studies in human populations, evidence of these pathways is accumulating and credible. The coming chapters provide detail on each specific mental health condition.

6   References

Bird, C.M., & Burgess, N. (2008). The hippocampus and memory: Insights from spatial processing. *Nature Neuroscience Reviews*, 9, 182-194.

Chang, Y.-T., Chen, Y.-C., Wu, C.-W., Lung Yu, L., Chen, H.-I., Chauying, J., & Kuo, J.Y.-M. (2008). Glucocorticoid signaling and exercise-induced downregulation of the mineralocorticoid receptor in the induction of adult mouse dentate neurogenesis by treadmill running. *Psychoneuroendocrinology*, 33, 1173-1182.

Cotman, C.W., Berchtold, N.C., & Christie, L.-A. (2007). Exercise builds brain health: Key roles of growth factor cascades and inflammation. *Trends in Neurosciences*, 30, 464-472.

Cotman, C.W., Nicole, C., & Berchtold, N.C. (2002). Exercise: A behavioural intervention to enhance brain health and plasticity. *Trends in Neurosciences*, 25, 295-301.

Ekstrand, J., Hellsten, J., & Tingström, A. (2008). Environmental enrichment, exercise and corticosterone affect endothelial cell proliferation in adult rat hippocampus and prefrontal cortex. *Neuroscience Letters*, 442, 203-207.

Evans, P., Forte, D., Jacobs, C., Fredhoi, C., Aitchison, E., Hucklebridge, F., & Clow, A. (2007). Cortisol secretory activity in older people in relation to positive and negative well-being. *Psychoneuroendocrinology*, 32, 922-930.

Huppert, F.A. (2009). A new approach to reducing disorder and improving well-being. *Perspectives in Psychological Science*, 4, 108-111.

Kempermann, G., Kuhn, H.G., & Gage, F.H. (1997). More hippocampal neurons in adult mice living in an enriched environment. *Nature*, 386, 493-495.

Lazarov, O., Mattson, M.P., Peterson, D.A., Pimplikar, S.W., & van Praag, H. (2010). When neurogenesis encounters aging and disease. *Trends in Neurosciences*, 33, 569-579.

Lupien, S.J., McEwen, B.S., Gunnar, M.R., & Heim, C. (2009). Effects of stress throughout the lifespan on the brain, behaviour and cognition. *Nature Reviews–Neurosciences*, 10, 434-445.

McEwen, B.S., & Milner, T.A. (2007). Hippocampal formation: Shedding light on the influence of sex and stress on the brain. *Brain Research Reviews*, 55, 343-355.

Neeper, S.A., Gomez-Pinilla, F., Choi, J., & Cotman, C. (1995). Exercise and brain neurotrophins. *Nature*, 373, 109.

Raichlen, D.A., Foster, A.D., Gerdeman, G.L., Seillier, A., & Giuffrida, A. (2012). Wired to run: Exercise-induced endocannabinoid signaling in humans and cursorial mammals with implications for the "runner's high." *Journal of Experimental Biology*, 215, 1331-1336.

Rose, G. (1992). *The strategy of preventive medicine*. Oxford: Oxford University Press.

Ryff, C.D., & Singer, B.H. (2008). Know thyself and become what you are: A eudemonic approach to psychological well-being. *Journal of Happiness Studies*, 9, 13-39.

Tong, L. (2001). Effects of exercise on gene expression profile in the rat hippocampus. *Neurobiology of Disease*, 8, 1046-1056.

Tortosa-Martínez, J., & Clow, A. (2012). Does physical activity reduce risk for Alzheimer's disease through interaction with the stress neuroendocrine system? *Stress*, 15, 243-261.

van Praag, H., Schinder, A.F., Christie, B.R., Toni, N., Palmer, T.D., & Gage, F.H. (2002). Functional neurogenesis in the adult hippocampus. *Nature*, 415, 1030-1034.

Yau, S.-Y., Lau, B.W.-M., & So, K.-F. (2011). Adult hippocampal neurogenesis: A possible way how physical exercise counteracts stress. *Cell Transplantation*, 20, 99-111.

Zhao, C., Deng, W., & Gage, F.H. (2008). Mechanisms and functional implications of adult neurogenesis. *Cell*, 132, 645-660.

Physical Activity Guidelines and National Population-Based Actions

Fiona Bull, PhD
University of Western Australia, Perth, Australia

Adrian Bauman, PhD
University of Sydney, Sydney, Australia

Chapter Outline

1. Population-Based Approach to Promoting Physical Activity
2. Physical Activity Guidelines
3. Development of the First National Physical Activity Guidelines
4. Current Best Practice in Developing Guidelines
5. Global, Regional and National Physical Activity Guidelines
6. Implementation and Influence of Physical Activity Guidelines
7. Summary
8. References

Editors' Introduction

Physical activity guidelines (PAGs) provide a crucial point of reference for all who are interested in promoting physical activity, whether at the individual or policy level. PAGs provide an authoritative, evidenced-based consensus on the types and levels of physical activity that are beneficial to health. However, dissemination of PAGs to target audiences is often poor. Greater use could be made of PAGs to help promote physical activity in mental health care settings. Although PAGs for specific mental health conditions do not exist, the general PAGs provide invaluable advice about appropriate types of physical activity that can benefit those in mental health care settings. This chapter discusses the multiple stages of generating PAGs and emphasises the need for enhanced communication to all who could benefit.

Physical inactivity is the fourth leading risk factor for noncommunicable diseases and contributed to more than 3 million preventable deaths globally in 2010 (World Health Organisation, 2011). Reducing physical inactivity is a global public health priority. However, most countries have not yet taken widespread action or created specific physical activity-related policy at the necessary scale (Bull & Bauman, 2011). To date, much of the focus on physical activity has related to obesity prevention, diabetes and cardiovascular disease (U.S. Department of Health and Human Services, 2008g) and less attention has been paid to the substantial benefits of physical activity in other areas of health promotion and disease prevention.

The association between physical activity and mental health outcomes is underrecognised in both adults and children (Biddle & Asare, 2011; Teychenne, Ball & Salmon, 2008). Evidence clearly shows the benefits of regular physical activity in preventing and treating anxiety and depression (Lawlor & Hopker, 2001) (see chapter 9). In addition, emerging evidence shows that regular physical activity benefits people with schizophrenia (Holley et al., 2011) (see chapter 11) and potentially benefits people with other mental health conditions, including social phobia (Saxena et al., 2005). Benefits can be direct or indirect (see chapter 1). For example, physical activity can improve outcomes by addressing medication-induced obesity and cardiometabolic disturbance in people with schizophrenia (Vancampfort et al., 2010).

Data consistently show that physical activity is positively associated with mental well-being and that it reduces the risk of psychosocial stress in the general population (Pawlowski, Downward & Rasciute, 2011; Pressman et al., 2009). Systematic reviews of these studies identify the relationship between physical activity and mental health and add to the plethora of benefits of physical activity in other areas of health (U.S. Department of Health and Human Services, 2008g).

Most PAGs seem to recommend at least 150 min/wk of moderate-intensity physical activity.

Additional intensity may contribute to further reductions in depression or dementia risk, but data are too sparse to make definitive conclusions. Physical activity and structured exercise may also benefit people with other mental health problems and may help manage clinical populations with mental health concerns. It appears that most of the benefit for people with mental health problems occurs with levels of activity that are below those needed to improve fitness (U.S. Department of Health and Human Services, 2008g). This suggests that physical activity at lower levels of intensity (i.e., below those of the usual exercise programme) enhances health and that total physical activity can be accumulated throughout the day in sessions of at least 10 continuous min. In terms of promoting mental health and preventing depression and anxiety, this means encouraging an active lifestyle, making choices to be physically active throughout the day, using active transport to get to and from places and regularly building in leisure-time physical activity.

Much of the evidence on the health and clinical benefits of physical activity is collected through population-based epidemiological studies. Evidence consistently points to the need for recommendations for physical activity as it relates to both health and mental health. PAGs summarise the evidence and provide a mechanism for interpreting scientific findings for use in practice and policy. These recommendations can then be incorporated into health services (including mental health) and programmes for health promotion and primary prevention. This chapter discusses the purpose of PAGs and how they are developed and provides examples of PAGs. The chapter also explores how PAGs can and should be used to influence physical activity promotion in general and the area of mental health specifically.

1   Population-Based Approach to Promoting Physical Activity

Many people are starting to understand that physical activity confers both physical and mental health benefits. However, at the whole-population level, participation in physical activity remains low. For this reason, it is necessary to target and motivate whole populations rather than just individuals (e.g., one on one, clinical settings, small groups) to become more physically active. Population-based strategies aim to reach many people and can be accessed by a large segment of the physically inactive population. Such strategies usually require the use of mass-reach programmes at the organisational or community levels. Campaigns often use paid and unpaid media (e.g., television, radio and print communications) to raise awareness and educate whole populations about the benefits of physical activity for health and wellness (Bauman & Chau, 2009).

A population-based approach can also aim to influence the built environment and the development of policies that assist people and make physical activity easier and more accessible. One example is the provision of free access (thus removing the cost barrier) to local, government-run swimming pools in the United Kingdom from 2006 to 2008. Another example is the provision, through policy, regulation or legislation, of bicycle paths, which provide safe environments for recreational travel and commuting.

The gap between what people believe about physical activity and their actual behaviour is a substantial challenge for public health practitioners as well as government and nongovernment agencies. Many theorists have proposed models and frameworks for changing physical activity behaviour (Glanz & Bishop, 2010). These models start with awareness and understanding of physical activity as a preventive health issue. People then need to move through stages of cognitive change, eventually trying the behaviour, and then to the regular adoption of physical activity behaviours (Bauman & Chau, 2009) (see figure 2.1). Initial approaches to physical activity promotion need to communicate the physical activity message, inform people of the health and other benefits of being active and indicate the amount, intensity and frequency of physical activity required for health. Once the community understands the message, persuasion is required to move them to think seriously about becoming physically active for their own health and

KEY CONCEPTS

- Reducing levels of physical inactivity is a global public health priority for preventing noncommunicable diseases, including mental health problems, and promoting health and well-being.

- PAGs are evidence-based statements on the preventive health benefits of physical activity. They provide a consensus about the "dose" of physical activity required to gain these benefits. The dose includes what type of physical activity should be undertaken (e.g., aerobic activity, strength training, weight bearing), the frequency (e.g., 3 days/wk), the duration (e.g., 30 min) and the intensity (e.g., moderate, vigorous).

- Current PAGs recommend 30 min of moderate-intensity physical activity on most days of the week. This is expressed as "at least 150 min/wk of moderate-intensity activity" in the most recent global, U.S. and U.K. recommendations.

- PAGs are an important component of a national population-based approach to increasing levels of participation. A population-based approach aims to reach many people and usually includes educational campaigns (e.g., television, radio and print communications) to raise awareness and understanding, programmes that provide opportunities for participation and actions aimed at influencing the built environment to assist people and to make physical activity the easy choice.

well-being. Normal stages of cognitive change include reassessing the pros and cons of being active, evaluating barriers and opportunities and revisiting how important the behaviour is to the individual. A shift in cognitive understanding can lead to attempts to increase physical activity behaviours. At this point, both supportive environments and policies and access to facilities and programmes are required. As this chapter demonstrates, the work of PAGs is to contribute to population change in the earlier phases of this process of behaviour change to increase physical activity (left side of figure 2.1).

2   Physical Activity Guidelines

PAGs are evidence-based summary statements on the health benefits of physical activity and represent a high level consensus on what the scientific evidence has demonstrated by describing, in a summary format, the "dose" of the behaviour required to gain the benefits. National guidelines aimed at the whole population (as opposed to specific populations defined by a medical condition) focus on the optimal amount of activity to prevent disease and promote

health and well-being. PAGs indicate the type (e.g., aerobic activity, strength training, weight bearing), frequency (e.g., 3 days/wk), duration (e.g., 30 min) and intensity (e.g., moderate, vigorous) (see figure 2.2) of physical activity to undertake and for what benefits. These detailed specifications reflect the latest science on the topic.

PAGs need to be updated periodically because evidence about the relationship between physical activity and health changes over time and knowledge grows. Some guidelines are more general in nature, whereas others provide very specific details; this usually reflects the state of knowledge at that time. Through a review and revision process, more specific details are added to PAGs when available. For example, in various national PAGs, guidelines relating to maintaining musculoskeletal strength have been revised over time and now include details on how much strength training is required for good health (World Health Organisation, 2010) and, specifically, for preventing falls and treating depression (Singh, Clements & Singh, 2001).

National guidelines are an important component of a population-based approach to address-

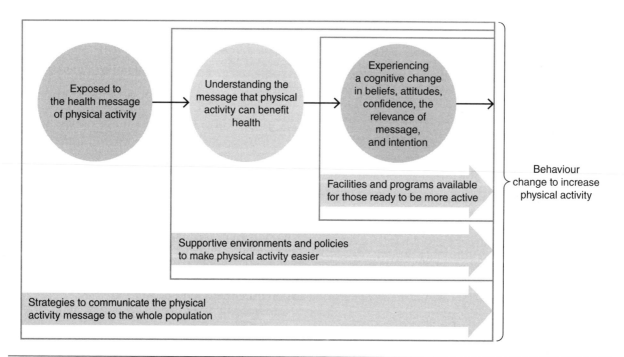

Figure 2.1   Population changes to physical activity.

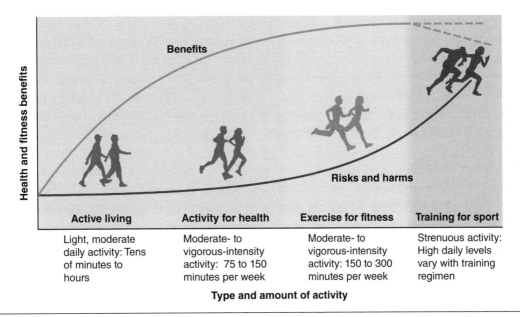

Figure 2.2   The dose–response relationship: Increasing benefits from increasing amounts (expressed in frequency, duration and intensity) of activity.

Reprinted, by permission, from I. Vuori, 1995, *Terveysliikunta* [Health and physical education]. UKK Institute for Health Promotion Research (Tampere, Finland).

ing any public health issue. First, such guidelines communicate a consensus on the scientific evidence of the importance of the issue. They describe the strength of the science in terms of the volume as well as the quality (determined based on the quality of study designs and research methods used) of the evidence. Communicating scientific consensus is important because it removes doubt and speculation about the validity of the health issue and its importance. This scientific consensus can also be used to advocate for resources and programmes. However, just because guidelines exist does not mean that everyone agrees about what the science says—far from it. However, these disagreements, or alternative interpretations of overall findings to date, are usually communicated in technical reports that accompany the publication of PAGs and are not fully accessible to the general public.

The process of developing PAGs usually involves leadership by a high-level institution. This adds credence to the message that the issue is important. For example, several national and international health agencies, such as the American Heart Association (Haskell et al., 2007), have developed guidelines on physical activity.

National governments, usually the ministry of health, often lead the development process and endorse national PAGs. This endorsement is very useful because it specifies the government's position on physical activity and thereby provides the opportunity for interested parties such as charities and public health directors to leverage the government into supporting further action and funding for programmes and services aimed at increasing physical activity. This might include government endorsement of counselling and clinical services for inactive patients, as has been trialled in the United Kingdom (Bull & Milton, 2011). Government involvement and endorsement can also prevent policy inaction. The absence of an official position on physical activity can block funding and further development of a national population-based approach.

One important role of PAGs is to direct community-level actions aimed at increasing physical activity in the whole population. The details in PAGs about the type, frequency, duration and intensity of activities required for different age groups can provide clinicians, health care practitioners and others with direction on what types of programmes to provide and promote to patients and the wider community.

PAGs should drive and direct action not just at the level of individuals and service providers but also at all levels—national, regional and local—of government. If the national government endorses PAGs, ideally with multiparty political support, the government should be held accountable when levels of physical activity are not improving and can be expected to include physical activity promotion as part of ongoing disease-prevention and health-promotion strategies. The role of PAGs and national surveillance of risk factors is discussed in more detail later in this chapter.

3   Development of the First National Physical Activity Guidelines

Epidemiological studies of exercise and health were well advanced by the 1970s. The American College of Sports Medicine released the first set of recommendations in 1975 and released another set in 1980 (American College of Sports Medicine, 1975, 1980). These recommendations were predominantly directed at cardiorespiratory fitness and suggested that people undertake vigorous-intensity aerobic exercise 3 times/wk for 20 min each time. This was a practical interpretation of the exact recommendation from 1975, which suggested that people undertake 20 to 45 min of physical activity 3 to 5 days/wk at 70% to 90% of heart rate (i.e., vigorous intensity) (American College of Sports Medicine, 1975). The focus on aerobic exercise for increasing fitness continued to dominate and influence health messages about physical activity until the early 1990s. However, guidelines began to recommend moderate-intensity physical activity rather than vigorous-intensity activity, and by the mid-1990s the focus shifted from cardiorespiratory fitness to health benefits. This new position on physical activity was communicated in a landmark set of recommendations from the office of the U.S. surgeon general in the report "Physical Activity and Health" (U.S. Centers for Disease Control and Prevention, 1996).

In the mid-1990s, epidemiological evidence started to show that people with different health conditions require slightly different amounts of physical activity. Although the recommendation for 30 min of moderate-intensity activity on most days remained valid for preventing heart disease and diabetes, studies showed that slightly more physical activity was recommended for preventing cancer. Further, studies identified that the amount of activity required for weight loss or preventing weight gain was greater than that required to prevent chronic disease (Haskell et al., 2007). For example, the International Association for the Study of Obesity recommendations made a clear distinction between the minimum physical activity required for health benefits and the amount required for preventing weight gain. The recommendations state that "45 to 60 min (60-90 min for formerly obese individuals) of moderate-intensity physical activity daily is needed to prevent the transition to overweight or obesity" (Saris et al., 2003). Furthermore, research has now shown that the amount of physical activity required by young people differs from that of adults. The overall amount of physical activity recommended for children is twice that recommended for adults and is usually expressed as "at least 60 min/day" (Canadian Society for Exercise Physiology, 2011a; Saris et al., 2003).

These different recommendations make the development of PAGs complex. However, a core and consistent interpretation of the evidence is that 30 min of moderate-intensity physical activity on most days of the week is associated with maximum overall population benefit and the prevention of major noncommunicable diseases. This same dose has been expressed as "at least 150 min/wk of moderate-intensity activity" in the most recent global, U.S. and U.K recommendations (Department of Health, 2011b; U.S. Department of Health and Human Services, 2008a; World Health Organisation, 2010).

4   Current Best Practice in Developing Guidelines

Figure 2.3 illustrates the process of developing guidelines. The first step is establishing the need for guidelines. This need is often defined by policymakers, public health scientists, advocates and, sometimes, the community. Then a process for guideline development needs to be agreed on by interested parties, with actions planned in sequence and, ideally, a linkage between the PAG development process and other aspects of national or regional physical activity policy and strategy development (step 1 in figure 2.3). The next stage comprises reviewing the scientific evidence and creating an updated summary of what the research says and how this information differs from that in previous guidelines. A number of countries, notably Canada and, most recently, the United Kingdom and United States, have undertaken this process. Tremblay and colleagues (2010) extensively discuss this process with reference to the recent Canadian guidelines along with frameworks and a checklist for auditing data quality in the review stage.

Once the science has been reviewed, the next stage is developing communication messages based on the evidence and testing these messages with the target audience for acceptability, comprehension and usefulness. This step is part of developing a communications strategy for disseminating the evidence (stages 3 and 4 in figure 2.3). It requires resources for conducting the qualitative and quantitative research and the involvement of communications and media specialists in framing the messages correctly so that they will have optimal impact on the target populations. The final stages (stages 5-7 in figure 2.3) involve disseminating the message to the community, professional groups and other stakeholders. Historically, those developing PAGs have put considerable effort into the technical and scientific stages and have often neglected message development and communication. Frequently, only informal and unpaid communication channels are used after the launch of PAGs. Thus, a very important step in PAG development and dissemination is the final public health promotion component.

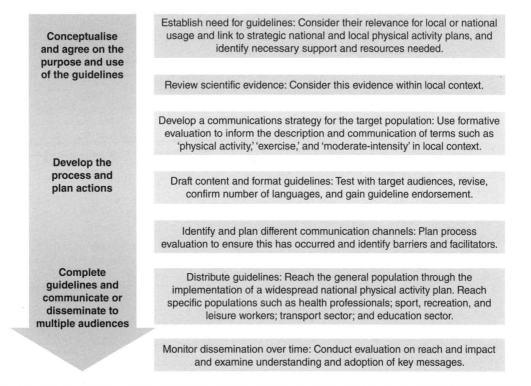

Figure 2.3 Framework for developing physical activity guidelines.
Adapted from Bauman et al. 2006.

5 Global, Regional and National Physical Activity Guidelines

Table 2.1 summarises the 2011 global PAGs and provides examples of regional (i.e., European and Western Pacific islands) and national guidelines. Quite a few countries in Europe have their own national PAGs, and many of these countries (e.g., Finland, Switzerland, the Netherlands, United Kingdom) have been engaged with implementing national population-based approaches for some time (Department of Health, 2011b; Ministry of Health, Welfare and Sport, 2011; Swiss Federal Office of Sports, 2006; UKK Institute, 2009). Other countries in Europe have officially or unofficially adopted the guidelines published by the U.S. Centers for Disease Control and Prevention in 1996 and the more recently updated 2008 version.

PAGs in other regions of the world are patchy. Australia (Department of Health and Ageing, 2005b) and New Zealand (Sport and Recreation New Zealand, 2005) have had national guidelines for some time. In Australia, guidelines exist for all ages, from young children (Department of Health and Ageing, 2004) to older adults (Department of Health and Ageing, 2005b), although all guidelines are more than 5 yr old and arguably are due for updating to reflect the latest science. Far fewer examples of PAGs exist in South America, Asia, the Middle East and Africa because physical activity promotion is relatively new in these regions. Countries in which national action on physical activity is beginning have often used the U.S. guidelines as an international benchmark. This has allowed the countries to develop an agenda of physical activity promotion without being hindered by the absence of PAGs. However, in some countries, adopting the PAGs of another country is not politically or culturally welcome or appropriate. Either these countries have developed their own PAGs (a recent example from the Middle East is Brunei; Ministry of Health, 2011) or very little physical activity promotion has occurred.

The absence of a set of official global guidelines did not hinder the World Health Organisation (WHO) from developing the Global Strategy on Diet, Physical Activity and Health in 2004 (World Health Organisation, 2004). Since the publication of the 2002 health report (World Health Organisation, 2002), the focus on the need for greater action to prevent noncommunicable disease and address mental health has increased. To address these issues, WHO commenced developing global guidelines in 2007. WHO launched the final global recommendations on physical activity in 2010 after a 2 yr process involving global and regional consultations (World Health Organisation, 2010). These global guidelines are now available for adoption and use by countries with no national PAGs. Because the guidelines are from WHO, the leading international health agency, the scientific quality and relevance of these guidelines are usually accepted.

Of interest is that the development process included significant review and consideration of the applicability of the research, which is conducted mostly with populations in high-income countries, to populations in low- and middle-income countries. Other reports have also considered this issue. Overall, assessments have shown that biological mechanisms and physical responses to physical activity are generalisable even though the types of physical activities undertaken vary according to culture, interests and geographical and climatic conditions (Armstrong et al., 2007; World Health Organisation, 2008).

Of particular importance is the role the 2010 global PAGs can play in countries with few resources and little or no scientific capacity to develop their own PAGs. Countries can now circumvent the time- and resource-intensive process of developing PAGs by formally adopting the global PAGs. PAGs developed at the regional level (e.g., the guidelines for the Western Pacific Islands or Brunei-Darussalam; Ministry of Health, 2011; World Health Organisation, 2008) can be tailored more specifically to characteristics of the region and country.

Table 2.1 Global, Regional and National Physical Activity Guidelines

Location	Activity level	Children	Adults	Older adults
GLOBAL				
Global (World Health Organisation, 2010)	Moderate to vigorous	60 min/day of moderate- to vigorous-intensity physical activity.	150 min/wk of moderate-intensity aerobic physical activity, or ≥75 min/wk of vigorous-intensity aerobic physical activity, or an equivalent combination of moderate- and vigorous-intensity activity. Perform aerobic activity in bouts of ≥10 min. For additional health benefits, increase moderate-intensity aerobic physical activity to 300 min/wk or engage in 150 min/wk of vigorous-intensity aerobic physical activity or an equivalent combination of moderate- and vigorous-intensity activity. Perform muscle-strengthening activities that involve major muscle groups ≥2 days/wk.	150 min/wk of moderate-intensity aerobic physical activity, or ≥75 min/wk of vigorous-intensity aerobic physical activity, or an equivalent combination of moderate- and vigorous-intensity activity. Perform aerobic activity in bouts of ≥10 min. For additional health benefits, increase moderate-intensity aerobic physical activity to 300 min/wk or engage in 150 min/wk of vigorous-intensity aerobic physical activity or an equivalent combination of moderate- and vigorous-intensity activity.
	Strength, balance and flexibility	Most daily physical activity should be aerobic. Incorporate vigorous-intensity activity, including those that strengthen muscle and bone, ≥3 days/wk.	—	Those with poor mobility should perform physical activity that enhances balance ≥3 days/wk to prevent falls. Perform muscle-strengthening activities that involve major muscle groups ≥2 days/wk. Those who cannot perform the recom-mended amount of physical activity due to health conditions should be as physically active as abilities and conditions allow.
REGIONAL				
European Union (European Union, 2008)	Moderate	60 min/day of moderate-intensity physical activity.	30 min/day of moderate-intensity physical activity.	30 min/day of moderate-intensity physical activity.
Western Pacific region (World Health Organisation, 2008)	Moderate to vigorous	—	30 min of moderate-intensity physical activity ≥5 days/wk. Enjoy regular vigorous-intensity activity for extra health and fitness benefits.	—

(continued)

Table 2.1 *(continued)*

Location	Activity level	Children	Adults	Older adults
NATIONAL				
Australia (Department of Health and Ageing, 2005a,b)	Moderate	—	—	(1999) 30 min of moderate-intensity physical activity most, preferably all, days. Those who cannot perform 30 min should start with 10 min once or twice/day and, after 2 wk, perform 15 min twice/day to accomplish 30 min/day.
	Moderate to vigorous	(2004) Ages 5-12 yr: 60 min/day to up to several hours/day of moderate- to vigorous-intensity physical activity.	(1999) 30 min of moderate-intensity physical activity most, preferably all, days. Enjoy regular vigorous-intensity activity for extra health and fitness benefits.	—
	Sedentary	Use electronic media (e.g., computer games, television, Internet) for entertainment, particularly during daylight hours, for no more than 2 h/day.	—	—
Brunei (Ministry of Health, 2011)	Moderate to vigorous	≥60 min/day of moderate- to vigorous-intensity physical activity. Activity should be mostly aerobic. Being physically active for >60 min/day provides additional health benefits.	≥150 min/wk of moderate-intensity aerobic physical activity spread over 3 days, or ≥75 min/wk of vigorous-intensity aerobic physical activity, or an equivalent combination of moderate- and vigorous-intensity activity. For additional health benefits, increase moderate-intensity aerobic physical activity to 300 min/wk or engage in 150 min/wk of vigorous-intensity aerobic physical activity or an equivalent combination of moderate- and vigorous-intensity activity.	≥150 min/wk of moderate-intensity aerobic physical activity spread over ≥3 days, or ≥75 min/wk of vigorous-intensity aerobic physical activity, or an equivalent combination of moderate- and vigorous-intensity activity. Perform aerobic activity in bouts of ≥10 min. For additional health benefits, increase moderate-intensity aerobic physical activity to 300 min/wk or engage in 150 min/wk of vigorous-intensity aerobic physical activity or an equivalent combination of moderate- and vigorous-intensity activity.
	Sedentary	Use electronic media (e.g., computer games, television, Internet) for no more than 2 h/day unless it is educational.	—	—
	Strength, balance and flexibility	Incorporate vigorous-intensity activities that strengthen muscles and bones 3 days/wk.	Perform muscle-strengthening activities that involve major muscle groups ≥2 days/wk.	Perform muscle-strengthening activities that involve major muscle groups ≥2 days/wk.

Location	Activity level	Children	Adults	Older adults
		NATIONAL *(continued)*		
Canada (Canadian Society for Exercise Physiology, 2011a)	Moderate to vigorous	Ages 5-11 yr: 60 min/day of moderate- to vigorous-intensity physical activity. Ages 12-17 yr: 60 min/day of moderate- to vigorous-intensity physical activity.	150 min/wk of moderate- to vigorous-intensity aerobic physical activity. Perform activity in bouts of ≥10 min.	150 min/wk of moderate- to vigorous-intensity aerobic physical activity. Perform activity in bouts of ≥10 min.
	Strength, balance and flexibility	Ages 5-11 yr: Perform vigorous-intensity activy ≥3 days/wk. Perform activities that strengthen muscle and bone ≥3 days/wk. Ages 12-17 yr: Perform vigorous-intensity activity ≥3 days/wk. Perform activities that strengthen muscle and bone ≥3 days/wk.	For additional benefits, perform muscle- and bone-strengthening activities that use major muscle groups ≥2 days/wk.	For additional benefits, perform muscle- and bone-strengthening activities that use major muscle groups ≥2 days/wk. Those with poor mobility should perform physical activity that enhances balance to prevent falls.
Finland (UKK Institute, 2009)	Moderate	Ages 7-18 yr: 1-2 h of physical exercise/day.	—	—
	Moderate to vigorous	—	≥150 min/wk of moderate activity or 75 min/wk of vigorous activity over several days.	—
	Strength, balance and flexibility	—	Increase muscle strength and improve balance ≥2 days/wk.	—
Ireland (Department of Health and Children, Health Service Executive, 2009)	Moderate to vigorous	≥60 min/day of moderate- to vigorous-intensity physical activity.	30 min/day of moderate-intensity activity 5 days/wk (or 150 min/wk).	30 min/day of moderate-intensity activity 5 days/wk (or 150 min/wk).
	Strength, balance and flexibility	Perform muscle-strengthening, flexibility and bone-strengthening exercises 3 days/wk.	—	Focus on aerobic activity, muscle strengthening and balance.
Japan (Office for Lifestyle-Related Diseases Control, 2006)	Moderate	—	Walk 8,000-10,000 steps/day. Those who rely on exercise for health promotion: 35 min/wk of jogging or playing tennis or 1 h/wk of brisk walking. Quantity of physical activity: (Equivalent of an activity lasting approximately 60 min/day at an intensity of 3 METs. If the activity mainly comprises walking, the quantity is equivalent to 8,000-10,000 steps/day). Quantity of exercise: 4 METs h/wk (e.g., 60 min of fast walking or 35 min of jogging or playing tennis).	—

(continued)

Table 2.1 *(continued)*

Location	Activity level	Children	Adults	Older adults
NATIONAL *(continued)*				
New Zealand (Sport and Recreation New Zealand, 2005)	Moderate to vigorous	—	30 min of moderate-intensity physical activity most, preferably all, days. Enjoy regular vigorous-intensity activity for extra health and fitness benefits.	—
Norway (Becker et al., 2004)	Moderate to vigorous	≥60 min/day of moderate- or vigorous-intensity physical activity.	≥30 min/day of moderate- or vigorous-intensity physical activity. This activity can be made up of several sessions, each lasting ≥10 min, during the day.	≥30 min/day of moderate- or vigorous-intensity physical activity. This activity can be made up of several sessions, each lasting ≥10 min, during the day.
Netherlands (Ministry of Health, Welfare and Sport, 2011).	Moderate	≥60 min/day of moderate-intensity physical activity [5 MET (e.g., aerobics, skateboarding) to 8 MET (e.g., running 8 km/h)]. Perform activity aimed at improving or maintaining physical fitness (power, agility and coordination) ≥2 days/wk.	≥30 min of moderate-intensity physical activity [4-6.5 MET; briskly walking (5 km/h) or cycling (16 km/h)] ≥5 days/wk.	≥30 min of moderate-intensity physical activity [3-5 MET; walking (4 km/h) or cycling (10 km/h)] ≥5 days/wk (preferably every day). Nonactive people with or without physical limitations: All extra physical exercise is significant regardless of intensity, duration, frequency and type.
Slovenia (Republic of Slovenia Ministry of Health, 2007)	Moderate	—	≥30 min of moderate-intensity activity ≥5 days/wk. Exercise should be as diverse as possible, balanced by type (50% aerobic exercise, 25% flexibility exercise and 25% strength exercise), and enjoyable. Exercise can be carried out in various settings (e.g., home, work, for transportation purposes).	—
Switzerland (Swiss Federal Office of Sports, 2006)	Moderate	≥60 min/day of physical activity (younger children even more).	≥30 min/day of moderate-intensity physical activity.	≥30 min/day of moderate-intensity physical activity.
	Strength, balance and flexibility	As part of or in addition to the 1 h minimum, perform for ≥10 min several days/wk activities that build strong bones, stimulate the heart and circulation, strengthen muscles, maintain flexibility and improve agility.	Perform endurance training for 20-60 min 3 days/wk. Perform strength and flexibility exercises 2 days/wk.	Perform endurance training for 20-60 min 3 days/wk. Perform strength and flexibility exercises 2 days/wk.

Location	Activity level	Children	Adults	Older adults
		NATIONAL *(continued)*		
United Kingdom (Department of Health, 2011b)	Moderate to vigorous	Ages under 5 yr: Physical activity should be encouraged from birth, particularly through floor-based play and water-based activities in safe environments. Those capable of walking unaided should be physically active for ≥180 min/day spread throughout the day. Minimise time spent restrained or sitting for extended periods (except time spent sleeping). Ages 5-18 yr: At least 60 min/day and up to several hours/day of moderate- to vigorous-intensity physical activity. Perform vigorous-intensity activities, including those that strengthen muscle and bone, ≥3 days/wk.	150 min/wk of moderate-intensity activity in bouts of 10 min or more (one way to approach this is to perform 30 min ≥5 days/wk), or 75 min/wk of vigorous-intensity activity, or a combination of moderate- and vigorous-intensity activity.	150 min/wk of moderate-intensity activity in bouts of 10 min or more (one way to approach this is to perform 30 min ≥5 days/wk). Those who are already regularly active at moderate intensity can perform 75 min/wk of vigorous-intensity activity or a combination of moderate- and vigorous-intensity activity.
	Strength, balance and flexibility	Avoid being sedentary for extended periods of time.	Perform physical activity that improves muscle strength ≥2 days/wk.	Perform physical activity that improves muscle strength ≥2 days/wk. Those at risk of falls should perform physical activity that improves balance and coordination ≥2 days/wk.
	Sedentary	—	Avoid being sedentary for extended periods of time.	Avoid being sedentary for extended periods of time.
United States (U.S. Department of Health and Human Services, 2008b)	Moderate to vigorous	—	≥150 min/wk of moderate-intensity aerobic physical activity or ≥75 min/wk of vigorous-intensity aerobic physical activity. Perform activity for bouts of at least 10 min at a time.	—
	Strength, balance and flexibility	—	Perform strengthening activities ≥ 2 days/wk.	—

Dash indicates no data.

MET = Metabolic equivalent.

6   Implementation and Influence of Physical Activity Guidelines

National PAGs have a number of applications in a comprehensive, population-based approach. For PAGs to be effective, they must be well disseminated. PAGs can be communicated to professionals and the general community as part of educational strategies, used to guide the national surveillance systems that monitor levels of physical activity over time and used to inform national policy and develop and support clinical and preventive practice and health promotion. The following sections explore these roles in more detail.

6.1   Dissemination

First and foremost, PAGs are a means of communicating to a population how much physical activity is needed to promote health and prevent disease. However, they are usually written in a detailed, often scientific, format and use terminology that may be unfamiliar to wider audiences. One of the first tasks after creating PAGs is developing a set of appropriate communication tools, a communication strategy and a dissemination plan (stages 6 and 7, refer to figure 2.3). Evidence to date suggests that this step is often overlooked. Too often, PAGs remain formal, seldom-used documents of which people in professional communities and the general public are unaware. To avoid this outcome, it is desirable to engage experts with backgrounds in communication when developing and testing ways to best communicate the key messages of the PAGs to different audiences. This is ideally undertaken concurrently with the final steps of PAGs development to allow a set of resources, targeted to multiple audiences and uses, to be available at the time of the formal launch of the PAGs.

When creating communications about PAGs, the level of detail and the medium used should be appropriate for the intended audiences. Brief pamphlets and handouts are particularly useful because they can be distributed to patient populations and placed in public locations. The amount of detail included depends on the space available. Recently, agencies have used pictures or schemas to try to convey the complex message of the different amounts and types of activity recommended. In Finland, the activity pie (figure 2.4) has been developed to show the multiple ways one can combine types and duration of activity to reach the recommended amount. In Switzerland physical activity recommendations are shown as a pyramid (figure 2.5). Several versions of this pyramid exist, and each has increasing level of detail. Fact sheets are popular because few professionals have time to read detailed scientific reports. The most recent PAGs from Canada, the United Kingdom and the United States have been launched with a set of fact sheets (Canadian Society for Exercise Physiology, 2011b; Department of Health, 2011c; U.S. Department of Health and Human Services, 2008d) (see figure 2.6).

An important question is whether the presence of PAGs has affected levels of physical activity in a country. Because few evaluations have been conducted to date, evidence is limited. Evaluation has, however, taken place is Canada, where PAGs were first released in 1998 by the health ministry in partnership with the Canadian Exercise Science Professional Society. One measure of success of PAGs is the level of unprompted awareness of the guidelines as recorded in population surveys. In Canada, rates of unprompted awareness in adults were initially low; only 5% to 7% of Canadian adults recalled the guidelines (Bauman, Craig & Cameron, 2005). Recall was highest among those who were more affluent or most physically active (Bauman, Craig & Cameron, 2005). In 2003, the results again showed that overall unprompted awareness remained low, although rates of prompted awareness were higher (approximately one third of Canadian adults; Bauman, Craig & Cameron, 2005; Cameron et al., 2007). In surveys measuring awareness, items ask whether the responder has heard of any campaigns and, if yes, asks the responder to list them (unprompted awareness). The items also ask whether the responder has

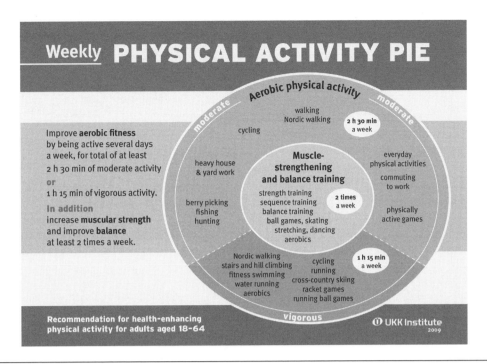

Figure 2.4   Physical activity pie from Finland.

Reprinted, by permission, from T. Vasankari (Tampere Finland: UKK Institute). ©UKK Institute.

heard of any of the specific campaigns listed (prompted awareness). The Canadian findings illustrate the importance of evaluating the reach and success of communicating PAGs to the target audience. Moreover, the experience in Canada illustrates how population-surveillance systems can be used to assess the reach and level of use of PAGs and their impact on physical activity

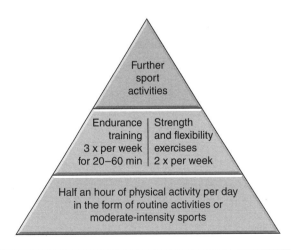

Figure 2.5   Activity pyramid from Switzerland.

Martin BW and Marti B. 1998, Swiss Federal Offices of Sport and Public Health 1999.

levels. Low levels of population awareness and penetration of PAGs, as shown in Canada in the 1990s, indicate that greater attention and effort are required to achieve dissemination of the message throughout the population.

Dissemination can be achieved through large-scale, sustained public education campaigns aimed at reaching the whole community with a clear message about being more active derived from the PAGs. A recent example from the United States shows how a set of diverse resources can support PAG dissemination. The 2008 launch of the U.S. PAGs was accompanied by a scientific report (>700 pages) providing full details of the findings of the 2 yr scientific review (U.S. Department of Health and Human Services, 2008g), the guidelines themselves in a report (79 pages) aimed at professional audiences (U.S. Department of Health and Human Services, 2008e), a website and toolkits (U.S. Department of Health and Human Services, 2008f), fact sheets for health professionals (U.S. Department of Health and Human Services, 2008d), how-to guides and a blog (U.S. Department of Health and Human

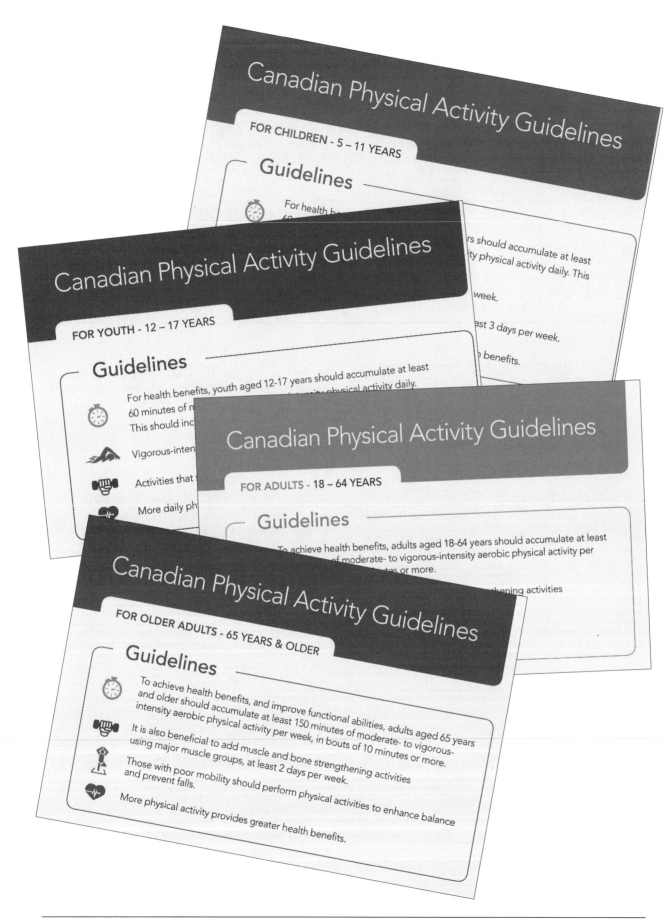

Figure 2.6 Canadian physical activity guideline fact sheets.

Services, 2008c). This suite of resources reflects a large-scale investment in communication and dissemination and should lead to better reach and awareness in the community. Ideally these actions would be accompanied by a good evaluation programme to assess outcome and effectiveness and to inform future implementation strategies.

PAGs should be communicated to relevant professional groups. This may involve tailoring the content to the contexts in which the professionals work and may require repeated annual communications until all of the target audience (e.g., general practitioners, clinicians) are aware of the PAGs, know the content and report using them in routine practice. The potential professional audience for PAGs extends beyond the health sector and can include those in the education sector (at all levels), transport sector and local government. For example, in the United Kingdom, resources were recently developed for disseminating the new PAGs for children under the age of 5 yr to childcare centres (Department of Health, 2011a).

PAGs will not achieve optimal reach and impact without a sustained dissemination strategy

Case Study: Mass-Media Campaigns

FIND THIRTY

Mass-media campaigns are a common strategy used to promote the health benefits of physical activity and encourage increased levels of participation. One of the first campaigns in Australia, launched over 35 yr ago, was called "Life. Be In It." After a long gap, the National Heart Foundation launched new campaigns in the early 1990s in response to increasing scientific evidence of the health benefits of increased physical activity. These campaigns included "Exercise: Make It Part of Your Day," aimed at all Australians aged 15 yr and older (Booth et al., 1992); "Exercise: Take Another Step," which built on the earlier campaign and emphasised walking (Owen et al., 1995); and "Exercise: You Only Have to Take it Regularly, Not Seriously" (Bauman et al., 2001), delivered only in New South Wales, which targeted adults who were motivated but who had not undertaken sufficient levels of activity.

In 2002, the first statewide physical activity campaign in Western Australia, "Find Thirty. It's Not a Big Exercise," commenced. The campaign was funded by the Health Department of Western Australia. Iterations of the "Find Thirty" slogan have run over the past 10 yr. Most recently, the campaign "Find Thirty Every Day" aimed to further promote the physical, mental and social health benefits of regular physical activity to adults aged 20 to 54 yr.

Mass-media campaigns can involve multiple communication channels, including television, radio, print media and billboards. The "Find Thirty Every Day" television commercials included 15- and 30-second advertisements featuring a montage of everyday physical activities, including parents playing with children, adults walking for recreation and transport, dancing or cycling and active domestic tasks such as raking leaves. The Australian PAGs were an important platform for the content and the core tag line "Find Thirty," and the involvement of scientific experts in the design, content and evaluation of mass-media campaigns ensured that mass-media communications were consistent with the science and best practice (Leavy et al., 2011).

AGITA SÃO PAULO

In 1996, the Studies Center of the Physical Fitness Research Laboratory of São Caetano do Sul and the São Paulo State Secretariat of Health launched the Agita São Paulo programme. It aimed to promote physical activity among the 37 million inhabitants of the state of São Paulo, Brazil. The verb *agita*, which means "to move the body," was used to suggest changing the way people were thinking about physical activity and to promote becoming a more active citizen. Rather than saying "sport is health" or "fitness is heath," the programme focussed on

(continued)

(continued)

the lifestyle changes people could make to gain the many health benefits that come from an active way of living.

The core message of the Agita São Paulo programme is that one should accumulate at least 30 min/day of moderate-intensity physical activity most days of the week. This focus was explicitly based on the then-new physical activity recommendations launched in the surgeon general's 1996 report. The programme logo has become widely known in Brazil and internationally.

The programme promotes the physical activity recommendations using a multilevel intervention and targets three main groups: students, workers and the elderly. It has a strong focus on using megaevents that reach and involve large numbers of people. Megaevents are used to launch a new programme components and reinforce existing activities. They generally coincide with cultural or seasonal events such as public holidays, carnivals or summer vacations. Megaevents can often attract broad media coverage from television, radio, magazines, newspapers and the Internet, which in turn increases awareness of the importance of an active lifestyle. This use of free media to gain widespread coverage of the physical activity recommendations has been very successful in Brazil. Megaevents can be targeted to and held on specific dates. For example, "Agita Melhori-

dade" ("Move, Elderly People") was launched on the National and International Day of Older Persons. Older people who joined in the activities received T-shirts, fans and hats printed with the Agita programme message (i.e., 30 min/day of physical activity). The programme also aims to establish partnerships with governmental and nongovernmental organisations to continue and expand activities aimed at physical activity. Partners can use and modify the Agita São Paulo logo for multiple purposes, thus increasing the dissemination and reach.

Since 1996, the Agita São Paulo programme has been widely copied throughout Brazil and in other countries in Latin America. In 2000, the Ministry of Health launched Agita Brasil, which retained the message of moving the body, changing the way of thinking and becoming a more active citizen (Brazil Ministério da Saúde, Secretaria de Políticas Públicas, 2002). In 2002, WHO adopted the core message for the 2002 World Health Day on physical activity and used the slogan "Agita Mundo" ("Move the World"). Agita São Paulo, a multilevel programme that has a clear scientific base and is consistent with current physical activity recommendation, is now widely promoted as a model for programmes in other low- and middle-income countries (Advocacy Council of the International Society for Physical Activity and Health, 2011).

aimed at both professional and community audiences. A variety of examples of strategies exist. However, to date, little good information is available to help evaluate the effectiveness of these approaches and guide future efforts.

6.2   Surveillance

An important link exists between PAGs and national surveillance systems for monitoring physical activity at the population level. Increasingly more countries are including physical activity levels in the national surveillance system in order to assess changes in physical activity over time. These usually involve serial (often annual) health surveys, conducted by telephone or in

person, of a representative population. Such surveys need to ask identical questions on physical activity so that trends are comparable (Carlson et al., 2009). As new guidelines are developed from new evidence or as guidelines change or become more specific, more demands are placed on the surveillance questions needed. For example, few surveillance systems include questions for assessing strength training or time spent in sedentary behaviours, yet emerging evidence and the most recent PAGs indicate that these questions may be necessary.

In addition to measuring and reporting the levels of physical activity in the population and presenting these data in ways that are aligned with the national PAGs, national surveillance systems can be used to assess the reach and understanding of PAGs in a population. As previously discussed, Canada is an example of a country that has used the national survey to evaluate the dissemination of PAGs.

6.3 Policy

An important component of a population-based approach to promoting physical activity is a national policy and action plan that outlines the intent, responsibilities and actions that must be undertaken within a specific period of time (Bull et al., 2004). PAGs are an important part of the process of developing policies and action plans in that they provide a summary of scientific evidence and a clear message on how much and what types of physical activity should be encouraged. PAGs can create a platform of consensus and provide the necessary catalyst for policy development. Policy can take the form of a standalone national policy on physical activity [e.g., that in Norway (Ministry of Health, 2005) or the United Kingdom (Department of Health, 2004)] or may be part of a wider policy document that addresses multiple health issues (e.g., healthy eating and physical activity, health lifestyles). Since the WHO global strategy in 2004 (World Health Organisation, 2004), considerable progress has been made in national policy development, particularly in the European region (Daugbjerg et al., 2009).

National policy and support for more detailed action plans on physical activity can give physical activity promotion coherence and visibility at the political level. Although PAGs can lead to policy, a national policy might be developed in advance of PAGs. Indeed, one of the first actions outlined in the policy itself may be the development of national PAGs or the endorsement of the now-available global PAGs.

PAGs help form the content of the policy and outline who should be involved. The details provided in PAGs about the types and amount of physical activity required can show how a variety of agencies and sectors can and should be involved in promoting physical activity to different groups. For example, one can accrue the recommended physical activity through different types of activity, including walking and cycling. This information can be used to highlight how sectors beyond health and sports and recreation, such as transport (promoting active commuting), the environment and national parks, should be engaged. PAGs allow agencies inside and outside of government to work together with coherent and consistent objectives and purpose.

6.4 Clinical Practice

PAGs are useful tools for practitioners because they specify the types and amount of physical activity one should perform to promote health and mange or prevent disease. They also allow practitioners to develop setting-specific programmes and interventions. Extensive work has been done in primary care settings to promote physical activity through counselling and advice from medical or allied health practitioners. PAGs are often used as the basis of the assessment and counselling, and simplified versions of PAGs can be provided to the patient in the form of health-education pamphlets. Strong evidence exists for the effectiveness of these approaches. However, PAGs have been underutilised in mental health promotion and in clinical care pathways for people with mental health problems. Physical activity has low salience among mental health professionals (Phongsavan et al., 2007) and is seldom part of care planning. Therefore, physical activity promotion for people with mental health problems could benefit from further evidence-based advocacy.

6.5 Recommendations on Physical Activity Interventions

Another important area of population-based approaches to promoting physical activity is the development of recommendations on which programmes and strategies effectively increase participation levels and how best to implement them. Considerable progress has been made in this area in recent years. Many investigators have

EVIDENCE TO PRACTICE

- General PAGs provide a useful point of reference for mental health practitioners.
- Developing PAGs is a multistep process that involves technical and scientific reviews, stakeholder and consumer consultation, message testing, and dissemination and evaluation.
- Dissemination of PAGs to multiple audiences is critical but often executed poorly and with few resources.
- Practitioners, including those in the mental health setting, can use PAGs to demonstrate evidence-based scientific agree-

ment and to advocate for resources and programmes aimed at addressing physical inactivity.
- PAGs provide practitioners with direction on the types of programmes to provide and promote to patients (including mental health patients) and the wider community.
- Practitioners can use PAGs to direct action at the levels of patients and clients and service providers and all levels—national, regional and local—of government.

led reviews of the literature (Bravata et al., 2007; Conn et al., 2009; Foster, Hillsdon & Thorogood, 2005; Li et al., 2008; Ogilvie et al., 2007; Pucher, Dill & Handy, 2010), and a number of nationally led efforts have assessed what works to increase rates of participation. These efforts can result in the creation of national guidance documents on physical activity interventions. Examples include the work in the United Kingdom led by the National Institute for Health and Clinical Excellence (NICE) and, in the United States, *The Guide to Community Preventive Services* (Zaza, Briss & Harris, 2005), which specifically includes physical activity (Kahn et al., 2002). NICE has produced a large number of guidance reports covering common approaches to physical activity interventions the environment and worksite settings (National Institute for Health and Clinical Excellence, 2006a,b, 2008a,b). These guidance statements are based on extensive systematic reviews of the selected approaches to promoting physical activity. In some cases this can also extend to including an assessment of cost effectiveness, which is an important and necessary argument to present in order to secure resources. PAGs that provide both information on the types and amount of activity required and guidance on interventions are core resources for effectively directing national population-based approaches.

7   Summary

This chapter explains the purpose of PAGs, their development and their role in a comprehensive, population-based approach to promoting physical activity. This chapter also discusses the history of the development of PAGs and their application and use in surveillance, practice and policy. A critical step in the development of PAGs is dissemination. However, this step is often overlooked and poorly resourced. PAGs provide the maximum benefit only if they are adequately communicated and disseminated to all relevant audiences. Few countries have disseminated guidelines well, although evidence suggests that the lessons of the past have led to better practice, as seen with the efforts to disseminate the most recent guidelines in the United Kingdom, United States and Canada. PAGs remain underused by clinical and allied health practitioners as part of therapy and preventive strategies, particularly in the area of mental health. Guidelines provide a focus for policymakers and practitioners to promote physical activity in individuals, communities and whole populations. The area of mental health promotion and treatment could include a stronger emphasis on promoting physical activity and could use existing guidelines to facilitate changes in practice in this area.

8 References

Advocacy Council of the International Society for Physical Activity and Health. (2011). *Noncommunicable disease prevention: Seven investments that work for physical activity.* Available: www.globalpa.org.uk/investmentsthatwork.

American College of Sports Medicine. (1975). *Guidelines for graded exercise testing and exercise prescription.* Philadelphia: Lea & Febiger.

American College of Sports Medicine. (1980). *Guidelines for graded exercise testing and exercise prescription.* Philadelphia: Lea & Febiger.

Armstrong, T., Bauman, A., Bull, F., Candeias, V., Lewicka, M., Magnussen, C., et al. (2007). *A guide for population-based approaches to increasing levels of physical activity: Implementation of the WHO global strategy on diet, physical activity and health.* Geneva, Switzerland: World Health Organisation.

Bauman, A., & Chau, J. (2009). The role of media in promoting physical activity. *Journal of Physical Activity and Health*, 6(Suppl. 2), S196-S210.

Bauman, A., Craig, C.L., & Cameron, C. (2005). Low levels of recall among adult Canadians of the CSEP/Health Canada physical activity guidelines. *Canadian Journal of Applied Physiology*, 30(2), 246-252.

Bauman, A.E., Bellew, B., Owen, N., & Vita, P. (2001). Impact of an Australian mass media campaign targeting physical activity in 1998. *American Journal of Preventive Medicine*, 21(1), 41-47.

Bauman, A.E., Nelson, D.E., Pratt, M., Matsudo, V., & Schoeppe, S. (2006). Dissemination of physical activity evidence, programs, policies, and surveillance in the international public health arena. *American Journal of Preventive Medicine*, 31(4), 57-65.

Becker, W., Lyhne, N., Pedersen, A.N., Aro, A., Fogelholm, M., Phórsdottir, I., et al. (2004). Nordic nutrition recommendations 2004—Integrating nutrition and physical activity. *Scandinavian Journal of Nutrition*, 48(4), 178-187.

Biddle, S.J.H., & Asare, M. (2011). Physical activity and mental health in children and adolescents: A review of reviews. *British Journal of Sports Medicine*, 45(11), 886-895.

Booth, M., Bauman, A., Oldenburg, B., Owen, N., & Magnus, P. (1992). Effects of a national mass-media campaign on physical activity participation. *Health Promotion International*, 7(4), 241-247.

Brasil Ministério da Saúde, Secretaria de Políticas Públicas. (2002). Projeto Promoção da Saúde. Programa nacional de atividade física "Agita Brasil": Atividade física e sua contribuição para a qualidade de vida. *Rev Saude Publica*, 36(2), 254-256.

Bravata, D.M., Smith-Spangler, C., Sundaram, V., Gienger, A.L., Lin, N., Lewis, R., et al. (2007). Using pedometers to increase physical activity and improve health. *Journal of the American Medical Association*, 298(19), 2296-2304.

Bull, F., & Milton, K. (2011). Let's Get Moving: A systematic pathway for the promotion of physical activity in a primary care setting. *Global Health Promotion*, 18(1), 59-61.

Bull, F.C., & Bauman, A.E. (2011). Physical inactivity: The "Cinderella" risk factor for noncommunicable disease prevention. *Journal of Health Communication*, 16(Suppl. 2), 13-26.

Bull, F.C., Bellew, B., Schöppe, S., & Bauman, A.E. (2004). Developments in national physical activity policy: An international review and recommendations towards better practice. *Journal of Science and Medicine in Sport*, 7(Suppl. 1), 93-104.

Cameron, C., Craig, C.L., Bull, F.C., & Bauman, A.E. (2007). Canada's physical activity guides: Has their release had an impact? *Applied Physiology, Nutrition, and Metabolism*, 32(Suppl. 2E), S161-S169.

Canadian Society for Exercise Physiology. (2011a). *Canadian physical activity guidelines.* Ottawa, Canada: Canadian Society for Exercise Physiology.

Canadian Society for Exercise Physiology. (2011b). *Canadian physical activity guidelines factsheets.* Ottawa, Canada: Canadian Society for Exercise Physiology. Available: www.csep.ca/english/view.asp?x=804.

Carlson, S.A., Densmore, D., Fulton, J.E., Yore, M.M., & Kohl, H.W. (2009). Differences in physical activity prevalence and trends from 3 U.S. surveillance systems: NHIS, NHANES, and BRFSS. *Journal of Physical Activity and Health*, 6(Suppl. 1), S18-S27.

Conn, V.S., Hafdahl, A.R., Cooper, P.S., Brown, L.M., & Lusk, S.L. (2009). Meta-analysis of workplace physical activity interventions. *American Journal of Preventive Medicine*, 37(4), 330-339.

Daugbjerg, S.B., Kahlmeier, S., Racioppi, F., Martin-Diener, E., Martin, B., Oja, P., et al. (2009). Promotion of physical activity in the European region: Content analysis of 27 national policy documents. *Journal of Physical Activity and Health*, 6, 805-817.

Department of Health. (2004). *At least five a week: Evidence on the impact of physical activity and its relationship to health*. London: Department of Health.

Department of Health. (2011a). *Physical activity guidelines for early years (under 5s)—For infants who are not yet walking*. London: Department of Health. Available: www.dh.gov.uk/prod_consum_dh/groups/dh_digitalassets/documents/digitalasset/dh_128142.pdf.

Department of Health. (2011b). *Start active, stay active: A report on physical activity for health from the four home countries' chief medical officers*. London: Department of Health.

Department of Health. (2011c). *UK physical activity guidelines: Factsheets 1-4*. London: Department of Health. Available: www.dh.gov.uk/en/PublicationsandstatisticsPublications/PublicationsPolicyAndGuidance/DH_127931.

Department of Health and Ageing. (2004). *Australia's physical activity recommendations for 5-12 year olds*. Canberra: Commonwealth Government of Australia.

Department of Health and Ageing. (2005a). *Active kids are healthy kids: Australia's physical activity recommendations for 5-12 year olds*. Canberra: Commonwealth Government of Australia.

Department of Health and Ageing. (2005b). *An active way to better health: National physical activity guidelines for adults*. Canberra: Commonwealth Government of Australia.

Department of Health and Children, Health Service Executive. (2009). *The national guidelines on physical activity for Ireland*. Dublin: Department of Health and Children, Health Service Executive.

European Union. (2008). *EU physical activity guidelines: Recommended policy actions in support of health-enhancing physical activity*. Brussels, Belgium: European Union.

Foster, C., Hillsdon, M., & Thorogood, M. (2005). Interventions for promoting physical activity. *Cochrane Database of Systematic Reviews*, 1. doi: 10.1002/14651858.CD003180.pub2.

Glanz, K., & Bishop, D.B. (2010). The role of behavioral science theory in development and implementation of public health interventions. *Annual Review of Public Health*, 31, 399-418.

Haskell, W., Lee, I., Pate, R., Powell, K., Blair, S., Franklin, B., et al. (2007). Physical activity and public health: Updated recommendation for adults from the American College of Sports Medicine and the American Heart Association. *Circulation*, 116, 1081-1093.

Holley, J., Crone, D., Tyson, P., & Lovell, G. (2011). The effects of physical activity on psychological well-being for those with schizophrenia: A systematic review. *British Journal of Clinical Psychology*, 50, 84-105.

Kahn, E., Ramsey, L., Brownson, R., Heath, G., Howze, E., Powell, K., et al. (2002). The effectiveness of interventions to increase physical activity: A systematic review. *American Journal of Preventive Medicine*, 22(4S), 73-107.

Lawlor, D.A., & Hopker, S.W. (2001). The effectiveness of exercise as an intervention in the management of depression: Systematic review and meta-regression analysis of randomised controlled trials. *British Medical Journal*, 322, 763.

Leavy, J.E., Bull, F.C., Rosenberg, M., & Bauman, A. (2011). Physical activity mass media campaigns and their evaluation: A systematic review of the literature 2003–2010. *Health Education Research*, 26(6), 1060-1085.

Li, M., Li, S., Baur, L.A., & Huxley, R.R. (2008). A systematic review of school-based intervention studies for the prevention or reduction of excess weight among Chinese children and adolescents. *Obesity Reviews*, 9(6), 548-559.

Ministry of Health. (2005). *The action plan on physical activity (2005-2009)*. Available: http://helsedirektoratet.no/publikasjoner/the-action-plan-on-physical-activity-2005-2009/Publikasjoner/the-action-plan-on-physical-activity-2005-2009.pdf.

Ministry of Health. (2011). *National physical activity guidelines for Brunei Darussalam*. Negara, Brunei Darussalam: Ministry of Health.

Ministry of Health, Welfare and Sport. (2011). *Dutch healthy exercise norm: NNGB*. Available: http://jeugdmonitor.cbs.nl/en-GB/menu/inlichtingen/begrippen/nngb.htm.

National Institute for Health and Clinical Excellence. (2006a). *Four commonly used methods to increase physical activity: Brief interventions in primary care, exercise referral schemes, pedometers and community-based exercise programmes for walking and cycling*. London: National Institute for Health and Clinical Excellence.

National Institute for Health and Clinical Excellence. (2006b). *Physical activity and the environment. Review 2: Urban planning and design*. London: National Institute for Health and Clinical Excellence.

National Institute for Health and Clinical Excellence. (2008a). *Promoting physical activity for children. Review 5: Active transport interventions.* London: National Institute for Health and Clinical Excellence.

National Institute for Health and Clinical Excellence. (2008b). *NICE public health guidance 8: Promoting and creating built or natural environments that encourage and support physical activity.* London: National Institute for Health and Clinical Excellence.

Office for Lifestyle-Related Diseases Control. (2006). *Exercise and physical activity guide for health promotion 2006: To prevent lifestyle-related diseases. Exercise guide 2006.* Japan: Office for Lifestyle-Related Diseases Control.

Ogilvie, D., Foster, C.E., Rothnie, H., Cavill, N., Hamilton, V., Fitzsimons, C.F., et al. (2007). Interventions to promote walking: Systematic review. *British Medical Journal, 334,* 1204.

Owen, N., Bauman, A., Booth, M., Oldenburg, B., & Magnus, P. (1995). Serial mass-media campaigns to promote physical activity: Reinforcing or redundant? *American Journal of Public Health, 85*(2), 244-248.

Pawlowski, T., Downward, P., & Rasciute, S. (2011). Subjective well-being in European countries—On the age-specific impact of physical activity. *European Review of Aging and Physical Activity, 8*(2), 93-102.

Phongsavan, P., Merom, D., Bauman, A., & Wagner, R. (2007). Mental illness and physical activity: Therapists' beliefs and practices. *Australian and New Zealand Journal of Psychiatry, 41*(5), 458-459.

Pressman, S.D., Matthews, K.A., Cohen, S., Martire, L.M., Scheier, M., Baum, A., et al. (2009). Association of enjoyable leisure activities with psychological and physical well-being. *Psychosomatic Medicine, 71*(7), 725-732.

Pucher, J., Dill, J., & Handy, S. (2010). Infrastructure, programs, and policies to increase bicycling: An international review. *Preventive Medicine, 50*(Suppl. 1), S106-S125.

Republic of Slovenia Ministry of Health. (2007). *National health enhancing physical activity programme 2007-2012.* Ljubljana, Slovenia: Ministry of Health.

Saris, W.H.M., Blair, S.N., Van Baak, M.A., Eaton, S.B., Davies, P.S.W., Di Pietro, L., et al. (2003). How much physical activity is enough to prevent unhealthy weight gain? Outcome of the IASO 1st Stock Conference and consensus statement. *Obesity Reviews, 4*(2), 101-114.

Saxena, S., Van Ommeren, M., Tang, K.C., & Armstrong, T.P. (2005). Mental health benefits of physical activity. *Journal of Mental Health, 14*(5), 445-451.

Singh, N.A., Clements, K.M., & Singh, M.A.F. (2001). The efficacy of exercise as a long-term antidepressant in elderly subjects: A randomized, controlled trial. *The Journals of Gerontology Series A: Biological Sciences and Medical Sciences, 56*(8), M497-M504.

Sport and Recreation New Zealand. (2005). *Guidelines for promoting physical activity to adults.* Wellington, New Zealand: Sport and Recreation New Zealand.

Swiss Federal Office of Sports. (2006). *Health-enhancing physical activity.* Zurich, Switzerland: Swiss Federal Office of Sports.

Teychenne, M., Ball, K., & Salmon, J. (2008). Physical activity and likelihood of depression in adults: A review. *Preventive Medicine, 46*(5), 397-411.

Tremblay, M.S., Kho, M.E., Tricco, A.C., & Duggan, M. (2010). Process description and evaluation of Canadian Physical Activity Guidelines development. *International Journal of Behavioral Nutrition and Physical Activity, 7,* 42.

UKK Institute. (2009). *Physical activity pie.* Available: www.ukkinstituutti.fi/filebank/64-physical_activity_pie.pdf.

U.S. Centers for Disease Control and Prevention. (1996). *Physical activity and health: A report of the surgeon general.* Atlanta: U.S. Department of Health and Human Services.

U.S. Department of Health and Human Services. (2008a). *2008 physical activity guidelines for Americans: Be active, healthy and happy!* Washington, D.C.: U.S. Department of Health and Human Services.

U.S. Department of Health and Human Services. (2008b). *Be active your way: A guide for adults.* Washington, D.C.: U.S. Department of Health and Human Services, Centers for Disease Control and Prevention.

U.S. Department of Health and Human Services. (2008c). *Be active your way* [blog]. Washington, D.C.: U.S. Department of Health and Human Services. Available: www.health.gov/paguidelines/blog.

U.S. Department of Health and Human Services. (2008d). *Physical activity guidelines for Americans* resources. *At-a-glance: A fact sheet for professionals.* Washington, D.C.: U.S. Department of Health and Human Services. Available: www.health.gov/paguidelines/factsheetprof.aspx.

U.S. Department of Health and Human Services. (2008e). *Physical activity guidelines for Americans resources.* Washington, D.C.: U.S. Department of Health and Human Services. Available: www.health.gov/paguidelines.

U.S. Department of Health and Human Services. (2008f). *Physical activity guidelines for Americans toolkit.* Washington, D.C.: U.S. Department of Health and Human Services. Available: www.health.gov/paguidelines/toolkit.aspx.

U.S. Department of Health and Human Services. (2008g). *Physical Activity Guidelines Advisory Committee report.* Washington, D.C.: U.S. Department of Health and Human Services. Available: www.health.gov/paguidelines/report/pdf/CommitteeReport.pdf.

Vancampfort, D., Knapen, J., Probst, M., van Winkel, R., Deckx, S., Maurissen, K., et al. (2010). Considering a frame of reference for physical activity research related to the cardiometabolic risk profile in schizophrenia. *Psychiatry Research,* 177(3), 271-279.

World Health Organisation. (2002). *Reducing risk, promoting healthy life.* Geneva, Switzerland: World Health Organisation.

World Health Organisation. (2004). *Global strategy on diet, physical activity and health.* Geneva, Switzerland: World Health Organisation.

World Health Organisation. (2008). *Pacific physical activity guidelines for adults: Framework for accelerating the communication of physical activity guidelines.* Manila, Philippines: World Health Organisation.

World Health Organisation. (2010). *Global recommendations on physical activity for health.* Geneva, Switzerland: World Health Organisation.

World Health Organisation. (2011). *Global status report on noncommunicable disease 2010.* Geneva, Switzerland: World Health Organisation.

Zaza, S., Briss, P.A., & Harris, K.W. (2005). *The guide to community preventive services: What works to promote health?* Oxford: Oxford University Press.

Challenges in Measuring Physical Activity in the Context of Mental Health

Natalie Taylor, PhD
University of Leeds, Leeds, United Kingdom

Chapter Outline

Editors' Introduction

Physical activity is a complex, multidimensional behaviour that is difficult to assess accurately. As a result, a plethora of assessment methods are available and each differs in validity and feasibility. Understanding the challenges in assessing physical activity is a vital starting point for this text. Such understanding provides the base from which to evaluate evidence and enables researchers to choose the most appropriate measurement method for use in their studies. This chapter provides a comprehensive and practical overview of the strengths and weaknesses of available approaches for measuring physical activity and discusses issues particularly relevant to a mental health context.

In the modern world of stress and inactivity, the need to assess the potential benefits of physical activity for mental health is increasing. Precise measurement of physical activity is required in order to identify current or changing levels of physical activity in different populations, relationships between physical activity and physical and mental health and the effects of physical activity interventions on components of physical and mental health. However, physical activity is a complex, multidimensional behaviour that is difficult to assess, and the appropriate method to use depends on various factors such as the number of individuals to be monitored, the time period of measurements and available finances. Increasing understanding of physical activity and exercise behaviour involves acquiring information about people's patterns of activity and exercise. These behaviours can be studied using a range of methods such as direct observation, measurement of activity using pedometers or accelerometers, use of indirect measures such as capacity for oxygen exchange or heart rate, analyses of self-reports of activity on questionnaires and measurement and analyses of sleep patterns and other periods of activity, inactivity and sedentariness (Spruijt-Metz et al., 2009).

This chapter first outlines important concepts and definitions that are useful for understanding the information presented. Next, it presents problems associated with measuring physical activity and covers the history of measurement, the purpose of measuring physical activity and factors that affect one's choice of measurement tool. This chapter also discusses the difficulties of assessing physical activity in the context of mental health and summarises how research in this area has been hindered. It also presents the methods available for measuring physical activity, advantages and disadvantages of these methods and examples of the use of these techniques in the context of mental health. Finally, this chapter includes recommendations for the use of measurement methods, particularly in the mental health arena.

The "Key Concepts" sidebar provides a list of definitions that are important when attempting to understand the subject of physical activity

measurement. In addition, the following sections define and describe the terms *physical activity*, *exercise* and *sedentariness* in detail. These three types of behaviour are very closely related, can be measured either separately or simultaneously by the same instrument or a combination of measures and are sometimes used interchangeably.

Caspersen, Powell & Christenson (1985) describe physical activity as "any bodily movement produced by skeletal muscles that results in energy expenditure" (p. 126). Physical activity is a complex set of behaviours, and its type, intensity, frequency and duration can be measured. Physical activity can take place in all areas of life, including daily chores, leisure activities and organised sports. It can be either planned specifically (e.g., booking a 1 h activity class at the gym) or unplanned (e.g., getting up to make a cup of tea) and can take place in either structured (e.g., refereed football match, supervised exercise session) or unstructured (e.g., walking to the shop) formats.

Exercise is a subcategory of physical activity and consists of planned, structured and repetitive bodily movement undertaken to promote and maintain components of physical fitness. Although the definition of the term *exercise* is different from that of *physical activity*, exercise is often captured in absolute measures of physical activity. However, for certain research projects or treatment programmes, it may be important to distinguish the two. For example, if a practitioner aims to increase the planned and structured exercise levels of his patients, measurement tools may need to identify the time participants have spent or the energy they have expended performing these types of activities compared with other unplanned or unstructured physical activities (e.g., taking a flight of stairs, doing chores).

Sedentary behaviour, inactivity and sleep involve the absence of movement. Sedentary behaviour may be an independent indicator that is related to ill health, obesity rates, reduced social interaction and reduced physical activity due to excessive lengths of time spent sitting in front of the computer at work or the television (also known as screen time). For these reasons, physical inactivity is included as a lifestyle-relevant domain. It can be measured by both physical activity tools and tools that specifically measure sedentary behaviour.

1 Types of Measurement Information

Attempts to understand what motivates individuals to become active and maintain a physi- cally active status have been complicated by the difficulty of measuring physical activity in various contexts. Measurement techniques existed as early as the 1600s, starting with the scientific study of animal respiration (which ultimately led to the gold standard method of indirect calorimetry). Recently, web-based self-reported measures of physical activity have been developed. Such a variation in available

KEY CONCEPTS

- **physical activity**—Any bodily movement produced by skeletal muscles that results in expenditure of energy. One can undertake physical activity during leisure time for enjoyment purposes, as part of an occupation, to complete home-based tasks or for active transport (e.g., walking to work instead of driving).

- **exercise**—Physical activity that is planned or structured. When exercising, one performs repetitive bodily movement in order to improve or maintain physical fitness.

- **sedentary behaviour**—Not engaging in physical activity (e.g., watching television, sitting at a work station).

- **energy expenditure**—The amount of energy (calories) that a person uses to breathe, circulate blood, digest food and be physically active. To prevent weight gain, energy intake (caloric intake) must be balanced with energy expenditure.

- **cardiorespiratory fitness**—The ability of the body's circulatory and respiratory systems to supply fuel and oxygen during sustained physical activity.

- **MET**—Standard metabolic equivalent. One MET equals the energy (oxygen) used by the body while sitting quietly. Activity intensity can be presented in METs.

- **intensity**—The effort exerted when performing a particular physical activity. Intensity, which can be either measured directly or estimated, is used as part of the calculation of energy expenditure.

- **light physical activity**—Activities that expend less than 3 METs/min.

- **moderate physical activity**—Activities that expend 3 to 6 METs/min.

- **vigorous physical activity**—Activities that expend more than 6 METs/min.

- **frequency**—The number of times physical activity or a particular activity of a particular intensity is performed.

- **duration**—The length of time physical activity or a particular activity of a particular intensity is performed.

- **type**—The mode of physical activity (e.g., running, badminton, swimming, skiing, surfing, dusting, vacuuming, lifting, climbing stairs).

- **context**—The environment in which one performs physical activity (e.g., park, home, leisure centre, path or walkway).

- **reliability**—The repeatability or consistency of results. (*Note:* Reliability does not indicate that results are valid.)

- **validity**—Determines whether the research tool measures what it intends to measure or how trustworthy the results are. Previously validated measures can be used to test the validity of new measures. Gold standard measures are considered the most valid.

measurement techniques has created a shifting pattern of strengths and weaknesses in the evidence supporting the claim that physical activity improves physical and mental health. Different health implications of measuring activity, gauging intensity and assessing fitness add to this complexity. Researchers have found developing accurate, valid and cost-effective techniques of quantifying physical activity under free-living conditions to be particularly challenging.

Researchers and practitioners often need to assess physical activity for a number of reasons. For example, a PhD student-researcher with limited funds may wish to test the relationship between psychological variables (e.g., self-efficacy, intention, symptoms of depression, symptoms of schizophrenia) and current levels of purposeful and structured moderate physical activity in a cross-sectional study of overweight and obese adults. This information may further understanding about mechanisms that influence the decision to participate in physical activity. A team of researchers may wish to test the efficacy of an intervention that targets certain psychological variables in order to increase habitual physical activity of employees in the workplace. Other researchers might have funds to assess the effect of a 6 wk rehabilitation programme on the time it takes for elderly patients to walk without aid after undergoing a knee-replacement operation. Health service practitioners may need to assess for service-improvement purposes the longitudinal impact of a certain type of physical activity recommended to and performed by adolescent patients diagnosed with depression or may need to understand the fitness levels of patients diagnosed with cardiovascular disease in order to design a rehabilitation programme. Another research team may wish to assess the effectiveness of an acute intervention for decreasing the energy expenditure (EE) of individuals diagnosed with exercise addiction. These examples demonstrate that the reasons for wanting to assess physical activity can differ widely depending on a range of factors, such as the population being studied (and therefore the problem being addressed), the aspect of physical activity of interest and the time or funds avail-

able. As such, researchers and practitioners must carefully consider what information is necessary for their research or practice purposes when choosing a measurement tool.

2   Factors That Affect Method Choice

Researchers should consider a number of important factors when making the decision to use a particular tool to measure physical activity. These factors include the research question and the physical activity domains of interest, the population type and logistics (i.e., number of participants, time period and available finances). Each of these factors is complex in itself and there are a multitude of ways in which they could combine. This means that it is impossible to recommend any one objective or subjective technique. However, taking the time to think about each of the three factors in turn before choosing a measurement tool should enhance the extent to which any current patterns or changes in specific physical activity-related behaviours can be evidenced . Researchers and practitioners can use the following checklist when faced with the need to choose a measurement instrument.

2.1   Research Question and Physical Activity Domains of Interest

The measurement tool should collect information that can sufficiently answer the research question or hypothesis. Crucial elements of a research question often relate to the type, frequency, duration and intensity of physical activity and the context in which physical activity is performed (see the "Key Concepts" sidebar for definitions of these factors). Interventionists attempting to increase physical activity among individuals in the workplace may wish to see an increase in the number of employees taking the stairs (context) as well as improvements in cardiovascular fitness (which can be indirectly represented by intensity). These outcomes might be measured effectively using step counters,

Checklist: Factors to Consider Before Choosing a Measurement Tool

1. What type of information do I need to collect?
   - ☐ Intensity
   - ☐ Frequency
   - ☐ Duration
   - ☐ Type
   - ☐ Context

2. What do I want to use the results for?
   - ☐ To test a theory or relationship
   - ☐ To evaluate a patient-treatment programme
   - ☐ To test an intervention for research purposes

3. How many people do I need to measure?
   - ☐ <10
   - ☐ 10-20
   - ☐ 20-100
   - ☐ 100-200
   - ☐ 200-500
   - ☐ >500

4. Who are my participants?
   - ☐ Age
   - ☐ Physical health status
   - ☐ Mental health status
   - ☐ Education level
   - ☐ Employment status
   - ☐ Time available

5. What is my budget for the following?
   - ☐ Participants

6. How long do I have to do the following?
   - ☐ Complete the project
   - ☐ Test each participant
   - ☐ Collect all data
   - ☐ Analyse all data

7. How accurate do I need my results to be in terms of the following?
   - ☐ Energy expenditure
   - ☐ Time spent
   - ☐ Physical activity patterns
   - ☐ Movement capabilities
   - ☐ Impact of the environment

From N. Taylor, 2013, Challenges to measuring physical activity in the context of mental health. In *Physical activity and mental health*, edited by A. Clow and S. Edmunds (Champaign, IL: Human Kinetics).

electronic information about use of the lift or stairs or a fitness test. On the other hand, those delivering a rehabilitation programme to elderly patients after a knee-replacement operation may look for steady increases in the frequency and duration of very low-intensity exercise in the context of a hospital stay and subsequent appointments. This might be best measured using a diary method or measures of strength. Alternatively, practitioners delivering counselling sessions to adolescent patients diagnosed with depression may wish to see an increase in social (context) physical activity types with a moderate level of intensity, such as dancing, team sports, hiking or orienteering. This may be best mea-sured via a questionnaire. Finally, researchers testing an intervention for individuals diagnosed with exercise addiction may wish to see a reduction in the frequency, intensity and duration of physical activity among their sample. This may be best measured using accelerometers. These examples show that the questions researchers or practitioners aim to answer require measurement of outcomes that can vary according to one or a combination of physical activity domains, and for each outcome the use of one tool may be more appropriate than the use of another. Table 3.1 summarises the measurement properties of some common physical activity measurement techniques.

Table 3.1   Measurement Properties of Physical Activity Measurement Techniques

Measurement technique	Type	Frequency	Context	Duration	Intensity	Feasibility	Validity
Doubly labelled water	No	Yes	No	Yes	Yes		
Direct observation	Yes	Yes	Yes	Yes	Yes		
Accelerometers	No	Yes	No	Yes	Yes	↓	↑
Indirect objective observation	No	Yes	No	Yes	Yes		
Pedometers	No	Yes	No	Yes	Yes		
Self-report	Yes	Yes	Yes	Yes	Yes		

The "Feasibility" and "Validity" columns are grouped under the heading MEASUREMENT OUTCOME.

2.2   Population Type

Problems may arise if a measurement technique is selected without considering the population in question. For example, asking young children to complete a questionnaire about their physical activity habits may produce differing levels of detail depending on the children's reading and writing capabilities. Expecting full-time employees to complete a detailed daily diary about their lifestyle physical activity might present difficulties in terms of the time required to complete the measure. Requesting patients diagnosed with certain mental health problems to remember to wear an accelerometer might introduce an additional stressor in their daily lives. Each of these potentially inappropriate decisions may affect the accuracy of the results and raises a number of issues about whether the requirements and expectations placed on the participants are fair. Therefore, when thinking about the suitability of a measurement technique for use with a particular population, researchers should consider demographics such as age, education level and employment status as well as more population-specific factors regarding physical and mental status.

2.3   Research Logistics

The number of individuals studied in a research project or assessed and treated by practitioners can vary depending on the research question being investigated or the problem being treated.

Scientifically validated objective data would be the ideal measure of current patterns of or changes in physical activity. However, in many instances these more accurate measures are not feasible due to factors such as the number of participants to be studied and the time and finances available. For example, it would be useful to use accelerometers to gather objective data regarding changes in physical activity among employees of a large organisation (e.g., university, health service, factory). However, this may be too expensive given the large numbers of participants who would need to be measured or the time it would take to analyse the masses of data these devices gather. It may be more appropriate to provide a validated questionnaire to all employees as the primary outcome measure and provide a subsample of the population with accelerometers. This method would provide a more objective measure for the subsample and could help validate the responses from the questionnaire. However, not all research projects or treatment regimens involve large-scale interventions or the assessment of physical activity patterns among communities. For example, studies of patients being treated for a particular condition (e.g., exercise addiction or depression) may involve a smaller number of participants and may require more accurate information about physical activity patterns in order to refine any treatment programmes or interventions with confidence. As such, gathering information through accelerometers or step counters may be more feasible here than in a large-scale intervention in terms of finances, cost and time. Daily diaries or questionnaires might also be used to supplement the objective data gathered because they can provide information such as context, mode of activity and feelings experienced.

3   Challenges in Measuring Physical Activity in a Mental Health Context

Complexity is a primary cause of the difficulties faced when attempting to measure physical activity in the mental health domain. Working with mental health populations presents a new set of factors to consider, which further complicates the task of measuring physical activity for the purposes of research studies and treatment programmes. Mental health encompasses two very distinct but closely related dimensions: mental well-being, which includes factors such as emotional well-being, life satisfaction, optimism, hope and a sense of purpose and belonging, and mental health problems, which refers to symptoms that meet criteria for clinical diagnosis of mental illness (e.g., depression, anxiety, schizophrenia). Individuals may have optimal mental well-being while experiencing diagnosable mental health problems and have minimal mental well-being while experiencing no diagnosable mental health problems (Tudor, 1996). Research or treatment in the area of mental health and physical activity should be very carefully planned and thought out given the potentially fragile and vulnerable nature of participants, especially those who have been diagnosed with mental health problems. For example, the ethical position of those working with patients diagnosed with health problems becomes more sensitive when testing physical activity treatment programmes. One must spend time identifying all the potential negative outcomes that may occur and create strategies for avoiding or dealing with these outcomes. As such, even the most carefully considered research in this area can be difficult because both mental health and physical activity are conceptually

complex and diverse and do not lend themselves to clearly structured and controlled trials that would highlight any definitive causal links (Whitelaw et al., 2008).

The complex nature of both physical activity and mental health has meant that research in this area continues to evolve at a modest pace. Work in this area has tended to be of an epidemiological nature and uses cross-sectional survey methods that establish correlational associations between physical activity and mental health rather than determine causality. This lack of information about cause and effect makes it very difficult to confidently design appropriate interventions that will help improve mental health or prevent psychological impairment. Of the available research, few large-scale population studies have been undertaken. The majority of the cross-sectional research available focusses on mental well-being. Of the relatively small amount of research available in the context of mental health problems, most focusses on the areas of anxiety and depression (Have, de Graaf & Monshouwer, 2011). A number of randomised controlled studies that have measured physical activity in the context of mental health have found that individuals with mental health disorders are more likely to drop out of the studies and not provide follow-up data. Consequently, attrition may have confounded results regarding changes in physical activity and mental health or any connections between the two. Furthermore, validation of physical activity measurement techniques is often demonstrated in the general population; very few studies validate these tools in populations suffering from a range of mental health conditions. Combined, these issues reduce researcher confidence in the validity of research in this area. This adds to the difficulties associated with designing effective physical activity interventions for mental health populations.

Even though discrepancies between self-report and objective measurement (outlined later) are evident, the majority of studies tend to use self-report measures of physical activity (Baumeister, Vohs & Funder, 2007). This is generally due to the difficulties associated with using objective measures, such as costs in terms of time and finances and the burden these tools can often place on participants. The use of self-report measures often decreases the accuracy of the results produced because they rarely correlate well with objective measures (Bussmann, Ebner-Priemer & Fahrenberg, 2009). Obtaining reliable self-reports is difficult, especially among populations diagnosed with mental health problems (Bezyak, 2011). Studies that use self-report measures have been criticised because physical activity and mental health measures may overlap conceptually (e.g., in the physical domains of health-related quality of life measures), which might inflate any relationships produced (Bize, 2007). Furthermore, many of these studies fail to measure the frequency and intensity of the exercise or the nature of the activity (e.g., team or individual sport, walking, swimming) because of the difficulties associated with recalling information of this nature, the accuracy of which varies among different mental health populations. As such, a lack of understanding exists about the optimal physical activity type and dose for enhancing psychological health, which is essential for designing effective interventions. The literature in the area has been recently summarised by a whole-population review on physical activity and the prevention of mental illness, dysfunction and deterioration:

> The limited numbers of studies and the range of aspects of physical activity measured, different measures used and the variety of outcome variables prevents the formulation of any firm conclusions about graded or threshold effects.
> *Fox & Mutrie, 2007, p. 10*

Despite these challenges, the past 15 to 20 yr have seen the development of a considerable body of literature that broadly suggests that physical activity has the potential to contribute to improvements in mental health (Whitelaw et al., 2008). As such, empirical research in this area must continue in order to overcome the challenges faced in establishing convincing links between physical activity and mental health.

4   Available Methods for Measuring Physical Activity

A range of methods are used in the assessment of physical activity, including self-report, systematic observation, motion sensors, cardiorespiratory fitness and free-living indirect calorimetry. Most are moderately correlated at best. Each method has its own strengths and limitations. Due to the complexity of physical activity, outlined previously, researchers and practitioners need to consider what is most important for their purposes when deciding to use a particular technique. Although no one measurement tool can be singled out as the most appropriate, recommendations for the most useful and practical measurement tools can be made after considering factors such as context, type, duration, frequency and intensity of physical activity as well as the constraints under which the research or treatment programme is operating. These techniques are presented in order of increasing feasibility but decreasing validity. Table 3.2 at the end of this section summarises the key advantages and limitations of each measurement technique.

4.1   Doubly Labelled Water

Doubly labelled water (DLW, or free-living indirect calorimetry) is a method commonly used to increase the precision and accuracy of physical activity measurement. DLW, which measures EE over several (4-21) consecutive days in a free-living person under normal life conditions (Schoeller, 1988), is the most widely accepted gold standard method by which to measure EE (Aadahl & Jørgensen, 2003). DLW measures EE of free-living, unrestricted subjects using water labelled with stable isotopes of oxygen and hydrogen (Schoeller & van Santen, 1982). It calculates activity-related EE by combining measurement of total EE with basal metabolic rate. The utility of the DLW method in measuring total EE is demonstrated by its use in a variety of settings, including all age groups, premature infants, hospitalised patients, pregnant women and the elderly (Ainslie, Reilly & Westerterp, 2003). As such, researchers who use this method to assess the relationship between physical activity and other psychological variables or to detect changes in physical activity as a result of interventions can be confident that the results produced regarding EE are accurate. Schoeller (1988) fully describes the validation of the DLW method.

Despite its level of precision, the DLW method is not without disadvantages, which include high cost, limitations for assessing brief periods of EE (Ainslie, Reilly & Westerterp, 2003) and additional demands on participants in terms of time and tasks required. The cost and availability of isotopes and the requirement for analysis by isotope ratio mass spectrometer prohibit DLW from being widely used in studies of large populations. The use of this method among populations with more severe mental health problems may likely present a set of ethical issues. Furthermore, although this technique provides an accurate measure of total EE, it cannot provide information about patterns of physical activity in terms of type, frequency, duration, intensity or context. Consequently, such an approach would not be feasible in a large natural-field experiment or in a test of the effect of interventions on changes in physical activity in both healthy populations and populations that suffer from mental health problems. However, this gold standard measure is believed to offer the most precise estimate of EE and is often used to validate many other types of tools that assess physical activity.

4.2   Direct Observation

Direct observation, one of the most basic approaches for acquiring information about behaviours, provides information about how people exercise and play, how environments shape the activities individuals participate in and how people use specific facilities (e.g., parks, leisure facilities, walking or cycling paths). It can take place using basic observation methods, systematic forms or sophisticated technology (e.g., lasers). Direct observation often involves a trained observer who codes physical activity behaviours (e.g., sitting, walking, running) undertaken by participants over time in vari-

ous settings (e.g., playground, park, home). A number of observation systems are available, such as SOPLAY (System for Observing Play and Leisure Activity in Youth), SOFIT (System for Observing Fitness Instruction Time), and the Systematic Pedestrian and Cycling Environmental Scan. The trained observer may either observe participants in person or review video media. Because it is time consuming, direct observation might be used only with small groups in specific settings (Dugdill & Stratton, 2007).

Advantages of direct observation include that self-report bias is eliminated, participants do not need to recall behaviour and the level of detail regarding behaviour patterns and context can be extremely accurate. Furthermore, practitioners may find some of these tools accessible. For example, clinical psychologists working with institutionalised individuals diagnosed with severe mental health conditions may find this type of measurement technique useful for assessing relationships between physical activity patterns or patterns of inactivity and specific mental illnesses because it can combine both context and behaviour to provide powerful data.

However, disadvantages include the time involved in recording and coding behaviour, the time involved in consolidating the plethora of data collected and the costs associated with training coders. Furthermore, the subjective bias of coders may lead to incorrect judgments about the intensities of specific activities, which would affect estimates of EE. As such, it would be important to consider whether information regarding patterns of behaviour combined with context or specific EE data are required to fulfill the aims of a research project or treatment programme.

4.3   Accelerometers

Motion sensors, such as pedometers and accelerometers, can be used to detect body movement and estimate physical activity (Spruijt-Metz et al., 2009). Accelerometers are devices that measure bodily movements in terms of acceleration. This measurement can then be used to estimate the intensity of physical activity, and therefore EE, over time (Burton et al., 2005; Chen & Basset, 2005). Accelerometers can measure human activity on vertical (uniaxial accelerometers), anterior–posterior and medial–lateral (triaxial accelerometers) planes. EE can then be then estimated from vector magnitude counts using a proprietary algorithm, which is a composite of counts from these planes of motion (Howe, Staudenmayer & Freedson, 2009). Accelerometers can be used repeatedly on numerous participants, are more accurate than pedometers and are less expensive (approximately £200 per device; ActiLife, 2009) than other objective methods such as DLW (approximately £200 per participant per procedure; Friedman & Johnson, 2002). However, they remain too expensive to use in studies that assess large numbers of people (Wood, 2000). Nevertheless, these devices are a more feasible and participant-friendly method of attempting to validate a self-report questionnaire than is DLW. They also provide the data necessary to allow researchers to distinguish between light, moderate and vigorous physical activity as well as between continuous and intermittent activity modes (Crouter, Clowers & Bassett, 2006). A recent review of accelerometers against DLW found ActiGraph (previously named CSA/MTI) models to be of the most valid types tested; they produce an average correlation of $r = .57$ (Plasqui & Westerterp, 2007). Limitations of accelerometers include the increased time required to analyse the large amount of data provided, participant burden of wearing the device, that they cannot be feasibly used to test large-scale interventions, and that they cannot provide information about the specific type of activity (e.g., playing football, going to the gym) or the context in which it is performed.

Some studies have attempted to validate accelerometers among populations diagnosed with mental health conditions. For example, Sharpe and colleagues (2006) conducted a study to assess the validity of the RT3 accelerometer against DLW in people with schizophrenia. They found that the accelerometer overpredicted energy expended on physical activity by an average of 148 kcal/day (standard deviation = 413

kcal/day); this varied from an underestimation of 614 kcal/day to an overestimation of 582 kcal/day. The authors suggested that the RT3 accelerometer is a poor tool for measuring activity EE in sedentary men with schizophrenia. As such, the results of studies that have used this measurement tool in mentally ill populations may be questionable. For example, the recent intervention study of Jerome and colleagues (2009) used the RT3 accelerometer to measure physical activity in persons with mental illness. The authors of this study concluded that participants were undertaking approximately 120 min/wk of moderate-intensity physical activity on average, which would equal approximately 70 kcal/day. Given that the results of the study by Sharpe and colleagues (2006) indicated that the RT3 accelerometer overpredicted EE, it is possible that the results found by Jerome and colleagues (2009) overestimate the amount of physical activity undertaken by participants. Consequently, this might affect the validity of the relationships found between physical activity and various mental health variables measured in this study. Sharpe and colleagues (2006) did, however, indicate that the RT3 appeared to be a valid measure of physical inactivity in men with schizophrenia. Therefore, it could be used for research or clinical purposes to quantify the contribution of sedentary behaviour to medical conditions associated with inactivity. Sharpe and colleagues (2006) also recommended that using the RT3 to validate questionnaires may not be appropriate until it is more robust.

4.4 Indirect Objective Measures

Indicators of the physiologic response to physical activity include heart rate and pulmonary gas exchange. Heart-rate monitoring is a promising measurement method because heart rate is a physiological parameter that correlates well with, and strongly predicts, EE (Strath et al., 2002). Most heart rate monitors include software that converts heart rate data into an estimate of EE. However, one of the limitations of heart rate monitoring is that training state and individual heart rate characteristics can affect the relationship between heart rate and oxygen consumption. Higher levels of accuracy can be obtained through a graded submaximal exercise test that calibrates participant heart rate to simultaneous oxygen consumption. This information allows for the construction of a calibration curve that estimates EE at moderate and strenuous levels of exercise. (A linear relationship exists between increasing heart rate and oxygen consumption; Freedson & Miller, 2000.) Measuring heart rate is a common method used to describe intensity and duration of physical activity and is a relatively inexpensive method of measuring EE. However, heart rate is affected by factors other than physical activity, such as emotional stress, temperature, humidity, dehydration, posture and illness (Ainslie, Reilly & Westerterp, 2003). These factors can influence heart rate without causing associated changes in oxygen consumption. Given the potentially increased fluctuations in emotions in individuals diagnosed with mental health conditions, this method may not be the most appropriate for obtaining accurate physical activity levels. Furthermore, the relationship between oxygen uptake and heart rate is weak at low levels of activity (Keim, Blanton & Kretsch, 2004). Evidence suggests that individuals suffering from mental health problems tend to perform less intensive physical activity than do members of the general population (e.g., Brown et al., 1999). Therefore, the heart rate method may not provide accurate information about the physical activity of mental health populations. Also, the heart rate method is unable to identify types of activity or the context in which physical activity is performed. Although heart rate is a physiological marker for physical activity and may provide a general picture of physical activity patterns, it may not be the best method available for obtaining an accurate estimate of EE.

4.5 Pedometers

Pedometers, which measure steps on a single axis as well as calories expended, are less expensive than some other types of motion sensors. As such, these devices are an attractive alternative to self-report in large observational or intervention studies. Public health campaigns have also promoted pedometers as a motivational tool for achieving the goal of 10,000 steps daily. A range of pedometers is available. The pedometer that is most suitable for a particular study may depend on factors such as the research question (outcome of interest), population, available funds, context and validity of the model. For example, when considering context, researchers or practitioners who wish to understand the types of physical activity being undertaken in a variety of settings would not gain this information using pedometers alone. When considering population, some pedometers are validated in healthy adults but not in other populations such as children, the elderly or those diagnosed with mental illness. Pedometers have demonstrated reduced accuracy in elderly populations because of the slow pace or shuffling nature with which elderly people walk (Cyarto, Myers & Tudor-Locke, 2004). Tudor-Locke and colleagues (2002) evaluated the validity of pedometers in a review of 25 studies and found a strong correlation between pedometer counts and accelerometer output (median of reported correlations is $r = .86$). However, evidence suggests that the validity of pedometers for measuring EE and distance in normal populations is questionable. The findings of a study testing the validity of 10 pedometers (Crouter et al., 2003) indicated that these devices overestimated distance at slower speeds and underestimated distance at faster speeds. Furthermore, in 8 of the pedometers tested, it was unclear whether the device was measuring gross EE (all the energy expended by an individual during a specific activity) or net EE (the energy expended by an individual during a specific activity minus the resting EE for the equivalent amount of time). The Yamax Digiwalker SW-200 was found to be the most reliable and accurate pedometer available (Crouter et al., 2003). This pedometer was used in a recent study by McKercher (2009) that assessed relationships between physical activity and depression in young adults. This study found that low levels of depression were significantly correlated with moderate levels of physical activity, as measured by the Yamax Digiwalker SW-200, among females. However, this device has not been validated in specific mental health populations, which may limit the validity of these results. It is important to validate physical activity devices among specific populations because patterns of physical activity in these populations may differ from those in the general population. For example, individuals with serious mental illness are significantly less active than the general population (Brown et al., 2004). As such, using a physical activity measure that has been validated with mental health populations in research on physical activity and mental health will increase the strength of the results produced.

4.6   Self-Report

Self-report methods for describing physical activity include questionnaires, interviews and activity diaries. Survey approaches for measuring physical activity vary in complexity and can range from self-administered single-item questions to interviewer-administered surveys of lifetime physical activity. Most questionnaires record frequency, duration or intensity of work-related, sport or leisure-time activities. Large-scale epidemiologic studies that aim to determine the relationship between activity and health typically use telephone- or computer-assisted surveys or written questionnaires to characterise population-level physical activity. In contrast, practitioners might use physical activity logs to monitor how well the client or patient has adhered to the physical activity programme. One must consider the detail required, how much time participants require to complete the survey and how labour intensive analysing the data gathered will be. For example, a diary method can potentially produce a plethora of information about activity patterns, but the information recorded is affected by participants' commitment to completing these detailed measures thoroughly. So participants' commitment ultimately affects the accuracy of the results.

The validity of survey measures also depends on both the ability of respondents to accurately recall the different aspects of physical activity

they have performed and the extent to which they respond honestly. Studies have identified problems with a number of previously designed self-report measures of physical activity. For example, Rzewnicki, Auweelw and De Bourdeaudhuij (2002) reported that the International Physical Activity Questionnaire (IPAQ; Craig et al., 2003)—perhaps the most widely used measure of physical activity—has a tendency toward overreporting, perhaps because it asks for average times and best estimates of frequencies and uses a perceived intensity of breathing as a means of categorising physical activity as moderate or vigorous intensity. Additionally, test–retest reliability has proven problematic for the light and moderate measures of physical activity taken from the Godin Leisure Time Exercise Questionnaire (Godin & Shephard, 1997) and all exercise-related aspects of the Seven-Day Physical Activity Recall Questionnaire developed by Blair and colleagues (1985) (Jacobs et al., 1993). Nonetheless, researchers have undertaken work to demonstrate the good measurement properties of these measures. For example, a mean Spearman's rho of .30 was found against the CSA (now ActiGraph) accelerometer in a study that assessed the validity of the IPAQ in 12 countries (Craig et al., 2003). Furthermore, the Godin Leisure Time Exercise Questionnaire demonstrated a significant correlation of .32 against Caltrac accelerometers and .56 against $\dot{V}O_2$max. Although these correlations are low, they are not dissimilar to those of many other studies that validate self-report measures of physical activity (Jacobs et al., 1993). Also, one of the main benefits of these types of questionnaires is that they are able to measure physical activity at a group or population level, which is something that more expensive objective measures cannot feasibly do. Perhaps the most recent work summarising the measurement properties of available self-report physical activity questionnaires, undertaken by van Poppel (2010), would be most useful when selecting a self-report tool for measuring physical activity. This systematic review indicated that 23 of the 87 physical activity questionnaires assessed were deemed accurate enough for the intended dimension measured. A list of these 23 questionnaires is provided here. References for each questionnaire on this list can be found in van Poppel (2010).

Physical Activity Questionnaires Deemed Appropriate

Bharati

European Perspective Investigation Into Cancer and Nutrition Questionnaire (EPIC Original Q)

European Prospective investigation of Cancer-Norfolk Physical Activity Questionnaire (EPIC-Norfolk; EPAQ2)

Harvard/College Alumnus Physical Activity Questionnaire

Long International Physical Activity Questionnaire (Long IPAQ)

Adapted International Physical Activity Questionnaire (Adapted IPAQ)

Kaiser Physical Activity Survey

Life After Cancer Epidemiology Study Physical Activity Questionnaire (LACE PA Q)

Leisure Time Physical Activity Questionnaire (LTPA)

Mail Survey of Physical Activity Questionnaire

Norman Questionnaire

New Zealand Physical Activity Questionnaire (NZPAQ-SF)

One-Week Recall Questionnaire

Physical Activity Frequency Questionnaire

Physical Activity History Questionnaire

Past Year Total Physical Activity Questionnaire (PYT-PAQ)

Singh Questionnaire

Short Questionnaire to Assess Health Enhancing Physical Activity (SQUASH)

Historical Walking, Running and Jogging Questionnaire

Neighbourhood Physical Activity Questionnaire (NPAQ)

Health Insurance Plan of New York

Tecumseh Occupational Questionnaire (TOQ)

London Physical Activity Questionnaire

The capacity of a questionnaire to perform well against validation measures appears to be based on the logic with which the questions are constructed rather than its length or attention to detail (Baranowski, 1988; Jacobs et al., 1993). One approach to determining EE from measuring physical activity by questionnaire is through the use of the Compendium of Physical Activities. This method is based on the concept that a metabolic equivalent (MET) unit can be used to express the intensity of every activity. This allows one to estimate EE for specific physical activities using the following equation: MET value of the activity $\times$ time spent engaging in the activity = estimated EE (Ainsworth et al., 2000). This estimate can be converted to kilocalories expended if the body weight of the individual is known. Questionnaires such as the IPAQ ask for information regarding light, moderate and vigorous activity. However, Jacobs and colleagues (1993) recommend that questions should focus on specific physical activity domains (e.g., walking) in the context in which people usually perform the activity (e.g., the workplace) and should use the language that is customarily used for that activity. Capturing this type of information enables types of activities (e.g., walking, running, tennis, football) to be distinguished from one another and therefore leads to more accurate calculations of EE.

Self-report questionnaires have a clear advantage over objective or observational measures when used in large population-based and epidemiological studies because they allow for group-level measurement of physical activity at low cost. With the exception of continual direct observation, self-report is the only method that provides information about the type, context and setting of physical activity. This level of information is important in informing aspects of public policy and helping shape urban design (Spruijt-Metz et al., 2009).

One disadvantage of questionnaires is that they lack precision in estimating levels of physical activity due to the need for participants to recall past behaviour. As such, measuring physical activity of people with mental health problems, in whom cognitive impairment and social and functional limitations are common, poses an additional set of challenges. For example, instruments developed for use in the general population have several limitations when used in predominantly sedentary adults, such as those with certain mental health conditions (e.g., schizophrenia). Given that inactive persons engage in less-intensive activities more frequently than moderate or vigorous activities and perform these activities on an irregular basis, their recall of physical activity is less accurate (Harada et al., 2001). This has been highlighted by Lindamer and colleagues (2008), who suggested that the IPAQ may not be appropriate for individuals with mental health conditions given that it does not inquire about light activities or provide cues for recall. Consequently, Lindamer and colleagues attempted to validate the self-report Yale Physical Activity Scale (DiPietro et al., 1993). Even though this measure employs prompts and cued recall and inquires about light activities and sedentary behaviour, it did not perform well against accelerometers in a population of individuals with schizophrenia. More specifically, results showed that persons with schizophrenia spent less than half the time engaged in physical activity and expended less than half of the kilocalories per week relative to a nonpsychiatric comparison group when measured using the Yale Physical Activity Scale, but no group differences were seen when the groups were measured using accelerometry. Consequently, the authors recommended that further work be required in developing methods that help participants with mental health conditions recall different types of activities of different intensities and suggested that the use of cards that visually depict different activities may assist in this process.

4.7 Self-Report Via the Internet

Self-reported assessment of physical activity has rapidly advanced due to the explosion of sophisticated computer technology. The number of people who have access to the Internet is steadily increasing across the globe. Miniwatts (2010) reported that 53% of people in Europe and 76.4% of people in the United Kingdom had Internet access in 2009. Consequently, the Internet can be an effective medium for collecting and exchanging information in research related to psychology and physical activity. Survey administration via the Internet is potentially superior to paper because it provides increased accessibility and the capability for dynamic and interactive forms that eliminate the viewing of irrelevant questions (Miller et al., 2002). For example, certain computer programmes (e.g., Finlay, 1999) provide a skip logic function that allows the researcher to construct a questionnaire that directs individuals to specific questions based on a previous answer. This eliminates the need for participants to read and respond to redundant questions. A review of nine studies comparing Internet and laboratory versions of self-report questionnaires demonstrated that results from the two methods yield a good level of agreement (Krantz, Ballard & Scher, 1997); this has been confirmed by subsequent studies (e.g., Birnbaum, 2004). For these reasons, an online approach might demonstrate advantages over paper-and-pencil self-report measures for assessing physical activity. More recently, mobile electronic devices have become affordable to a wide range of people in Western society and have been used to gather and assess self-reported information about physical activity and other psychological factors in real time (Stone et al., 2007). Another advantage of electronically measuring self-reported physical activity is the ability to stamp the assessment with the date and time. This can be useful for learning more about adherence or times at which certain exercises are performed—information that would be valuable when designing effective interventions. Electronic self-report methods also provide the opportunity to gather more ecologically valid information because data can be collected in closer temporal proximity to when activities occur (Spruijt-Metz et al., 2009). In addition, gathering data electronically eliminates the need for labourious data entry because the information can be transported from the online system into analysis packages in a matter of seconds.

Finally, the ability to integrate electronic self-report data with that collected using objective methods becomes possible. As such, researchers are now using the Internet to electronically gather and store self-reported physical activity information.

However, measuring self-reported physical activity electronically does not eliminate some of the limitations generally associated with the self-report method and presents a new set of challenges. For example, issues such as participants' ability to accurately recall the frequency, duration and intensity of activities performed remain. New challenges, such as lack of access to the Internet for certain populations and potentially failing technology, are likely to affect the precision of the results collected. Although time may be saved in the area of data entry, the plethora of information collected makes for extremely large data sets that can be labourious and difficult to manage and that may require sophisticated analysis skills to accurately identify patterns in behavioural, psychological, social, environmental and other contextual variables about physical activity that may have been collected.

One example of a recent online questionnaire used to collect information about physical activity is the Online Self-Reported Walking and Exercise Questionnaire (OSWEQ; Taylor et al., 2012). The OSWEQ is constructed so that participants can select via drop-down boxes the type, frequency and number of minutes and hours spent on each type of activity. (See figures 3.1 and 3.2 for illustrations of the web-based measure.) Each of the 188 activities included in the questionnaire possesses its own MET value, taken from the previously mentioned compendium of physical activities (Ainsworth et al., 2000). As such, the OSWEQ allows for calculation of total METs after completion of the questionnaire as well as calculation of METs for specific activity domains (e.g., team sports, working out at the gym) and specific activities (e.g., netball, running at 8 km/h, volleyball) across the week. This online measure of physical activity demonstrated good test–retest reliability (correlations ranged from $r = .71$ to $r = .77$) and good concurrent validity

against the criterion measure of ActiGraph GT3X accelerometers for total moderate and vigorous physical activity (MVPA) minutes [$r = .39$, $p < .05$, mean difference = 367 min/wk, prediction interval (PI) = −435, 1169] and average daily MVPA MET minutes [$r = .44$, $p < .05$, mean difference = 150.4, PI = −328, 628] compared with an online version of the IPAQ [MVPA activity minutes: $r = .13$, $p > .05$, mean difference = 434.7, PI = −427, 1297; average daily MVPA MET minutes: $r = .08$, $p > .05$, mean difference = 247.5, PI = −231, 725]. However, because this study relied on a voluntary sample of university staff and students, the results obtained may not be generalisable to the wider population or mental health populations.

The difficulties of electronically measuring self-reported physical activity are further amplified in the context of mental health. For example, individuals may not have access to the Internet at home or via a mobile device, which may limit the populations from which researchers can collect information in this manner. Ability to use the Internet or understand the content of the online questionnaires may also be limited in populations with particular mental health conditions, given the increased potential for cognitive impairment among these populations. This might affect the accuracy of the results collected or negatively affect participants by causing confusion or distress. The potential issues raised here further increase the need for researchers to carefully consider whether the Internet is an appropriate medium for collecting information about physical activity patterns in the context of mental health, especially among those diagnosed with certain mental health conditions.

5 Summary

This chapter highlights the challenges associated with choosing an appropriate method by which to assess physical activity. Researchers often choose self-report measures over objective measures. The reasons for this and the limitations that result have been discussed in this chapter. Furthermore, some of the ways in which

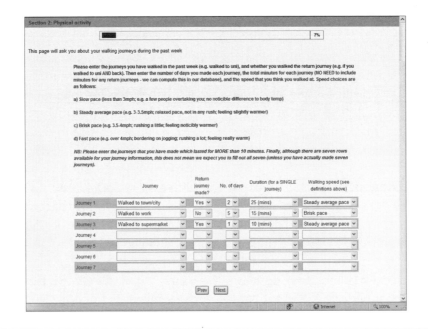

Figure 3.1 Online Self-Reported Walking and Exercise Questionnaire walking tables.

Reprinted, by permission, from N.J. Taylor et al., 2012, "Development and validation of the online Self-Reported Walking and Exercise Questionnaire," *Journal of Physical Activity and Health*. In press.

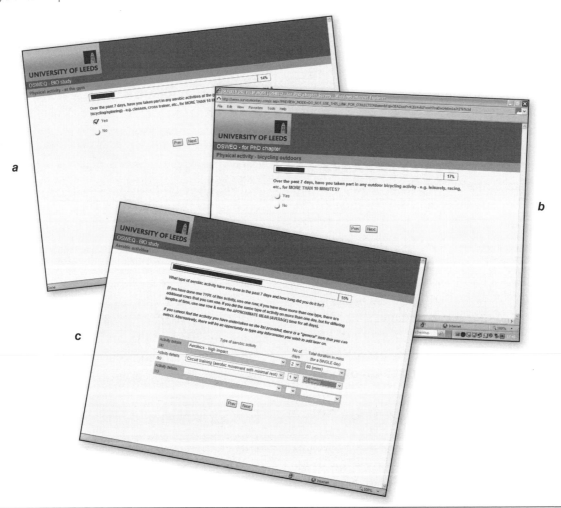

Figure 3.2 Online Self-Reported Walking and Exercise Questionnaire (OSWEQ) activity tables. *(a)* First question about specific activity type. *(b)* Second question about specific activity type. *(c)* Sample question about specific activity details.

Reprinted, by permission, from N.J. Taylor et al., 2012, "Development and validation of the online Self-Reported Walking and Exercise Questionnaire," *Journal of Physical Activity and Health*. In press.

Table 3.2   Advantages and Limitations of Physical Activity Measurement Techniques

Measurement technique	Explanation	Advantages	Limitations
Doubly labelled water	Measures EE over several consecutive days in a free-living person under normal life conditions.	• Accuracy (gold standard measure of EE). • Measures EE in the real world. • Can be used to validate other measures of physical activity.	• Expensive equipment. • Places demands on participants in terms of wearing equipment. • Cannot provide information on type or context of activity.
Direct observation	Provides information about how people exercise and play, how environments shape the activities individuals participate in and how people use specific facilities (e.g., parks, leisure facilities).	• Does not rely on participant recall. • Provides accurate information about type and context of physical activity. • Provides understanding about the impact of the environment.	• Expensive—need trained observers or sophisticated technology. • Time consuming—labourious observations and coding. • Subjective bias of observers.
Accelerometer	Measures body movements in terms of acceleration along vertical (uniaxial), anterior–posterior and medial–lateral planes.	• Can detect differences in intensity of activity (i.e., light, moderate, vigorous). • Can provide specific information about duration and frequency of activities. • Can distinguish between continuous and intermittent activity.	• Complex data analysis and large data sets. • Participant burden due to wearing the device for several days. • Cannot provide information about type or context of activity.
Indirect objective observation	Measures indicators of the physiological response to physical activity (e.g., heart rate, pulmonary gas exchange).	• Inexpensive. • Correlates well with EE. • Can provide higher levels of accuracy through graded submaximal exercise for individual participant calibration.	• Affected by non-activity-related fluctuations in heart rate. • Cannot identify type or context of activity. • Higher accuracy requires more expense in terms of equipment and labour.
Pedometer	Measures steps on a single axis. Some can measure calories expended.	• Less expensive than accelerometers. • Simple to use. • Less complicated analysis than accelerometers.	• Too expensive to use in large-scale interventions. • Accuracy is reduced in some populations. • Cannot provide information about type or context of activity. Provides limited information about frequency, intensity and duration of activity.
Self-report	Questionnaires, interviews and diary methods for recording physical activity behaviours.	• Low cost makes this method feasible for testing large-scale interventions. • Potential for large amounts of information. • Can provide information on type and context of physical activity.	• Relies on participant memory. • Possibility of social desirability bias. • Subjective participant judgment of intensity.

EE = energy expenditure.

EVIDENCE TO PRACTICE

Based on the evidence presented for the various methods of measuring physical activity, it appears that the biggest challenge for researchers and practitioners is choosing the tool that best fits the purpose given the constraints in which they are working. Difficulties arise when researchers have to decide on the most valid, accurate and reliable tools with which to measure physical activity while remaining realistic about available time and cost. Diaries, self-report questionnaires, pedometers, heart rate monitors, accelerometers, behavioural observation and indirect calorimetry techniques move from high to low feasibility and low to high validity (refer to table 3.1). The key issue is practicality and realism (Dugdill, Crone & Murphy, 2009). In the context of testing a large-scale intervention or working with patients in health services under tight budgets, it is often deemed unfeasible and unrealistic to use objective measures (Ainslie, Reilly & Westerterp, 2003). Although not ideal, the decision to use a self-report tool is therefore supported due to the practical value this type of measure has in monitoring current patterns and changes in both individual and population-level physical activity (Shephard, 2003). The confidence in the results that self-report measures provide may be enhanced if additional information is collected regarding change in biological markers that realistically could be measured simultaneously. Positive effects of physical activity interventions have been associated with improvements in blood pressure (Whelton et al., 2002), resting heart rate (Rennie et al., 2003) and body fat percentage (Dunn et al., 1999), each of which can help decrease the risk of health problems (e.g., cardiovascular disease, obesity, some cancers) and increased psychological well-being (Department of Health, 2004; Severson et al., 1989).

Markers such as these can be relatively simple and inexpensive to measure, although measuring blood pressure and body fat percentage would require meeting participants in person, which is not always realistic.

The challenges faced are further enhanced when measuring physical activity in the context of mental health. However, regardless of the reason for measuring physical activity (e.g., for research, for practice, in the context of mental or physical health), if one takes the time to carefully consider the factors associated with the research question, population and logistics (see "Checklist: Factors to Consider Before Choosing a Measurement Tool" earlier in this chapter), one will likely make the most appropriate decision for the objectives to be achieved. However, to increase the validity of research in the area of physical activity and mental health, two important research progressions should be made. First, current physical activity measures should be validated among a wider range of mental health populations. This will ensure that the results are as accurate as possible when relationships between mental health constructs and physical activity are tested. Second, measures of physical activity (particularly self-report measures, given their practicality and increasing use in research and practice) should be developed with mental health populations in mind, and existing measures should be adapted appropriately for use with individuals diagnosed with mental health conditions. Tailoring measures to mental health populations should increase the accuracy of the results these measures provide. As such, claims regarding the effectiveness of physical activity interventions on mental health outcomes or interventions to improve physical activity and mental health may be more convincing.

noninvasive and low-cost measures of other health indicators (e.g., blood pressure, resting heart rate, body fat percentage self-report measures) have been identified in this chapter. The key to the decision about which physical activity measure to use for a particular research study is the balance between feasibility (i.e., ease and cost) and validity (i.e., complexity and expense) and finding an appropriate middle ground between scientific rigour and practicality.

6   References

Aadahl, M., & Jørgensen, T. (2003). Validation of a new self-report instrument for measuring physical activity. *Medicine and Science in Sports and Exercise*, 35(7), 1196-1202.

ActiLife. (2009). ActiGraph (Version 4.4.1). Penascola, Florida Manufacturing Technology, Inc. (MTI).

Ainslie, P.N., Reilly, T., & Westerterp, K.R. (2003). Estimating human energy expenditure: A review of techniques with particular reference to doubly labelled water. *Sports Medicine*, 33, 683-698.

Ainsworth, B.E., Haskell, W.L., Whitt, M.C., Irwin, M.L., Swartz, A.M., Strath, S.J., et al. (2000). Compendium of physical activities: An update of activity codes and MET intensities. *Medicine and Science in Sports and Exercise*, 39(9), S498-S516.

Baranowski, T. (1988). Validity and reliability of self-report measures of physical activity: An information-processing perspective. *Research Quarterly for Exercise and Sport*, 59, 314-332.

Baumeister, R.F., Vohs, K.D., & Funder, D.C. (2007). Psychology as the science of self-reports and finger movements: Whatever happened to actual behavior? *Perspectives in Psychological Sciences*, 2, 396-403.

Bezyak, J.L., Berven, N.L., & Chan, F. (2011). States of change and physical activity among individuals with severe mental illness. *Rehabilitation Psychology*, 56(3), 182-190.

Birnbaum, M.H. (2004). Human research and data collection via the internet. *Annual Review of Psychology*, 55, 803-832.

Bize, R., Johnson, J.A., & Plotnikoff, R.C. (2007). Physical activity level and health-related quality of life in the general adult population: A systematic review. *Preventive Medicine*, 45, 401-415.

Blair, S.N., Haskell, W.L., Ho, P., Paffenbarger, R.S. Jr., Vranizan, K.M., Farquhar, J.W., et al. (1985). Assessment of habitual physical activity by a seven-day recall in a community survey and controlled experiments. *American Journal of Epidemiology*, 122, 794-804.

Brown, D.W., Brown, D.R., Health, G.W., Balluzi, A., Giles, W.H., Ford, E.S., et al. (2004). Associations between physical activity dose and health-related quality of life. *Medicine and Science in Sports and Exercise*, 36(5), 890-896.

Brown, S., Birtwistle, J., Roe, L., & Thompson, C. (1999). The unhealthy lifestyle of people with schizophrenia. *Psychological Medicine*, 29, 697-701.

Burton, W.N., McCalister, K.T., Chen, C.Y., & Edington, D.W. (2005). The association of health status, worksite fitness center participation, and two measures of productivity. *Journal of Occupational and Environmental Medicine*, 47(4), 343-351.

Bussmann, J.B.J., Ebner-Priemer, U.W., & Fahrenberg, J. (2009). Ambulatory activity monitoring: Progress in measurement of activity, posture, and specific motion patterns in daily life. *European Psychologist*, 14(2), 142-152.

Caspersen, C.J., Powell, K.E., & Christenson, G.M. (1985). Physical activity, exercise, and physical fitness: Definitions and distinctions for health-related research. *Public Health Reports*, 100(2), 126-130.

Chen, K.Y., & Basset, D.R.J. (2005). The technology of accelerometry based activity monitors: Current and future. *Medicine and Science in Sports and Exercise*, 37(11 Suppl.), S491-S500.

Craig, C., Marshall, A.L., Sjöstrom, M., Bauman, A.E., Booth, M.L., Ainsworth, B.E., et al. (2003). International physical activity questionnaire: 12-country reliability and validity. *Medicine and Science in Sports and Exercise*, 35(8), 1381-1395.

Crouter, S.E., Clowers, K.G., & Bassett, D.R.J. (2006). A novel method for using accelerometer data to predict energy expenditure. *Journal of Applied Physiology*, 100, 1324-1331.

Crouter, S.E., Schneider, P.L., Karabulut, M., & Bassett, D.R.J. (2003). Validity of 10 electronic pedometers for measuring steps, distance, and energy cost. *Medicine and Science in Sports and Exercise*, 35, 1455-1460.

Cyarto, E.V., Myers, A.M., & Tudor-Locke, C.E. (2004). Pedometer accuracy in nursing home- and community-dwelling older adults. *Medicine and Science in Sports and Exercise*, 36, 205-209.

Department of Health. (2004). At least five a week: Evidence on the impact of physical activity and its relationship to health: A report from the Chief Medical Officer. London: Department of Health.

DiPietro, L., Caspersen, C.J., Ostfeld, A.M., & Nadel, E.R. (1993). A survey for assessing physical activity amongst older adults. *Medicine and Science in Sports and Exercise*, 25, 628-642.

Dugdill, L., Crone, D., & Murphy, R. (2009). *Physical activity and health promotion: Evidence based applications to practice*. London: Blackwell.

Dugdill, L., & Stratton, G. (2007). *Evaluating sport and physical activity interventions*. London: Department of Health.

Dunn, A.L., Bess, M., Kampbert, J.B., Garcia, M.E., Khol, H.W., & Blair, S. (1999). Comparison of lifestyle and structured interventions to increase physical activity and cardiorespiratory fitness. *Journal of the American Medical Association*, 281, 327-334.

Finlay, R. (1999). SurveyMonkey. Available: www.surveymonkey.com.

Fox, K., Mutrie, N., & O'Donovan, K. (eds) (2010). Physical activity and the prevention of mental illness, dysfunction, and deterioration. *BASES guidelines on physical activity in the prevention of chronic disease*. Champaign, IL: Human Kinetics.

Freedson, P.S., & Miller, E.T. (2000). Objective measurement of physical activity using motion sensors and heart rate. *Research Quarterly for Exercise and Sport*, 71(Suppl. 2), S21-S29.

Friedman, A.B., & Johnson, R.K. (2002). Doubly labelled water: New advances and applications for the practitioner. *Nutrition Today*, 37(6), 243-249.

Godin, G., & Shephard, R.J. (1997). Godin Leisure-Time Exercise Questionnaire. *Medicine and Science in Sports and Exercise*, 29(June Suppl.), S36-S38.

Harada, N.D., Chiu, V., King, A.C., & Stewart, A.L. (2001). An evaluation of three self-report physical activity instruments for older adults. *Medicine and Science in Sports and Exercise*, 33, 962-970.

Have, M., de Graaf, R., & Monshouwer, K. (2011). Physical exercise in adults and mental health status: Findings from the Netherlands Mental Health and Incidence Survey Study (NEMISIS). *Journal of Psychosomatic Research*, 71(5), 342-348. doi: 10.1016/j.jpsychores.2011.04.001.

Howe, C., Staudenmayer, J.W., & Freedson, P.S. (2009). Accelerometer prediction of energy expenditure: Vector magnitude versus vertical axis. *Medicine and Science in Sports and Exercise*, 41(12), 2199-2206.

Jacobs, D.R.J., Ainsworth, B.E., Hartman, T.J., & Leon, A.S. (1993). A simultaneous evaluation of 10 commonly used physical activity questionnaires. *Medicine and Science in Sports and Exercise*, 25(1), 81-91.

Jerome, G.J., Young, D.R., Laferriere, D., Chen, C., Vollmer, W.M., Jerome, G.J., et al. (2009). Reliability of RT3 accelerometers among overweight and obese adults. *Medicine and Science in Sports and Exercise*, 41(1), 110-114.

Keim, N.L., Blanton, C.A., & Kretsch, M.J. (2004). America's obesity epidemic: Measuring physical activity to promote an active lifestyle. *Journal of the American Dietetic Association*, 104(9), 1398-1409.

Krantz, J.H., Ballard, J., & Scher, J. (1997). Comparing the results of laboratory and world-wide web samples on the determinants of female attractiveness. *Behaviour Research Methods, Instruments and Computers*, 29, 264-269.

Lindamer, L.A., McKibbin, C., Norman, G.J., Jordan, L., Harrison, K., Abeyesinhe, S., et al. (2008). Assessment of physical activity in middle aged and older adults with schizophrenia. *Schizophrenia Research*, 104, 294-301.

McKercher, C.M., Schmidt, M.D., Sanderson, K.A., Patton, G.C., Twyer, D., & Venn, A.J. (2009). Physical activity and depression in young adults. *American Journal of Preventive Medicine*, 36(2), 161-164.

Miller, E.T., Neal, D.J., Roberts, L.J., Baer, J.S., Cressler, S.O., Metrik, J., et al. (2002). Test-retest reliability of alcohol measures: Is there a difference between Internet-based and traditional methods? *Psychology of Addictive Behaviours*, 16, 56-63.

Miniwatts. (2010). *Internet world stats: Usage and population statistics*. Available: http://www.internetworldstats.com.

Plasqui, G., & Westerterp, K.R. (2007). Physical activity assessment with accelerometers: An evaluation against doubly labelled water. *Obesity*, 15(10), 2371-2379.

Rennie, K.L., Hemingway, H., Kumari, M., Brunner, E., Malik, M., & Marmot, M. (2003). Effects of moderate and vigorous physical activity on heart rate variability in a British study of civil servants. *American Journal of Epidemiology*, 158, 135-143.

Rzewnicki, R., Auweelw, Y.V., & De Bourdeaudhuij, I. (2002). Addressing overreporting on the international physical activity questionnaire (IPAQ) telephone survey with a population sample. *Public Health Nutrition*, 6(3), 299-305.

Schoeller, D.A. (1988). Measurement of energy expenditure in free living humans by using doubly labelled water. *Journal of Nutrition*, 118, 1278-1289.

Schoeller, D.A., & van Santen, E. (1982). Measurement of energy expenditure in humans by doubly labeled water method. *Journal of Applied Physiology*, 53, 955-959.

Severson, R.K., Nomura, A.M.Y., Grove, J.S., & Stemmerman, G.N. (1989). A prospective analysis of physical activity and cancer. *American Journal of Epidemiology*, 130, 522-529.

Sharpe, J.K., Stedman, T.J., Byrne, N.M., Wishart, C., & Hills, A.P. (2006). Energy expenditure and physical activity in clozopine use: Implications for weight management. *Australian and New Zealand Journal of Psychiatry*, 40, 810-814.

Shephard, R.J. (2003). Limits to the measurement of habitual physical activity by questionnaires. *British Journal of Sports Medicine*, 37, 197-206.

Spruijt-Metz, D., Berrigan, D., Kelly, L.A., McConnell, R., Dueker, D., Lindsey, G., et al. (2009). Measures of physical activity and exercise. In D.B. Allison & M.L. Baskins (Eds.), *Handbook of assessment methods for eating behaviors and weight related problems: Measures, theory and research* (2nd ed.) (pp. 187-253). Thousand Oaks, CA: Sage.

Stone, A., Shiffman, S., Atienza, A.A., & Nebeling, L. (2007). *The science of real-time data capture: Self-reports in health research*. New York: Oxford University Press.

Strath, S.J., Swartz, A.M., Bassett, D.R. Jr., O'Brien, W.L., King, G.A., & Ainsworth, B.E. (2002). Evaluation of heart rate as a method for assessing moderate intensity physical activity. *Medicine and Science in Sports and Exercise*, 32(9), S465-S470.

Taylor, N.J., Crouter, S.E., Lawton, R.J., Conner, M., & Prestwich, A. (2012). Development and valida-tion of the Online Self-Reported Walking and Exercise Questionnaire (OSWEQ). *Journal of Physical Activity and Health*. 3 (Dec).

Tudor, K. (1996). *Mental health promotion paradigms and practice*. London: Routledge.

Tudor-Locke, C.E., Williams, D.M., Reis, J.P., & Pluto, D. (2002). Utility of pedometers for assessing physical activity: Convergent validity. *Sports Medicine*, 32, 795-808.

van Poppel, M.N.M., Chinapaw, M.J.M., Mokkink, L.B., van Mechelen, W., & Terwee, C.B. (2010). Physical activity questionnaires for adults: A systematic review of measurement properties. *Sports Medicine*, 40(7), 565-600.

Whelton, S.P., Chin, A., Xin, X., & He, J. (2002). Effect of aerobic exercise on blood pressure: A meta-analysis of randomised controlled trials. *Annals of Internal Medicine*, 136, 493-503.

Whitelaw, S., Swift, J., Goodwin, A., & Clark, A. (2008). *Physical activity and mental health: The role of physical activity in promoting mental well-being and preventing mental health problems*. Glasgow: University of Glasgow & NHS Scotland.

Wood, T. (2000). Issues and future directions in assessing physical activity: An introduction to conference proceedings. *Research Quarterly for Exercise and Sport*, 71(Suppl. 2), ii-vii.

Factors Influencing the Interaction Between Mental Health and Physical Activity

A range of factors, both social and biological, can affect the benefits of physical activity on well-being and mental health. Part II explores these factors and provides insight into the links between physical activity and mental health.

Chapter 4 examines the evidence that adverse socioeconomic position is linked with lower physical activity and greater sedentary behaviour and discusses how this might accentuate the damaging effects of psychosocial stress. Insufficient physical activity is possibly one of the key mechanisms underpinning social health inequalities. Chapter 4 provides advice for targeting interventions to socially deprived groups. Chapter 5 describes the bidirectional relationship between physical activity and self-esteem. Participation in physical activity is thought to enhance self-esteem through skill development, and greater perceived competence for physical activity leads to greater participation in that behaviour. This chapter also provides practical advice for maximising benefits in clients with low self-esteem (e.g., by creating an exercise environment that highlights personal improvement in terms of physical skill and condition).

Physical activity and exercise at mild to moderate levels have proven beneficial for mental health. However, contrary to what may be expected when training load is increased beyond a certain point, this relationship changes. When overtraining, athletes stress the body above what is normally required for general fitness in order to maximise performance gains. However, some athletes respond in a negative manner to this increase in training volume and instead suffer from what is known as overtraining syndrome. Chapter 6 provides insight into this condition and highlights the role of mood disturbance in overtraining syndrome.

Chapters 7 and 8 discuss the evidence that physical activity is beneficial for mental well-being as well as physical health in older people and in those living with long-term conditions, respectively. These topics are particularly relevant given that in many Western countries the population is aging and the prevalence of people living with long-term conditions is increasing. These chapters provide practical suggestions for practitioners working with older adults and those with long-term conditions (namely chronic obstructive pulmonary disease, diabetes and cancer), each of which presents its own challenges and benefits with regard to physical activity.

Social Class Relationships in Physical Activity and Mental Health

Mark Hamer, PhD

University College London, London, United Kingdom

Chapter Outline

Editors' Introduction

This chapter examines the parallel population distributions of well-being and mental health and physical activity and how they are both related to socioeconomic status: lower socioeconomic status is associated with less physical activity and worse mental health. It reviews the evidence that physical inactivity is a major contributor to social inequalities in health and well-being and examines the pathways by which they may interact. This chapter is vital reading for those who are interested in public health and social inequalities in health. It highlights the need to target physical activity interventions in socially deprived groups and provides practical advice about how to do so.

W ell-being is a complex measure comprising physical, mental and social factors. Measures of subjective well-being, such as self-rated health and quality of life, have consistently been predictive of future objective health outcomes, such as mortality, and are thought to provide a wider evaluation of health status compared with that performed by a physician or evaluation instruments. Regular exercisers enjoy higher levels of well-being (Bize, Johnson & Plotnikoff, 2007) and have lower risk of many chronic diseases. However, opportunities to be physically active in everyday life are decreasing due to motorised transport and technological advances that allow more and more people to remain sedentary throughout their daily lives. This issue appears to be particularly relevant in socially deprived and ethnic minority groups. This chapter describes the key evidence linking socioeconomic status with physical activity behaviour and describes how socioeconomic status patterns in physical activity may be responsible, in part, for the well-described social gradients in health and well-being. In particular, the dysfunction of key physiological systems, including the sympathetic nervous system and hypothalamic–pituitary–adrenal axis (reviewed in chapter 1), have been implicated in psychosocial adversity. Exercise may play a crucial role in blunting harmful exposures to psychosocial stressors in lower socioeconomic status groups.

1 Inequalities in Social Health

Wide socioeconomic disparities exist in many of the most common health problems in the modern world, including coronary heart disease, depression, type 2 diabetes, hypertension, lung disease and many cancers (Marmot & Wilkinson, 2005). These disparities are reflected in the steep social gradient in life expectancy (figure 4.1). Effects are apparent for several markers of socioeconomic status (SES), including income, educational attainment and occupational status or prestige. In each case, lower-status individuals are at higher risk. For most diseases there exists an SES gradient and not just a difference between high and low SES groups; people of intermediate status have an intermediate risk. Thus, the crucial determinant of risk is not poverty or serious deprivation but relative deprivation and factors distributed throughout the population.

1.1 Whitehall Studies

Seminal work in the area of SES, health and behavior has come from the Whitehall epidemiological studies that are described throughout

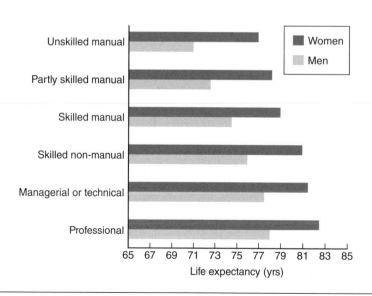

Figure 4.1 Occupational-class differences in life expectancy in England and Wales, 1997-1999.

this chapter. The original Whitehall study of British civil servants, begun in 1967, showed a steep inverse association between social class, as assessed by grade of employment, and mortality from a wide range of diseases. The Whitehall II study was later established in 1985 to identify causal pathways linking socioeconomic position with pathophysiological changes and clinical disease. The Whitehall II is an ongoing prospective cohort study of 10,308 British white-collar workers employed in the civil service (Marmot & Brunner, 2005). The study is primarily interested in the underlying psychological, biological and behavioural pathways associated with workplace social inequalities (e.g., job strain) and health-related behaviours (e.g., physical activity, smoking and diet). Data are collected at regular intervals through a combination of self-administered questionnaires and clinical examination. In the 20 years separating the two studies, social class difference in morbidity has not diminished and an inverse association remains between employment grade and prevalence of common diseases such as heart disease, cancer and respiratory disease.

1.2   SES and Health Gradient Factors

Several factors might underlie the SES gradient in health and well-being, starting with childhood socioeconomic experiences. One study of middle-aged men in Scotland showed a marked gradient in death from coronary heart disease, stroke, lung cancer and stomach cancer that was related to the occupational status of participants' fathers (Davey Smith et al., 1998). After the participants' own SES was taken into account statistically, an influence of childhood SES on mortality remained for stroke and stomach cancer. Another important factor in some health systems is variation in access to primary care services and prioritisation in secondary hospital care.

Stress processes are also related to SES. Various studies have indicated that participants from lower social classes are more vulnerable to stress than those in higher classes. For example, in a study of Japanese workers, job strain was associated with a higher risk of stroke in men from lower occupational classes, but no association was seen in men in higher-status white-collar and managerial positions (Tsutsumi, Kayaba & Ishikawa, 2011). The mechanisms that explain why people from disadvantaged backgrounds are more vulnerable to stress than are those of higher SES are poorly understood. A number of laboratory studies have measured psycho-physiological responses. (Psychophysiology is the study of biological responses to differences or changes in psychological state.) However, these studies have shown that relationships between SES and stress reactivity are consistent only in children, where those in lower SES groups appear to be more reactive in adults (Steptoe & Marmot, 2002). One reason for these inconsistencies in adults may be that the studies have

KEY CONCEPTS

- A strong and well-established social gradient exists in health and well-being.
- Adverse socioeconomic position is linked with lower physical activity and greater sedentary behaviour. This association appears to be largely driven by poorer education.
- Physical activity is known to have numerous beneficial effects on physical and mental health, increase life expectancy and promote healthy aging.
- In particular, physical inactivity in the socially deprived might accentuate the effects of psychosocial stress.
- Insufficient physical activity is possibly one of the key mechanisms linking lower socioeconomic status with poorer well-being

emphasised stress reactivity rather than recovery. In the Whitehall psychophysiology study, white-collar workers from higher, intermediate and lower occupational grades were sampled. Occupational grade was closely related to both income and educational attainment. The results showed that SES groups did not differ markedly in cardiovascular stress reactivity. However, poststress recovery of systolic blood pressure, diastolic pressure and heart rate variability was impaired in lower SES groups (Steptoe et al., 2002). These effects were substantial. For example, lower SES participants were 3 times more likely than higher SES participants to have incomplete diastolic blood pressure recovery 45 minutes poststress after accounting for age, sex, baseline blood pressure and task reactivity. Lower SES groups also had slower recovery in factors related to blood clotting, such as plasma viscosity, and larger stress responses of the inflammatory cytokine interleukin (IL)-6 (Brydon et al., 2004). Thus, poorer recovery in cardiovascular and biological parameters after acute stress might over time contribute to disease pathology.

Naturalistic monitoring studies have shown that salivary cortisol (a key marker of hypothalamic–pituitary–adrenal [HPA] axis function; see chapter 1) has a disturbed circadian pattern of secretion (slightly elevated over the day accompanied by a reduced decline in secretion from the typical morning high to the expected evening low concentration) in lower SES individuals compared with higher SES individuals (Cohen et al., 2006; Kumari et al., 2010). Heart-rate variability (a measure of autonomic nervous system activation) is reduced in lower SES groups; this is indicative of reduced vagal stimulation and autonomic imbalance (Lampert et al., 2005). Some evidence also suggests that variation in systemic peripheral biological function may be coupled with differences in central neurotransmitter activity in the brain. Matthews and colleagues (2005) studied serotonergic activity of the central nervous system by measuring the increase in prolactin after administration of the serotonin agonist fenfluramine. Lower SES participants showed blunted serotonin respon-

sivity; this may be related to depression and risk of substance abuse. More recently, research has found that people living in lower SES communities (defined by income, educational disadvantage and housing costs) also had reduced brain serotonergic responsivity, even after individual SES characteristics such as occupational grade and educational attainment had been taken into account (Manuck et al., 2005). Other important mechanisms might be related to cellular aging processes, which appear to be accelerated in less-educated participants (Steptoe et al., 2011). Evidence suggests that a wide range of biological processes play a role in the social health gradient.

2   Social Class and Exercise

Research has extensively explored the SES gradient in health-related behaviours such as smoking, binge drinking, physical activity and fruit and vegetable intake. The majority of this evidence comes from large epidemiological studies using samples of the population, where measures of SES and physical activity are available. These studies have assessed levels of physical activity using validated questionnaires that require participants to recall amounts and types of activity over the past week, month or year (see chapter 3 for a review of physical activity measurement). These studies most commonly assess leisure-time physical activity, which might include activities such as sport, exercise and walking for pleasure plus other relevant domains of activity, such as domestic activity (e.g., heavy housework, home-improvement work, gardening) and active commuting (e.g., cycling or walking to work). Intentional exercise performed in one's leisure time is possibly most relevant to SES. Leisure-time physical activity has consistently been associated with education in a number of studies across a range of countries, including the United States (Simpson et al., 2003), Canada (Barnett et al., 2007) and several European countries (Borodulin et al., 2008; Lynch, Kaplan & Salonen, 1997; Martínez-González et al., 2001; Vaz de Almeida et al., 1999). The SES gradient in physical activity appears to be established, to a large degree, in childhood. Among a cohort of approximately 6,000 adolescents from 36 London schools, differences in physical activity between SES groups were present at 11 years of age and did not evolve over the teenage years (Brodersen et al., 2007). Relatively little, however, is known about changes in physical activity behaviour over the life course, although social position may be an important influence. Adverse socioeconomic position across the life course has been associated with an increased cumulative risk of low physical activity in older age, as demonstrated in the British Women's Heart and Health Study (Hillsdon et al., 2008). Also, in an Australian cohort study, upward social mobility from childhood to adulthood (defined in this study as reaching a higher level of educational attainment than one's parents) was associated with greater likelihood of increasing activity and fitness over the life course (Cleland et al., 2009). It is possible that the influence of social position on physical activity across the life course is changeable at each life stage, although relatively little research has examined this. Transition from

primary to secondary school (Garcia, Pender & Antonakos, 1998), transition from high school to college or university (Burke, Beilin & Dunbar, 2004), marriage (Raymore, Barber & Eccles, 2001), becoming a parent (McIntyre & Rhodes, 2009) and retirement (Allender, Foster & Boxer, 2008) have all been suggested as important periods for change in physical activity behaviour and might be heavily influenced by social status.

2.1 SES Indicator Type

The social gradient of physical inactivity seems to be apparent regardless of the type of SES indicator used. In a representative sample of the Scottish population, Stamatakis and colleagues (2009) observed consistent graded associations between a range of SES indicators and sedentary behaviour as indexed by time spent watching television. Figure 4.2 shows age-standardised means and 95% confidence limits of self-reported daily time spent viewing television and other screen-based entertainment in relation to various indicators of social position. Wardle and Steptoe (2003), however, suggest that the social

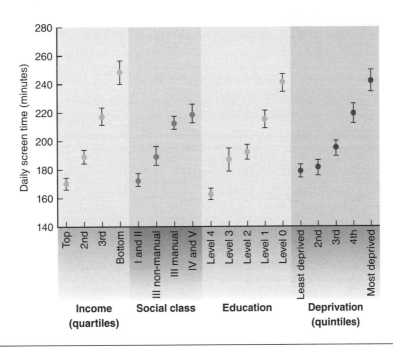

Figure 4.2 Age-standardised means and 95% confidence limits of self-reported daily time spent viewing television and other screen-based entertainment.

Data are from 7,940 Scottish adults who participated in the 2003 Scottish Health Survey.

Reprinted, by permission, from E. Stamatakis et al., 2009, "Television viewing based entertainment in relation to multiple socioeconomic status indicators and area deprivation: The Scottish health survey 2003," *Journal of Epidemiology & Community Health* 63(9): 734-740.

gradient in leisure-time physical activity can primarily be attributed to better knowledge of health that is gained during longer educational careers. A recent study across 12 European countries (Mäkinen et al., 2012) examined the association between leisure-time physical activity and three SES markers: occupational class, employment status and educational level. The findings suggest that, among working-age participants, occupational class and employment status contribute only modestly to educational differences in leisure-time physical activity in Europe. This supports the concept that education is the prime driver of physical activity behaviour. Nevertheless, these findings must be viewed alongside evidence that suggests that educational interventions alone tend to be ineffective for promoting physical activity in either children or adults (van Sluijs, McMinn & Griffin, 2007).

2.2 Measurement Limitations

One of the major limitations of the body of work exploring associations between social class and exercise to date has been the use of self-reported measures of physical activity (see chapter 3), which might introduce reporting biases. This could be particularly relevant when comparing physical activity behaviour across SES groups. The development of small, solid-state accelerometer devices (as discussed in chapter 3) now permits researchers to objectively assess physical activity over several days at low cost and to feasibly incorporate such measures in large-scale population studies. In the recent 2008 Health Survey for England, physical activity was measured objectively over 7 days using these devices (Craig, Mindell & Hirani, 2009). Interestingly, the SES trends in physical activity previously observed in studies that employed self-reported measures were not replicated in the Health Survey for England, which used objective assessments. Those in the highest income tertile recorded more sedentary time (591 min/day in men and 585 min/day in women) than those in the middle and lowest income tertiles (approximately 570 min/day). Conversely, those in the middle and lowest income tertiles spent

more time on average performing light-intensity activity compared with those in the highest income tertile. No differences existed in levels of moderate- to vigorous-intensity activity across household income groups (see figure 4.3). These contrasting data suggest that physical activity measurement is a crucial aspect in understanding potential SES differences. Further large-scale population studies with objective measures of physical activity are therefore required to further investigate variations in physical activity across social groups.

2.3 Compensatory Behaviour and Occupational Characteristics

One possible explanation for the observed relationship between physical activity and social class is that those who spend most of their working day in manual tasks compensate by sitting more during leisure time. Previous reports have shown that occupational physical activity may moderate the relationship between SES and physical activity (Macintyre & Mutrie, 2004). Manual labourers engaged in heavy physical activity at work may compensate by doing less physical activity in their leisure time (Macintyre & Mutrie, 2004). A cross-sectional study of 1,048 working adults in Australia that assessed the mediating

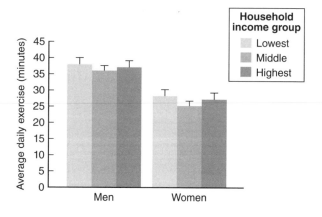

Figure 4.3 Objectively assessed levels of moderate- to vigorous-intensity physical activity across tertiles of equivalised household income. Data are from 979 men and 1,154 women aged 16 years and older.

Data from 2008 Health Survey for England.
Adapted from Cotman et al. 2002.

effect of sitting time on socioeconomic differences in rates of overweight and obesity reported that the association between SES and sitting time varied according to the day of the week and the type of sitting (Proper, Cerin & Brown, 2007). Respondents with low education living in deprived neighbourhoods spent less time sitting on weekdays, whereas low education was associated with more time spent sitting on weekend days. Also, a greater number of working hours per week was associated with more time spent sitting during weekdays and weekend days but less time spent sitting during leisure time. The differences in sitting on weekdays and weekend days suggest that workers who spent most of their working day sitting compensated by sitting less during leisure time. However, other studies have not found evidence of compensatory behaviour. An Australian cross-sectional study found no difference in leisure-time physical activity by level of occupational sitting (Mummery, Schofield & Steele, 2005). In a cross-sectional study of Dutch workers, sitting time at work varied considerably by type of occupation but sitting during leisure time did not (Jans, Proper & Hildebrandt, 2007). In this study, adjustment for occupational physical activity did not remove the association between social class and sitting time. In fact, 78% of men in social class III and 89% of men in social classes I and II reported no or only light physical activity at work, suggesting that few adults are engaged in heavy manual work that necessitates resting during leisure time. Taken together, the association between occupational physical activity and physical activity behaviour appears to vary according to how both types of activity are assessed. Indeed, in a recent review, white-collar workers reported higher levels of leisure-time physical activity than did blue-collar workers, although a positive association existed between occupational physical activity and leisure-time physical activity (Kirk & Rhodes, 2011). Thus, using only occupational grade as a proxy of occupational physical activity might produce misleading results.

Other occupational characteristics linked with social status might be important. Passive, nonchallenging, nondemanding jobs in which employees feel low control over work may encourage passive lifestyles. In the Whitehall II study of British civil servants, participants working in passive jobs were particularly likely to be physically inactive in their leisure time (Gimeno et al., 2009). However, other studies have failed to observe an association between these work characteristics and physical activity (Landsbergis, Schnall & Deitz, 1998; van Loon, Tijhuis & Surtees, 2000).

2.4 Income and Environment

It is possible that adults living on lower incomes cannot afford to engage in recreational activities such as going to a gym or leisure centre or playing sports. In the United Kingdom, household expenditure on recreation and culture increases with each decile of household income (Dunn, 2007). Households on lower incomes are more likely to report that money is a barrier to participation in physical activity (Chinn, White & Harland, 1999). It is also possible that low-income households spend what disposable income they have on screen-based entertainment in the home. However, data on family spending in the United Kingdom show that households in the lowest spending decile are far less likely to own a computer or satellite receiver than are households in the top decile (Dunn, 2008). Low-income households are also less likely to own a car that would allow them to travel to destinations that might encourage physical activity.

Neighbourhood SES might play a crucial role in explaining social patterns in physical activity behaviour. Existing research has largely focussed on the influence of neighbourhood characteristics on broader health outcomes of its residents rather than on individual health behaviours. However, data from a recent large U.S. cohort study demonstrated robust longitudinal associations between neighbourhood deprivation and lower physical activity. According to study results, levels of physical activity in the most-deprived areas were 16% lower than those in the least-deprived areas after accounting for individual SES (Boone-Heinonen et al., 2011). Neighbourhood deprivation may account for multiple synergistic pathways through which physical activity is influenced, including inequitable distribution of the built environment (e.g., facilities), social cues and social support for physical activity. Facilities that offer affordable physical activity (e.g., leisure centres, gyms, swimming pools) are fewer in poorer neighbourhoods, thus reducing opportunities for some forms of physical activity (Hillsdon, Panter & Foster, 2007; Panter, Jones & Hillsdon, 2008). Ironically, low-income households appear to have good access to unaffordable private-sector gyms (Panter, Jones & Hillsdon, 2008). It is not always true that more deprived neighbourhoods have less access to resources that promote physical activity. A study in Scotland showed that people living in deprived neighbourhoods have better access to public green space and children's play areas than do people living in more affluent neighbourhoods (Macintyre, 2007). A recent study of 13,927 participants from the United Kingdom that explored associations between physical activity and objectively measured geographical information found no association between physical activity and access to green space, although people were less likely to cycle for leisure in areas of high traffic density (Foster et al., 2009). It may be that access to facilities is mediated by concerns about personal safety. Negative perceptions of neighbourhood safety may also discourage people from spending time outside the home. Concerns about personal safety, which are frequently associated with low levels of physical activity, are greater in lower SES groups (U.S. Centers for Disease Control and Prevention, 1999). Furthermore, evidence shows that time spent viewing television is more valued in low SES women than in high SES women (Ball, Salmon & Giles-Corti, 2006). Of course, a major limitation of existing research examining neighbourhood influences on health and related behaviours is potential bias resulting from the drift of existing low active residents into low SES neighbourhoods, rather than neighborhoods themselves having the negative effect on physical activity. Thus, researchers must account for factors that influence residential mobility and location decisions when interpreting the findings. For example, one noncausal explanation for associations between neighbourhood SES and physical activity might

Physical Activity Behaviour and Risk of Coronary Heart Disease in Ethnic Minorities

Physical activity appears to be an important factor in determining health outcomes among ethnic minority groups, who tend to be socially disadvantaged and reside in more socially deprived areas. We recently investigated physical activity behaviour and risk of coronary heart disease among South Asian communities in the United Kingdom using the Health Survey for England. The results showed that levels of self-reported leisure-time physical activity were consistently lower in South Asians than in Caucasian participants (Williams et al., 2011b). This difference was consistent across men and women, age groups and subgroups and was independent of covariates, including self-reported health, adiposity and indicators of SES. These results might be explained by ethnic differences in knowledge about, attitudes toward and resources for engaging in healthy lifestyles. In further analyses we linked the survey data of the 15,412 participants (13,293 Caucasians and 2,120 South Asians) with mortality records in order to perform a prospective study that examined the association between physical activity and mortality risk among South Asians and the general Caucasian population. In these analyses, physical inactivity accounted for one fourth of the excess coronary heart disease mortality in South Asians compared with Caucasians even after adjusting for potential confounding variables (Williams et al., 2011a).

be that individuals who begin new jobs have less time for leisure-time physical activity and move to more urbanised, lower SES neighbourhoods that are closer to the workplace. However, poorer individuals often have limited choice about the neighbourhoods they live in.

3   Nature Versus Nurture

The links between social class, physical activity and well-being might have a genetic basis. This hypothesis can be tested using twin studies. The twin study design allows one to estimate the contribution of environmental factors and genetic factors by comparing effects in monozygotic (identical) and dizygotic (nonidentical) twin pairs. For example, if monozygotic twins are more similar in physical activity levels than are dizygotic twins, this would imply a substantial genetic influence with the remainder of the variability attributed to environment influences. Several twin studies have provided conflicting evidence on the contribution of genetics to physical activity behaviour. In a large study using data from 7 European twin registries of more than 37,000 adult twin pairs, self-reported leisure-time physical activity was largely explained by genetic influences (Stubbe et al., 2006). However, data from the Twins Early Development Study that collected objective measures of physical activity in 234 children showed that the shared environment was the dominant influence on children's activity levels (Fisher et al., 2010). Nevertheless, Fisher and colleagues (2010) provided evidence that suggests that enjoyment of activity was predominantly influenced by genetic factors. This is highly plausible because enjoyment of physical activity is influenced by physical ability, which itself is influenced by genetics. For example, genes related to muscle performance and muscle blood flow have been linked with exercise participation (De Moor et al., 2007). Exercise ability might affect exercise behaviour. The discrepancy in results between adults and children might reflect changes in genetic contribution across the life course. In childhood, the influence of teachers and parents might have

a stronger effect on certain behaviours such as physical activity. Indeed, other data suggest that the environment for exercise behaviour in adolescents is generation-specific involving shared environmental influences such as the neighbourhood, SES or environmental factors that are specific to the adolescent generation (e.g., the influence of siblings, friends, peers or the school or a combination of these factors) (De Moor et al., 2011).

It is also feasible that the association between physical activity and measures of well-being, such as depression and anxiety, is explained by common genetic factors. In a study of 6,000 twins from a Dutch twin registry, identical (monozygotic) twins discordant for exercise (one defined as sedentary and the other defined as active) displayed no differences in prevalence of depressive and anxious symptoms, suggesting that the link between exercise and mood might not be causal. These data suggest that a third factor, such as common genetic vulnerability, might determine exercise behaviour and mental health in the population (De Moor et al, 2008). It is unknown which genes might be involved in voluntary exercise behaviour and in the risk for anxiety and depression. However, genes involved in regulating the dopaminergic, norepinephrenergic, opioidergic or serotonergic neurotransmitter pathways of the brain are among those that may simultaneously affect the regulation of exercise drive and mood. This might partly explain why genetic contributions to exercise behaviour become stronger across the life course. People who do not experience positive affect from taking part in physical activities are unlikely to pursue them in their leisure time.

4   SES Mechanisms Linking Physical Activity and Health

Numerous mechanisms likely explain the social gradient in health and well-being. Physical inactivity in the socially deprived might accentuate the effects of psychosocial stress and partly account for the established social disparities in health and well-being.

4.1   Behavioural Mechanisms

The higher prevalence of unhealthy behaviours in lower SES individuals is seen as one of the key mechanisms linking lower SES with poorer well-being. Other factors such as cognitive and physical function, access to health care, psychosocial adversity and biological mechanisms have also been investigated. The combination of unhealthy behaviours, including lack of exercise, smoking, excess alcohol intake and poor diet, has been shown to explain up to 50% of the SES difference in mortality (Lantz et al., 1998; Stringhini et al., 2010). Self-reported physical activity was specifically shown to account for more than one third of the social gradient in mortality risk in participants from the Whitehall II cohort study that were followed up over 20 years (Stringhini et al., 2010). The Whitehall II cohort study also explored common causal explanations for social inequalities in other markers of well-being such as mental and physical health. The civil service employment grade is commonly used as a measure of SES in the Whitehall II study because it reflects both income and status. Employment grade is consistently associated with depressive symptoms and measures of physical function in a graded fashion (Stansfeld et al., 2003). The social gradient in these markers of well-being can again be partly explained by differences in health behaviours. Marked differences in physical inactivity exist between those in higher (6.6% are inactive) and lower (35.4% are inactive) grades. Individuals in lower social position are more resistant to changing their health behaviours, which might explain why poor lifestyle habits are a potent risk factor across the life course in disadvantaged participants.

4.2   Stress Processes

Stress processes have been related to SES and might play a key role in health and well-being. Individuals of lower SES are likely to experience greater psychosocial adversity in the form of lower job control, financial strain, marital conflict and poorer living conditions. These factors are known to contribute to daily wear and tear on the body's stress systems, such as the sympathetic nervous system and HPA axis, and over time result in gradual changes to physiological set points. Heightened daily reactivity to stressors might therefore be a clinically relevant health risk factor. For example, as described earlier in this chapter, compared with higher-grade workers, participants from the lowest employment grade in Whitehall II demonstrate slower recovery from laboratory-induced stressors in factors related to blood clotting, such as plasma viscosity, and larger stress responses of the inflammatory cytokine IL-6 (Brydon et al., 2004). Similarities between central and peripheral responses to exercise and mental stressors have led to the theory of cross-stressor adaptation, which posits that adaptations resulting from regular exercise lead to improved cardiovascular regulation both during exercise and in response to mental stressors (Sothmann et al., 1996). Thus, exercise may play a crucial role in blunting harmful exposures to psychosocial stressors in lower SES groups. Much of the existing psychophysiological work relating to the effects of physical exercise has focussed on cardiovascular stress responses. In particular, acute exercise has been associated with buffering blood pressure and cardiac responses to standardised mental stressors in the laboratory (Hamer, Taylor & Steptoe, 2006), although inconsistencies about the effects of chronic exercise training exist in the literature. Far less work has focussed on the psychobiological effects of acute and chronic exercise.

4.3   Chronic Stress and Exercise

Long-term voluntary exercise in animals causes an increase in adrenal mass as a response to increased glucocorticoid secretion (Droste et al., 2007) and adaptation in HPA responses to acute exercise, including a higher threshold of activation. This results in a blunted response to exercise at the same absolute intensity but greater responses to maximal exercise. For example, trained rats demonstrate greater corticosterone responses to forced swimming than do untrained rats. In humans, physically trained and unfit women demonstrate similar cortisol responses to high-intensity exercise, although during recovery the physically trained women have a greater rate of recovery of the glucocorticoid secretagogue adrenocorticotrophic hormone (ACTH) and higher cortisol levels (Traustadóttir et al., 2004). This finding suggests that physical training increases sensitivity of the adrenal glands to ACTH. Other evidence suggests that trained individuals demonstrate increased tissue sensitivity to glucocorticoids after a bout of acute exercise (Duclos, Gouarne & Bonnemaison, 2003); this may be a mechanism for preventing excessive muscle inflammatory responses. Some evidence suggests that basal levels of cortisol are reduced after prolonged physical training via a reduction in glucocorticoid receptor sensitivity, which might be beneficial in terms of chronic HPA activation (Silva et al., 2008). However, some studies have not demonstrated reduced corticotropic sensitivity to negative feedback by chronic exercise stress; this inconsistency might be explained by individual variability in exercise-training responses. In addition, animal data suggest that glucocorticoid receptor adaptation to exercise might be tissue

specific, resulting in decreases in glucocorticoid action in skeletal muscle and increased action in visceral fat.

Recent studies have consistently demonstrated blunted HPA responses to mental stressors in physically trained individuals (Rimelle et al., 2009). In a cross-sectional study, inflammatory cytokine (IL-6 and tumor necrosis factor-α) responses to acute mental stress are attenuated in individuals who are more physically fit and have been demonstrated to be independent of age, sex, SES, smoking, alcohol consumption and basal levels of inflammatory markers (Hamer & Steptoe, 2007), shown in figure 4.4. Associations with alcohol consumption and inflammatory markers are particularly relevant because disturbances in inflammatory and HPA stress responses have been associated with markers of subclinical cardiovascular disease (Ellins et al., 2008; Hamer et al., 2010) and may thus be important mechanisms in disease progression. Studies in animals appear to suggest stress-specific effects occur in relation to exercise training. Trained animals demonstrate exaggerated corticosterone responses to physical

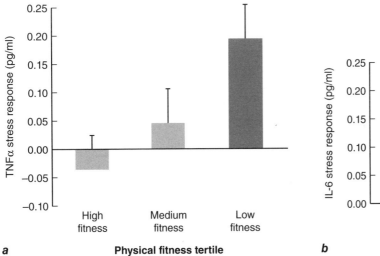

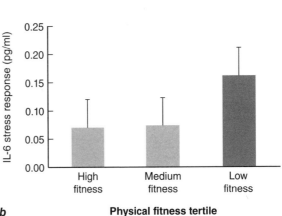

a   **Physical fitness tertile**   *b*   **Physical fitness tertile**

Figure 4.4.   The association between physical fitness and the change in (*a*) TNFα and (*b*) IL-6 between baseline and post-stress samples. Participants were 207 men and women (52 ± 3 yrs) drawn from the Whitehall II epidemiological cohort. Data are presented as mean ± SEM, adjusted for age, sex, body mass index, employment grade, smoking, alcohol, and basal levels of inflammatory cytokines. Physical fitness tertiles are based on heart rate response to cycling ergometry exercise at a standardized workload.

Reprinted, by permission, from M. Hamer and A. Steptoe, 2007, "Association between physical fitness, parasympathetic control, and proinflammatory responses to mental stress," *Psychosomatic Medicine* 69(7): 660-666.

stressors such as forced swimming but reduced responses to novel, anxiety-promoting stressors (Droste et al., 2007). This apparent stress-specific response might be explained by a dissociation of ACTH and glucocorticoids under certain stress conditions, although such effects have not been replicated in humans. Further data have also shown that exercise-trained animals demonstrate better HPA habituation to repeated noise stress (Sasse et al., 2008). This may be a critical adaptation because the inability to adequately adapt to chronic stressors may have long-term consequences on health. Adaptations to key stress-response systems might be a crucial mechanism in explaining the social gradient in disease risk, and exercise is a potential preventive tool for protecting disadvantaged individuals from the effects of excessive exposure to stress.

5   Public Health Interventions

The ever-widening gap in health between rich and poor has initiated developing lifestyle interventions that tackle social health inequalities. The numerous barriers to changes in physical activity in deprived areas include unsafe streets, dilapidated parks and lack of resources and facilities. Changing health behaviours in low-income groups can therefore be challenging and complex and requires a collaborative approach between partners (see Schwarte et al., 2010). Available evidence on the efficacy of community-based physical activity interventions is limited, although the current evidence generally does not support the hypothesis that multicomponent community-wide interventions effectively increase population levels of physical activity (Baker, Francis & Soares, 2011; Hillsdon, Foster & Thorogood, 2005; Marcus et al., 2006). Indeed, physical activity interventions typically produce small effects that are difficult to sustain over the long term. The effects of delivering brief verbal advice on changing physical activity behaviour in the primary care setting have been disappointing (Kinmonth et al., 2008), although programmes that are tailored to the individual and contain multiple components (e.g., goal setting, problem

solving, self-monitoring, supervised exercise) are generally more effective. Worksite interventions have generally demonstrated limited success because they are typically attended only by those who are already exercising or highly motivated. Recent reviews of workplace interventions have demonstrated small to moderate effect sizes of physical activity interventions on absenteeism, job stress and job satisfaction (Conn et al., 2009), although others have observed limited effects on markers of overall well-being (Brown et al., 2011). Similarly, mass-media campaigns show mixed results and often do not target the most deprived groups that have the greatest need. Another approach involves modifying the environment to make habitual activity easier. For example, the design and layout of towns and cities can encourage active transport, and the location and design of buildings can encourage the use of stairs. This is particularly relevant for individuals living in socially deprived inner-city areas. However, from the current evidence it is difficult to ascertain the effectiveness of environmental interventions on physical activity change, mainly because of the limitations of current research (e.g., lack of control groups, lack of appropriate physical activity assessment, insufficient follow-up). Furthermore, little is known about how the effects of interventions vary by SES.

One example of a recent community-based physical activity intervention programme is the Central California Regional Obesity Prevention Program in the United States, which targets low-income, disadvantaged ethnic and rural communities and has created a community-driven policy and environmental change model for obesity prevention (Schwarte et al., 2010). A range of interventions for increasing physical activity were introduced, including making public places safer for exercise, installing new walking paths and creating walking school bus programmes. These types of interventions are promising, although further work is required to better understand effective approaches to eradicating social inequalities in lifestyle and well-being.

EVIDENCE TO PRACTICE

- Physical activity interventions need to be targeted to socially deprived groups.
- It is important to understand the environmental barriers to physical activity change in deprived areas.
- Physical activity programmes that are tailored to the individual and contain multiple components (e.g., goal setting, problem solving, self-monitoring, supervised exercise) are generally more effective than those that do not.
- Changing health behaviour in low-income groups can be challenging and complex and requires a collaborative approach between partners.

6 Summary

Physical activity plays a crucial role in maintaining health and well-being. The evidence consistently demonstrates that a social gradient exists in physical activity behaviour. This gradient is established to a large extent in childhood and prevails across the life course. Physical inactivity in the socially deprived might accentuate the effects of psychosocial stress and partly account for the established social disparities in health and well-being. Numerous barriers to change in physical activity in lower SES groups exist and continue to make intervention a challenging area for researchers and public health workers. Further work is crucial for better understanding effective approaches to improving lifestyle in the socially deprived and eradicating social inequalities in health and well-being.

7 References

Allender, S., Foster, C., & Boxer, A. (2008). Occupational and nonoccupational physical activity and the social determinants of physical activity: Results from the Health Survey for England. *Journal of Physical Activity and Health*, 5, 104-116.

Baker, P.R., Francis, D.P., & Soares, J. (2011). Community wide interventions for increasing physical activity. *Cochrane Database Systematic Review*, 4, CD008366.

Ball, K., Salmon, J., & Giles-Corti, B. (2006). How can socio-economic differences in physical activity among women be explained? A qualitative study. *Women Health*, 43, 93-113.

Barnett, T.A., Gauvin, L., Craig, C.L., & Katzmarzyk, P.T. (2007). Modifying effects of sex, age, and education on 22-year trajectory of leisure-time physical activity in a Canadian cohort. *Journal Physical Activity and Health*, 4, 153-166.

Bize, R., Johnson, J.A., & Plotnikoff, R.C. (2007). Physical activity level and health related quality of life in the general adult population: A systematic review. *Preventive Medicine*, 45, 401-415.

Boone-Heinonen, J., Diez Roux, A.V., Kiefe, C.I., Lewis, C.E., Guilkey, D.K., & Gordon-Larsen, P. (2011). Neighborhood socioeconomic status predictors of physical activity through young to middle adulthood: The CARDIA study. *Social Science and Medicine*, 72, 641-649.

Borodulin, K., Laatikainen, T., Lahti-Koski, M., Jousilahti, P., & Lakka, T. (2008). Association of age and education with different types of leisure time physical activity among 4437 Finnish adults. *Journal of Physical Activity and Health*, 5, 242-251.

Brodersen, N.H., Steptoe, A., Boniface, D.R., & Wardle, J. (2007). Trends in physical activity and sedentary behaviour in adolescence: Ethnic and socioeconomic differences. *British Journal of Sports Medicine*, 41, 140-144.

Brown, H.E., Gilson, N.D., Burton, N.W., & Brown, W.J. (2011). Does physical activity impact on presenteeism and other indicators of workplace well-being? *Sports Medicine*, 41, 249-262.

Brydon, L., Edwards, S., Mohamed-Ali, V., & Steptoe, A. (2004). Socioeconomic status and stress-induced increases in interleukin-6. *Brain, Behavior, and Immunity*, 18, 281-290.

Burke, V., Beilin, L.J., & Dunbar, D. (2004). Changes in health-related behaviours and cardiovascular risk factors in young adults: Associations with living with a partner. *Preventive Medicine*, 39, 722-730.

Chinn, D.J., White, M., & Harland, J. (1999). Barrier to physical activity and socioeconomic position: Implications for health promotion. *Journal of Epidemiology and Community Health*, 53, 191-192.

Cleland, V.J., Ball, K., Magnussen, C., Dwyer, T., & Venn, A. (2009). Socioeconomic position and the tracking of physical activity and cardiorespiratory fitness from childhood to adulthood. *American Journal of Epidemiology*, 170, 1069-1077.

Cohen, S., Schwartz, J.E., Epel, E., Kirschbaum, C., Sidney, S., & Seeman, T. (2006). Socioeconomic status, race, and diurnal cortisol decline in the Coronary Artery Risk Development in Young Adults (CARDIA) Study. *Psychosomatic Medicine*, 68, 41-50.

Conn, V.S., Hafdahl, A.R., Cooper, P.S., Brown, L.M., & Lusk, S.L. (2009). Meta-analysis of workplace physical activity interventions. *American Journal of Preventive Medicine*, 37, 330-339.

Craig, R., Mindell, J., & Hirani, V. (2009). *On behalf of the Joint Health Surveys Unit. The Health Survey for England 2008. Volume 1: Physical activity and fitness. Chapter 3: Accelerometry in adults.* Available: www.ic.nhs.uk/pubs/hse-08physicalactivity.

Davey Smith, G., Hart, C., Blane, D., & Hole, D. (1998). Adverse socioeconomic conditions in childhood and cause specific adult mortality: Prospective observational study. *British Medical Journal*, 316, 1631-1635.

De Moor, M.H., Boomsma, D.I., Stubbe, J.H., Willemsen, G., & de Geus, E.J. (2008). Testing causality in the association between regular exercise and symptoms of anxiety and depression. *Archives of General Psychiatry*, 65, 897-905.

De Moor, M.H., Posthuma, D., Hottenga, J.J., Willemsen, G., Boomsma, D.I., & De Geus, E.J. (2007). Genome-wide linkage scan for exercise participation in Dutch sibling pairs. *European Journal of Human Genetics*, 15, 1252-1259.

De Moor, M.H., Willemsen, G., Rebollo-Mesa, I., Stubbe, J.H., De Geus, E.J., & Boomsma, D.I. (2011). Exercise participation in adolescents and their parents: Evidence for genetic and generation specific environmental effects. *Behavior Genetics*, 41(2), 211-222.

Droste, S.K., Chandramohan, Y., Hill, L.E., Linthorst, A.C., & Reul, J.M. (2007). Voluntary exercise impacts on the rat hypothalamic-pituitary-adrenocortical axis mainly at the adrenal level. *Neuroendocrinology*, 86, 26-37.

Duclos, M., Gouarne, C., & Bonnemaison, D. (2003). Acute and chronic effects of exercise on tissue sensitivity to glucocorticoids. *Journal of Applied Physiology*, 94, 869-875.

Dunn, E. (2007). *Family spending 2006.* London: Office for National Statistics.

Dunn, E. (2008). *Family spending 2007.* London: Office for National Statistics.

Ellins, E., Halcox, J., Donald, A., Field, B., Brydon, L., Deanfield, J., et al. (2008). Arterial stiffness and inflammatory response to psychophysiological stress. *Brain, Behavior, and Immunity*, 22, 941-948.

Fisher, A., van Jaarsveld, C.H., Llewellyn, C.H., & Wardle, J. (2010). Environmental influences on children's physical activity: Quantitative estimates using a twin design. *PLoS One*, 5, e10110.

Foster, C., Hillsdon, M., Jones, A., Grundy, C., Wilkinson, P., White, M., et al. (2009). Objective measures of the environment and physical activity: Results of the environment and physical activity study in English adults. *Journal of Physical Activity and Health*, 6(Suppl. 1), S70-S80.

Garcia, A.W., Pender, N.J., & Antonakos, C.L. (1998). Changes in physical activity beliefs and behaviors of boys and girls across the transition to junior high school. *Journal of Adolescent Health*, 22, 394-402.

Gimeno, D., Elovainio, M., Jokela, M., De Vogli, R., Marmot, M.G., & Kivimäki, M. (2009). Association between passive jobs and low levels of leisure-time physical activity: The Whitehall II cohort study. *Occupational Environmental Medicine*, 66, 772-776.

Hamer, M., O'Donnell, K., Lahiri, A., & Steptoe, A. (2010). Salivary cortisol responses to mental stress are associated with coronary artery calcification in healthy men and women. *European Heart Journal*, 31, 424-429.

Hamer, M., & Steptoe, A. (2007). Association between physical fitness, parasympathetic control, and proinflammatory responses to mental stress. *Psychosomatic Medicine*, 69, 660-666.

Hamer, M., Taylor, A., & Steptoe, A. (2006). The effects of acute aerobic exercise on stress related blood pressure responses: A systematic review and meta-analysis. *Biological Psychology*, 71, 183-190.

Hillsdon, M., Foster, C., & Thorogood, M. (2005). Interventions for promoting physical activity. *Cochrane Database Systematic Review*, 1, CD003180.

Hillsdon, M., Lawlor, D.A., Ebrahim, S., & Morris, J.N. (2008). Physical activity in older women: Associations with area deprivation and with socioeconomic position over the life course: Observations in the British Women's Heart and Health Study. *Journal of Epidemiology and Community Health, 62*, 344-350.

Hillsdon, M., Panter, J., & Foster, C. (2007). Equitable access to exercise facilities. *American Journal of Preventive Medicine, 32*, 506-508.

Jans, M.P., Proper, K.I., & Hildebrandt, V.H. (2007). Sedentary behavior in Dutch workers: Differences between occupations and business sectors. *American Journal of Preventive Medicine, 33*, 450-454.

Kinmonth, A.L., Wareham, N.J., Hardeman, W., Sutton, S., Prevost, A.T., Fanshawe, T., et al. (2008). Efficacy of a theory-based behavioural intervention to increase physical activity in an at-risk group in primary care (ProActive UK): A randomised trial. *Lancet, 371*, 41-48.

Kirk, M.A., & Rhodes, R.E. (2011). Occupation correlates of adults' participation in leisure-time physical activity: A systematic review. *American Journal of Preventive Medicine, 40*, 476-485.

Kumari, M., Badrick, E., Chandola, T., Adler, N.E., Epel, E., Seeman, T., et al. (2010). Measures of social position and cortisol secretion in an aging population: Findings from the Whitehall II study. *Psychosomatic Medicine, 72*, 27-34.

Lampert, R., Ickovics, J., Horwitz, R., & Lee, F. (2005). Depressed autonomic nervous system function in African Americans and individuals of lower social class: A potential mechanism of race- and class-related disparities in health outcomes. *American Heart Journal, 150*, 153-160.

Landsbergis, P.A., Schnall, P.L., & Deitz, D.K. (1998). Job strain and health behaviors: Results of a prospective study. *American Journal of Health Promotion, 12*, 237-245.

Lantz, P.M., House, J.S., Lepkowski, J.M., Williams, D.R., Mero, R.P., & Chen, J. (1998). Socioeconomic factors, health behaviors, and mortality: Results from a nationally representative prospective study of U.S. adults. *Journal of the American Medical Association, 279*, 1703-1708.

Lynch, J.W., Kaplan, G.A., & Salonen, J.T. (1997). Why do poor people behave poorly? Variation in adult health behaviours and psychosocial characteristics by stages of the socioeconomic lifecourse. *Social Science and Medicine, 44*, 809-819.

Macintyre, S. (2007). Deprivation amplification revisited; Or, is it always true that poorer places have poorer access to resources for healthy diets and physical activity? *International Journal of Behavioral Nutrition and Physical Activity, 4*, 32.

Macintyre, S., & Mutrie, N. (2004). Socio-economic differences in cardiovascular disease and physical activity: Stereotypes and reality. *Journal of the Royal Society Promotion of Health, 124*, 66.

Mäkinen, T.E., Sippola, R., Borodulin, K., Rahkonen, O., Kunst, A., Klumbiene, J., et al. (2012). Explaining educational differences in leisure-time physical activity in Europe: The contribution of work-related factors. *Scandinavian Journal of Medicine Science Sports, 22*(3), 439-447.

Manuck, S.B., Bleil, M.E., Petersen, K.L., Flory, J.D., Mann, J.J., Ferrell, R.E., et al. (2005). The socioeconomic status of communities predicts variation in brain serotonergic responsivity. *Psychological Medicine, 35*, 519-528.

Marcus, B.H., Williams, D.M., Dubbert, P.M., Sallis, J.F., King, A.C., Yancey, A.K., et al. (2006). Physical activity intervention studies: What we know and what we need to know. A scientific statement from the American Heart Association Council on Nutrition, Physical Activity, and Metabolism (Subcommittee on Physical Activity); Council on Cardiovascular Disease in the Young; and the Interdisciplinary Working Group on Quality of Care and Outcomes Research. *Circulation, 114*, 2739-2752.

Marmot, M., & Brunner, E. (2005). Cohort profile: The Whitehall II study. *International Journal of Epidemiology, 34*, 251-256.

Marmot, M., & Wilkinson, R.G. (Eds.). (2005). *Social determinants of health* (2nd ed.). Oxford: Oxford University Press.

Martínez-González, M.A., Varo, J.J., Santos, J.L., De Irala, J., Gibney, M., Kearney, J., *et al. (2001).* Prevalence of physical activity during leisure time in the European Union. *Medicine Science Sports Exercise, 33*, 1142-1146.

Matthews, K.A., Flory, J.D., Muldoon, M.F., & Manuck, S.B. (2005). Does socioeconomic status relate to central serotonergic responsivity in healthy adults? *Psychosomatic Medicine, 62*, 231-237.

McIntyre, C.A., & Rhodes, R.E. (2009). Correlates of leisure-time physical activity during transitions to motherhood. *Women Health, 49*, 66-83.

Mummery, K.W., Schofield, G.M., & Steele, R. (2005). Occupational sitting time and overweight and obesity in Australian workers. *American Journal of Preventive Medicine, 29*, 91-97.

Panter, J., Jones, A., & Hillsdon, M. (2008). Equity of access to physical activity facilities in an English city. *Preventive Medicine, 46*, 303-307.

Proper, K.I., Cerin, E., & Brown, W.J. (2007). Sitting time and socio-economic differences in overweight and obesity. *International Journal of Obesity, 31*, 169-176.

Raymore, L., Barber, B., & Eccles, J. (2001). Leaving home, attending college, partnership and parenthood: The role of life transition events in leisure pattern stability from adolescence to young adulthood. *Journal of Youth and Adolescence, 30*, 197-223.

Rimmele, U., Seiler, R., Marti, B., Wirtz, P.H., Ehlert, U., & Heinrichs, M. (2009). The level of physical activity affects adrenal and cardiovascular reactivity to psychosocial stress. *Psychoneuroendocrinology, 34*, 190-198.

Sasse, S.K., Greenwood, B.N., Masini, C.V., Nyhuis, T.J., Fleshner, M., Day, H.E., et al. (2008). Chronic voluntary wheel running facilitates corticosterone response habituation to repeated audiogenic stress exposure in male rats. *Stress, 11*, 425-437.

Schwarte, L., Samuels, S.E., Capitman, J., Ruwe, M., Boyle, M., & Flores, G. (2010). The Central California Regional Obesity Prevention Program: Changing nutrition and physical activity environments in California's heartland. *American Journal of Public Health, 100*, 2124-2128.

Silva, T.S., Longui, C.A., Faria, C.D., Rocha, M.N., Melo, M.R., Faria, T.G., et al. (2008). Impact of prolonged physical training on the pituitary glucocorticoid sensitivity determined by very low dose intravenous dexamethasone suppression test. *Hormone Metabolism Research, 40*, 718-721.

Simpson, M.E., Serdula, M., Galuska, D.A., Gillespie, C., Donehoo, R., Macera, C., *et al.* (2003). Walking trends among U.S. adults: The Behavioral Risk Factor Surveillance System, 1987-2000. *American Journal of Preventive Medicine, 25*, 95-100.

Sothmann, M.S., Buckworth, J., Claytor, R.P., Cox, R.H., White-Welkley, J.E., & Dishman, R.K. (1996). Exercise training and the cross-stressor adaptation hypothesis. *Exercise Sport Science Reviews, 24*, 267-287.

Stamatakis, E., Hillsdon, M., Mishra, G., Hamer, M., & Marmot, M. (2009). Television viewing and other screen-based entertainment in relation to multiple socioeconomic status indicators and area deprivation: The Scottish Health Survey 2003. *Journal of Epidemiology and Community Health, 63*, 734-740.

Stansfeld, S.A., Head, J., Fuhrer, R., Wardle, J., & Cattell, V. (2003). Social inequalities in depressive symptoms and physical functioning in the Whitehall II study: Exploring a common cause explanation. *Journal of Epidemiology and Community Health, 57*, 361-367.

Steptoe, A., Feldman, P.M., Kunz, S., Owen, N., Willemsen, G., & Marmot, M. (2002). Stress responsivity and socioeconomic status: A mechanism for increased cardiovascular disease risk? *European Heart Journal, 23*, 1757-1763.

Steptoe, A., Hamer, M., Butcher, L., Lin, J., Brydon, L., Kivimäki, M., et al. (2011). Educational attainment but not measures of current socioeconomic circumstances are associated with leukocyte telomere length in healthy older men and women. *Brain, Behavior, and Immunity, 25*, 1292-1298.

Steptoe, A., & Marmot, M. (2002). The role of psychobiological pathways in socio-economic inequalities in cardiovascular disease risk. *European Heart Journal, 23*, 13-25.

Stringhini, S., Sabia, S., Shipley, M., Brunner, E., Nabi, H., Kivimaki, M., et al. (2010). Association of socioeconomic position with health behaviors and mortality. *Journal of the American Medical Association, 303*, 1159-1166.

Stubbe, J.H., Boomsma, D.I., Vink, J.M., Cornes, B.K., Martin, N.G., Skytthe, A., et al. (2006). Genetic influences on exercise participation in 37,051 twin pairs from seven countries. *PLoS One, 1*, e22.

Traustadóttir, T., Bosch, P.R., Cantu, T., & Matt, K.S. (2004). Hypothalamic-pituitary-adrenal axis response and recovery from high-intensity exercise in women: Effects of aging and fitness. *Journal of Clinical Endocrinology Metabolism, 89*, 3248-3254.

Tsutsumi, A., Kayaba, K., & Ishikawa, S. (2011). Impact of occupational stress on stroke across occupational classes and genders. *Social Science Medicine, 72*, 1652-1658.

U.S. Centers for Disease Control and Prevention. (1999). Neighborhood safety and the prevalence of physical inactivity—Selected states, 1996. *Journal of the American Medical Association, 281*, 1373.

van Loon, A.J., Tijhuis, M., & Surtees, P.G. (2000). Lifestyle risk factors for cancer: The relationship with psychosocial work environment. *International Journal of Epidemiology, 29*, 785-792.

van Sluijs, E.M., McMinn, A.M., & Griffin, S.J. (2007). Effectiveness of interventions to promote physical activity in children and adolescents: Systematic review of controlled trials. *British Medical Journal*, 335, 703.

Vaz de Almeida, M.D., Graca, P., Afonso, C., D'Amicis, A., Lappalainen, R., & Damkjaer, S. (1999). Physical activity levels and body weight in a nationally representative sample in the European Union. *Public Health Nutrition,* 2(1A), 105-113.

Wardle, J., & Steptoe, A. *(2003).* Socioeconomic differences in attitudes and beliefs about healthy lifestyles. *Journal of Epidemiology and Community Health*, 57, 440-443.

Williams, E.D., Stamatakis, E., Chandola, T., & Hamer, M. (2011a). Physical activity behaviour and coronary heart disease mortality among South Asian people in the UK: An observational longitudinal study. *Heart*, 97, 655-659.

Williams, E.D., Stamatakis, E., Chandola, T., & Hamer, M. (2011b). Assessment of physical activity levels in South Asians in the UK: Findings from the Health Survey for England. *Journal of Epidemiology and Community Health*, 65, 517-521.

Physical Activity and Self-Esteem

Magnus Lindwall, PhD
University of Gothenburg, Gothenburg, Sweden

F. Hülya Aşçı, PhD
Başkent University, Ankara, Turkey

Chapter Outline

Editors' Introduction

Self-esteem, a multidimensional and hierarchical construct that is important for well-being and mental health, is strongly influenced by one's physical self-perception. The relationship between self-esteem and physical activity is bidirectional: Participation in physical activity increases self-esteem, and greater self-esteem is associated with increased physical activity. This chapter examines mechanisms underlying these relationships and proposes a biopsychosocial model that includes a role for biological and psychological factors. This chapter is of interest to researchers and students who are interested in mental health theory as well as practitioners who wish to use physical activity to enhance clients' self-esteem as a route to better well-being and mental health.

Few psychological constructs have received as much research attention as self-esteem. High self-esteem has been associated with emotional stability and adjustment to life demands; subjective well-being, happiness, life satisfaction and resilience to stress; and healthy behaviours. Low self-esteem, on the other hand, has been closely related to mental illness and psychopathology such as depression, anxiety and eating disorders. Self-esteem is a critical component of human functioning and performance and is highly relevant to well-being and mental health.

The terminology used in the academic literature to describe the self and self-esteem can be confusing. A number of disciplines have influenced the theoretical understanding of the self over time. As a result, a variety of terms tend to be used interchangeably to refer to the same or conceptually overlapping constructs (e.g., *self-esteem*, *self-worth*, *self-concept*, *self-perception*). This remains the case despite the efforts of several authors to provide clarification and define each term uniquely.

Early researchers used the term *self-concept* and defined it as "the individual as known by the individual" (Murphy, 1947, p. 996). The self-concept was considered to be a broad construct that included cognitive, affective and behavioural aspects. It is still often used as an umbrella term that includes more specific concepts such as *self-esteem* and *self-efficacy*.

More recently, researchers have made a distinction between a descriptive or cognitive component of self (i.e., answering the question "Who am I?") and an evaluative or affective component (i.e., answering the question "How do I feel about who I am?"). The descriptive or cognitive component is referred to as *self-description*, and the evaluative or affective component is referred to as *self-esteem*. Self-esteem is viewed as an evaluative component of the self (see Byrne, 1996) and as more specific than self-concept. A related definition of self-esteem is "the awareness of good possessed by self" (Campbell, 1984, p. 9). However, in practice the self-description and self-esteem components

of the self are inexorably intertwined, and the terms are often used interchangeably in research because it is difficult to describe the self without linking it to affect and evaluation.

1 Multidimensional Hierarchical Model of Self-Concept

Although several multidimensional models of self-concept have been proposed over the past 20 yr (see Marsh & Hattie, 1996), the model that has gained the greatest amount of empirical support is the multidimensional model of Shavelson, Hubner and Stanton (1976). It proposed a global or overarching conception of self-concept that comprises evaluations made by individuals in a number of areas of life (i.e., academic, social, emotional and physical). Individuals may evaluate themselves highly in some areas of life and low in others; global self-concept draws on experiences and evaluations across all these areas.

Shavelson, Hubner and Stanton (1976) also proposed that self-concept has a hierarchical structure and used the analogy of the root system of a tree to explain this structure in more detail. In this analogy, global self-concept is the relatively stable trunk at the top (or apex) of the root system, which divides into academic, social, emotional and physical self-concepts (see figure 5.1). These subdomains may be further divided into more specific self-concepts situated at a lower hierarchical level in the model. For example, the academic self-concept consists of self-concept for subjects such as English, mathematics and science. According to the model, global self-concept at the top level should be more stable over time compared with the more situation-specific self-concepts at the lower levels. This multidimensional, hierarchical model of the self has received wide support in the research literature (Marsh & Craven, 2006).

2 Physical Self

One domain of the multidimensional model of self-concept that is very relevant to physical

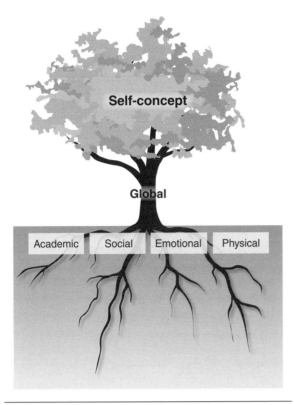

Figure 5.1 Multidimensional, hierarchical model of the self.

activity is the *physical self*. The physical self has been defined as an individual's perceptions of him, or herself in the physical domain. Based on the hierarchical structure of self-concept, the physical self may be further divided into several subdomains of physical competence and appearance, such as perceptions of strength, endurance, sport ability and body attractiveness (Fox & Corbin, 1989). Perceived competence in each subdomain can be further broken down into competence in a number of facets, subfacets and specific situations. For example, perceived sport ability (subdomain) includes perceived soccer competence, which includes perceived shooting ability, which includes scoring efficacy in a specific match (see figure 5.2). The relationship between global self-esteem and these levels of the physical self depends on where they are situated in the root-like hierarchy of the model. For example, physical self-worth at the domain level should be more closely related to global self-esteem than should scoring efficacy, which is lower down at the situation-specific level.

Physical self-worth is considered to be an important psychological outcome, correlate and antecedent of physical activity behaviour and is viewed as an important contributor to global perceptions of self-esteem (Marsh & Sonstroem, 1995). According to Fox (2000a, p. 230), "the physical self has occupied a unique position in the self-esteem system because the body, through its appearance, attributes and abilities, provides the substantive interface between individuals and the world." Sonstroem and Potts (1996)

KEY CONCEPTS

- Self-esteem is a multidimensional and hierarchical construct.
- Overall self-esteem, also known as global self-esteem, is strongly influenced by physical self-worth, and physical self-worth is strongly influenced by perceived body attractiveness.
- The importance of the body is reinforced by cultural pressures to be thin and have an athletic physique.
- General self-esteem increases from mid-adolescence, peaks around 50 to 60 yr of age, and declines during old age.

- A bidirectional relationship exists between physical activity and self-esteem; this relationship is described by two hypotheses. The skill-development hypothesis posits that participation in physical activity enhances self-esteem through increased competence in specific domains. The self-enhancement hypothesis posits that greater perceived competence for physical activity leads to greater participation in that behaviour.

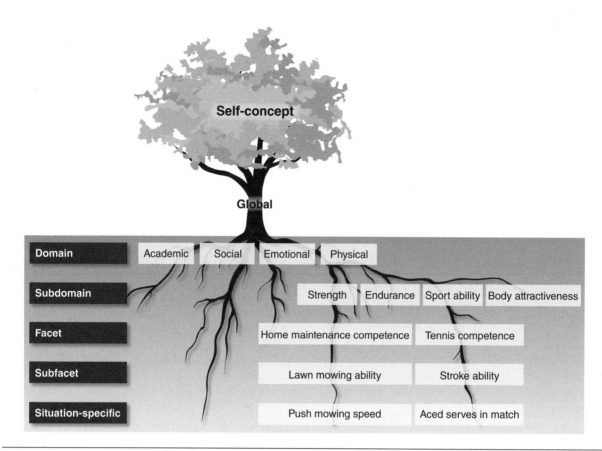

Figure 5.2   The link between self-esteem and physical self-perceptions.

note that the physical self affects social communication and interaction and is associated with aspects of life adjustment such as depression, mood and reported physical and psychological health.

2.1 Physical Self-Perception Profile

Fox and Corbin (1989) developed a multidimensional, hierarchical model of physical self-perception and used this model as the basis for the Physical Self-Perception Profile, a multidimensional instrument that measures perceptions of the physical self. In this model, global self-esteem is a superordinate domain above the more specific but global domain of physical self-worth, which, in turn, is hierarchically above the more differentiated subdomains of sport competence, body attractiveness, physical strength and physical conditioning (figure 5.2). Physical self-worth is proposed to mediate the relation-

ship between these specific (subdomain) physical self-perceptions and general (global) feelings of self-esteem (Fox, 1990). The subdomains are viewed as specific and changeable aspects of the self, and perceptions become more general and enduring at each higher level of the hierarchy. Furthermore, according to the model, these four subdomains account for the process, product and confidence aspects of an individual's physical self-concept. Studies have provided strong evidence that supports the validity and reliability of this model and the hierarchical nature of its underlying constructs in adults (Fox, 1990; Sonstroem, Speliotis & Fava, 1992) and children (Eklund, Whitehead & Welk, 1997; Welk, Corbin & Lewis, 1995; Whitehead, 1995).

2.2 Physical Self and Global Self-Esteem

As explained previously, multiple areas or domains of life influence global self-esteem.

Research has demonstrated that the physical self has the greatest influence on global self-esteem (e.g., Harter, 1993, 1999) and is thereby the component that is most predictive of global self-esteem.

As a multidimensional construct, physical self-worth can be differentiated into the subdomains of sport competence, body attractiveness, physical strength and physical conditioning. Of these four subdomains, bodily attractiveness is reported to be the most strongly related to physical self-worth; correlations in most studies are typically around $r = .7$ (see Fox, 1997). On the other hand, relationships between global self-esteem and the other three domains of physical self-worth have generally been found to be low to moderate in strength ($r = .15 - .40$). Results from a recent cross-national study that included more than 1,800 university students from England, Sweden, Turkey and Portugal showed that body attractiveness was the physical self-perception domain most strongly related to global self-esteem (Lindwall et al., 2011). This is consistent with the findings that average correlations between appearance and global self-esteem have typically been as high as $r = 0.8$ (Harter, 1993). The relationship between physical appearance and global self-esteem seems to be particularly strong in children, adolescents and young adults.

According to Sonstroem (1997), these strong relationships between global self-esteem, physical self-worth and body attractiveness, can be interpreted from at least three viewpoints: An attractive body is, in the eyes of many people, synonymous with physical self-worth and self-esteem; an attractive body is perceived as being synonymous with health, and health is perceived as closely related to self-esteem and self-worth; and the instruments used to measure global self-esteem, physical self-worth and body attractiveness overlap due to the use of similar phrases in the individual questions on each of these scales.

Many people view being physically fit and having an attractive body as important. As long ago as 1890, William James proposed that self-esteem is affected by perceptions of competence in domains the individual deems highly important, whereas perceived competence in domains interpreted as unimportant will have little impact on global self-esteem. Although debated, this idea has received support in modern research (e.g., Lindwall et al., 2011). It suggests that the perceptions an individual holds of his or her competence linked to the physical self will be most strongly related to global self-esteem if he or she also feels that the physical self is important. For example, if having well-developed muscles or a toned or slim body is important to a person, as it often is to young adults in the commercialised Western world, the perceptions of failure to achieve this will most likely have a negative effect on global self-esteem (for a review on the muscular ideal, see Cafri et al., 2005). However, if the person does not feel that body appearance or fitness is important, negative perceptions of one's competence linked to the body will probably have negligible effect on self-esteem.

2.3 Sociocultural Perspectives on the Body and Self-Esteem

Social and cultural ideals are adopted and integrated into the self-system through early socialisation and hence influence its function. Individuals' physical self-perceptions and global self-esteem are closely linked to these ideals. It has been suggested that the focus on exercise and body maintenance, at least from an individualistic perspective, reflects the development of modern society, culture and, more specifically, the central values and attitudes of present-day Western lifestyles (e.g., Featherstone, 1991; Turner, 1992). Diet and nutrition, exercise and plastic surgery are the most commonly used tools in the pursuit of the highly valued fit and attractive body (i.e., the athletic ideal) (Brownell, 1991a).

Two assumptions are made in the search for the better body: that the body is malleable (i.e., with the right training or programme everybody can succeed) and that the effort will be worthwhile in the end (i.e., substantial rewards await). The latter notion is empirically supported by the fact that physical attractiveness and outer appearance are, in the eyes of many people, naturally associated with highly prized personality traits and characteristics such as social competence, potency and adjustment (Eagly et al., 1991; Feingold, 1992; Langlois et al., 2000). The perfect, or fit, body stands as a symbol of control and discipline, which are two highly esteemed virtues in modern society (Brownell, 1991a,b). Through incorporating these ancient virtues into the lifestyle, the individual may control, discipline and sculpt the body to conform to the overarching body ideals of the modern era (i.e., slender, slim, muscular and fit), thus ensuring substantial internal and external rewards (see Leary, 1992; Martin Ginis et al., 2007). Moreover, research has shown that information regarding people's exercise habits affects the impressions that others form of them (Hodgins, 1992). More specifically, targets described as fit and regular exercisers were rated more favourably on a variety of personality variables than were people described as not regular exercisers and not fit, resulting in a form of positive exercise stereotype (Lindwall & Martin Ginis, 2006, 2008; Martin Ginis et al., 2007).

3 Global Self-Esteem and Physical Self-Esteem Across the Life Span

A number of studies have investigated differences in global self-esteem across various ages and how self-esteem changes across the life span. In terms of age differences, a large meta-analytic review (Twenge & Campbell, 2001) based on data from 355 samples found that self-esteem decreases slightly during early adolescence but generally increases after this age. The results also suggest that the decrease during adolescence may be linked to important transitions (in this case to junior high school). Similarly, a longitudinal study (Erol & Orth, 2011) that followed a sample of 7,100 individuals aged 14 to 30 yr over a 14 yr period found that self-esteem increased during adolescence and continued to increase,

although more slowly, in young adulthood. Therefore, the development of self-esteem displayed a curvilinear trend from midadolescence to early adulthood. Fewer longitudinal studies have examined change in self-esteem across the adult life span. However, those that have generally show a consistent pattern (e.g., Orth, Robins & Widaman, 2012; Orth, Trzesniewski & Robins, 2010). Self-esteem increases from about age 25 yr and reaches a peak around 50 or 60 yr (Orth et al., 2010; Orth et al., 2012). Thus, global self-esteem can be described as following a quadratic trajectory across the adult life span.

A further meta-analysis (Trzesniewski, Donnellan & Robins, 2003) examined the stability of global self-esteem in individuals aged 6 to 83 yr. Self-esteem showed a substantial degree of stability over time, but a robust developmental trend could be identified: the stability of self-esteem was lowest during childhood (ages 6-11 yr), increased during adolescence (12-17 yr) and young adulthood (18-29 yr) and declined in midlife (30-39 yr) and old age (60-82 yr). In other words, global self-esteem appears to be most susceptible to change during childhood, early adolescence and old age.

Looking more specifically at the physical self and physical self-perceptions, most published studies have demonstrated that physical self-esteem remains fairly stable across adolescence (Crocker et al., 2006; Kowalski et al., 2003; Morgan, Graser & Pangrazi, 2008; Raudsepp, Kais & Hannus, 2004; (Raustorp, Mattsson, Svensson & Ståhle, 2006; Raustorp, Archer, Svensson, Perlinger, & Alricsson, 2009). However, there are exceptions. For example, Lintunen (1995) examined the change of physical self-perceptions in adolescent boys and girls over 4 yr and found that the stability and change of self-perceptions varied considerably depending on the specific domain and sex. Perceptions of fitness for both boys and girls were very stable, whereas perceptions of appearance decreased for girls but increased for boys over the follow-up period. Unfortunately, no study to date has examined whether physical self-esteem remains stable during adulthood and into old age.

4 Causality of the Relationship Between Physical Activity and Self-Esteem

Controversy exists among researchers about the causality of the relationship between self-esteem and physical activity. More specifically, researchers are interested in whether achievement in sport and physical activity leads to enhanced self-esteem or whether self-esteem influences achievement in sport and physical activity. This issue is described in two major hypotheses (figure 5.3): the self-enhancement hypothesis and the skill-development hypothesis (Sonstroem, 1998). This debate about causality can be informed with reference to two other models that aim to explain the relationship between physical activity and self-esteem: the psychological model for physical activity and the exercise and self-esteem model.

4.1 Self-Enhancement Hypothesis

The self-enhancement hypothesis focuses on the influence of self-esteem on the environment. According to the self-enhancement hypothesis, individuals tend to act as they perceive themselves to be. Because society rewards achievement, individuals engage in activities that they believe will lead to success, thus enhancing self-esteem. This view suggests that people tend to behave and interpret their experiences in ways that preserve or confirm self-judgements and expectations. For example, people with positive perceived athletic competence will be more likely than those with negative perceived athletic competence to participate in endurance training.

The majority of cross-sectional and correlational studies on physical activity and self-esteem have supported the positive association between physical activity, sport and self-esteem. For example, studies have shown that individuals who participate in sport or who are physically active have higher self-esteem than those who do not participate or who are physically inactive (Aşçı, Koşar & İşler, 2001; Bowker, 2006). A positive link between physical self-perceptions and physical activity level has been demonstrated in children (e.g., Crocker, Eklund & Kowalski, 2000; Raudsepp, Liblik & Hannus, 2002), adolescents and university students (e.g., Aşçı, 2004; Lindwall & Hassmen, 2004) and adults (e.g., Sonstroem, Speliotis & Fava, 1992). Guyot, Fairchild and Hill (1981) and Harter (1982) concluded that participation in organised sport and physical activity increases feelings of confidence and adequacy in athletic endeavours, which in turn increase the desire to participate. Further studies have compared the physical self-perceptions of high-level athletes with those of their nonathlete counterparts, and all reported that elite and high-level athletes scored significantly higher on a number of the physical-self subdomains (Aşçı, 2004; Marsh, 1998; Marsh et al., 1997). This specific subpopulation, whose pursuit of achievement in sport is particularly high, has significantly

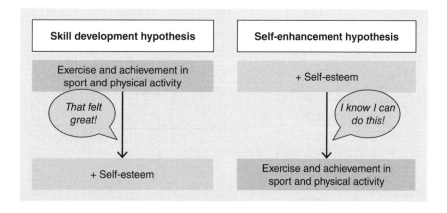

Figure 5.3 The relationship between exercise and self-perception from two perspectives.

higher perceptions of physical ability or sport competence than do normal populations.

Lindwall and Hassmen (2004) examined the relationship between frequency and duration of exercise participation and physical self-perception. They reported that exercising more frequently and for a longer duration on each occasion was related to higher physical self-perception. Fox and Corbin (1989) showed a relationship between physical activity type preferences and physical self-perception. For example, sport-competence perceptions were linked with participation in ball sports in both females and males; participation in endurance activities and calisthenics was positively associated with perceived condition competence and body attractiveness in females; and weight training was tied closely to perceived strength, condition competence and body attractiveness in males. These results predict that perceptions of high level of competence or adequacy in a domain lead to involvement in behaviours in which those abilities can be demonstrated. In other words, the results significantly support the self-enhancement hypothesis.

A few longitudinal studies have also examined the relationship between physical activity and the physical self, thus filling a gap in understanding the nature of the relationship between the physical self and physical activity over time. The study, which followed Canadian adolescent females aged 14 to 17 yr over a 3 yr period, identified that 12.9% of the decrease in physical activity during that time was attributable to change in physical self-perception. More specifically, perception of sport competence and physical condition were longitudinal predictors of physical activity (Crocker et al., 2006). This result indicated that perception of conditioning and sport competence play a role in the adoption or maintenance of future physical activity behaviour.

Two recent studies have further examined changes in physical activity and physical self-perception of adolescents over time. Knowles and colleagues (2009) examined adolescent girls over 12 mo and reported a significant correla-tion between changes in physical activity and changes in physical self-perception. A subscale of physical self-perception, perceived physical conditioning, was the only significant individual predictor of physical activity. On the other hand, Raustorp and colleagues (2009) reported weak relationships between subdomains of physical self-perception and physical activity at three time points over a 5 yr follow-up study of adolescent boys and girls.

McAuley and colleagues (2005) investigated the relationship between physical self-esteem and physical activity in older adults over a 4 yr period. They reported significant associations between physical activity and perceived physical condition, body attractiveness and strength. Over time, older adults who reported greater reductions in self-esteem and physical activity also reported greater reduction in subdomains of physical self-esteem.

In summary, the cross-sectional studies reviewed here clearly indicate that regularly taking part in sport, physical activity or exercise is moderately associated with more positive physical self-perceptions. Furthermore, exercise frequency, preference and mode and level of physical activity influence how individuals perceive themselves in the psychomotor domain. Most cross-sectional evidence supports the prominent role of perceived sport competence and conditioning in predicting physical activity behaviours. Longitudinal studies on adolescents indicate that developing high perceived physical condition and high perceived sport competence is important for initiating and maintaining participation in level of participation in physical activity. The positive perception of sport abilities and physical condition is an important determinant of physical activity behaviour during the transition from childhood to adolescence.

4.2 Skill-Development Hypothesis

The skill-development hypothesis focuses on the influence of environmental activities and forces on self-esteem. The skill-development hypothesis suggests that experiencing success and receiving rewards makes people feel better about themselves and strengthens their perceived competence. In relation to physical activity and exercise, the skill-development hypothesis holds that improvements in physical fitness or skills that result from participating in an exercise programme lead to enhanced self-esteem. Self-esteem is seen as an inherent consequence of successfully mastering motor skills (Sonstroem, 1998).

Several researchers (Fox, 2000a,b; Leith, 1994; Sonstroem, 1984; Sonstroem & Morgan, 1989) have identified self-esteem as the psychological variable with the most potential to reflect psychological benefits as a result of regular participation in physical activity. Upon the recognition of the multidimensionality of the self and the development of new instruments for measuring the unique and specific aspects of self-esteem, researchers began to examine the role of exercise interventions on specific aspects of self-esteem such as the physical self. Fox (2000a), who emphasised the mental health properties of the physical self, indicated that the physical self may be a legitimate and practically important outcome variable in exercise interventions as far as mental well-being is considered and that it should be a key target of exercise programmes. From this perspective, many researchers have used instruments developed specifically to assess the physical self to examine this construct as an outcome variable in exercise interventions.

4.2.1 Individual Intervention Studies

Different types of exercise and physical activity programmes have been used in determining the effect of physical activity on self-esteem. For example, the effect of participation in aerobic dance on the self-esteem of females has been widely investigated (Jasnoski et al., 1981; McInman & Berger, 1993; Plummer & Koh, 1987). The findings of these studies clearly indicate that self-esteem significantly improves after different lengths of participation in aerobic dance. Marsh, Richards and Barnes (1986a,b) found that participation in an Outward Bound programme

produced increases in multiple dimensions of self-concept over a 26-day interval; this increase was maintained 18 mo after the completion of the programme (Marsh, Richards & Barnes, 1986a).

Studies have also investigated the effect of other types of exercise on self-esteem, including skipping (Hatfield, Vaccara & Benedict, 1985), swimming (Miller, 1989), baseball (Hawkins & Gruber, 1982), creative-dance movement activities (Blackman et al., 1988), competitive and cooperative physical fitness programmes (Marsh & Peart, 1988), basketball, field hockey (Olu, 1990) and strength training (Tucker, 1983, 1987). These studies generally indicate that exercise is an effective intervention for improving self-esteem. Most of the studies revealed significant improvement in the sport-specific aspect of the self that was assessed (e.g., physical self, sport ability or physical appearance). However, results for general self-concept were inconsistent. Some of the studies reported significant improvement, whereas others reported no change.

The majority of intervention studies that have investigated the link between physical activity and physical self-concept have been conducted on adolescent females because they are at high risk for participating in low levels of physical activity, thus leading to an elevated risk of chronic disease, and because self-appraisal and physical appearance play a central role in adolescents' self-esteem. Lindwall and Lindgren (2005) examined the effects of a 6 mo exercise-intervention programme on physical self-perceptions of 110 adolescent Swedish girls who were previously physically inactive. They found a positive effect of exercise: The intervention group showed a more positive change in physical self-perception compared with the control group. Burgess, Grogan and Burwitz (2006) examined the impact of 6 wk of aerobic dance activity on physical self-perceptions of 50 British girls aged 13 to 14 yr. The results indicated a change in perceived body attractiveness and physical self-worth, although these improvements were not sustained. In contrast, a recent study found that a 9 mo school-based physical activity intervention among sedentary adolescent females was not effective for enhancing overall physical self-concept despite an increase in self-reported vigorous physical activity and significant improvement in cardiovascular fitness in the intervention group (Schneider, Dunton & Cooper, 2008).

Some intervention studies have examined the relationship between physical activity and physical self-concept in adult females and older adults. For example, Anderson and colleagues (2006) compared the effects of an 8 wk programme of regular brisk walking with the effects of abdominal electrical stimulation and no exercise in 37 sedentary adult females. They found significantly greater changes in the perceived physical condition of the walking group compared with the group that received abdominal electrical stimulation. No changes at higher subdomain levels of physical self-worth or body attractiveness occurred after 8 wk, and changes in physical strength and sport competence were minimal (Anderson et al., 2006). In adults aged 50 yr and older, participation in a 14 wk moderate-intensity physical activity programme resulted in significant and positive changes in perceived physical fitness (Stoll & Alfermann, 2002). Similarly, in a controlled 10 wk primary care exercise-referral intervention for adults aged 40 to 70 yr, the exercise group became more positive about their physical self-worth, physical condition and physical health compared with a control group (Taylor & Fox, 2005).

In one of the first studies that investigated the effects of exercise on the physical self-perception of males, Özdemir, Çelik and Aşçı (2010) examined the effects of a 12 wk exercise intervention (swimming, running and cycling) on physical self-perceptions of male university students. The study reported improvement in the mean scores of the exercise-intervention group compared with the control group for perceived sport competence, strength, body attractiveness and conditioning and improvement in the physical self-worth scales from before measurement to after measurement, but these increments did not reach statistical significance.

Aşçı (2002) examined the effect of sex on the relationship between participation in step dance and physical self-perception. In this study, 73 female and 65 male university students aged 18 to 27 yr were randomly assigned to step dance and control groups; a balance of sexes was maintained in each group. The experimental group attended 50 min sessions of step dance 3 days/wk for 10 wk, whereas subjects in the control group did not participate in any regular physical activity. Participants in the experimental group improved more on all subdomains of the physical self-perception profile than did participants in the control group. However, change in physical self-perception over the 10 wk did not differ by sex.

4.2.2 Reviews and Meta-Analyses

In addition to the experimental studies described previously, reviews by Sonstroem (1984) and Leith (1994) clearly indicate that participation in exercise programmes is linked to increased self-esteem scores. Furthermore, Fox (2000a) conducted a comprehensive review of exercise-intervention studies published since 1971 that had measured self-perception and self-esteem outcomes. The review identified 37 randomised controlled studies, including 9 unpublished theses and dissertations, and considered 42 nonrandomised controlled studies. The major conclusions drawn from this review include the following:

- Exercise can be used to promote physical self-worth and other important physical self-perceptions, such as body image.
- 78% of studies indicated positive changes in self-esteem, especially in the physical self.
- One half of the studies showed no changes in global self-esteem, although improvements did occur.
- All age groups can experience positive effects.
- Both males and females can experience positive effects.
- Effects are greater for those with low self-esteem.

- Several types of exercise are effective in changing self-perceptions, although most evidence exists for aerobic exercise and weight training.

Ekeland, Heian and Hagen (2005) reviewed 23 randomised controlled trials conducted with children and young people between the ages of 3 and 20. The review indicated that exercise has positive short-term effects on self-esteem.

Several meta-analyses of the effects of exercise on self-esteem have also been conducted. In a meta-analysis of play and physical education programmes for children, Gruber (1986) calculated the effect sizes of 27 controlled experimental studies and reported positive effects of .41. His paper provided strong empirical evidence that structured play or physical education (or both) caused an increase in children's self-esteem. Gruber (1986) reported that the effects of physical activity on self-esteem were stronger for children with physical and mental disabilities and for participants involved in fitness-oriented programmes. A further meta-analysis of 37 studies that explored aerobic fitness training and its effect on self-concept in adults found that exercise leads to a significant and positive increase in self-concept (McDonald & Hodgdon, 1991). The magnitude of the effect for self-concept [effect size (ES) = 0.56] was significantly larger than that found in the same meta-analysis for changes in state anxiety due to exercise (ES = −0.28).

A more recent meta-analysis by Spence, McGannon and Poon (2005) further examined the effect of exercise on self-esteem and included 113 studies. Based on the assumptions of the exercise and self-esteem model (see section 4.4), Spence, McGannon and Poon hypothesised that exercise participants who experience changes in physical fitness should also experience larger changes in self-esteem, that individuals who are less physically fit should experience larger changes in self-esteem compared with those who are more fit, that individuals with lower initial self-esteem should experience the most change due to exercise and that larger doses of exercise (i.e., exercise of higher frequency,

intensity and duration) should be related to larger changes in self-esteem. Overall they found that participation in exercise led to a small but significant improvement in self-esteem. Significant changes in physical fitness were related to greater changes in self-esteem, supporting their first hypothesis. Moreover, although the finding was not statistically significant, individuals with lower initial self-esteem and physical fitness demonstrated larger changes in self-esteem compared with individuals starting with higher levels of self-esteem and physical fitness. Similarly, a nonsignificant trend was found whereby exercising more frequently resulted in larger gains in self-esteem compared with exercising less frequently.

In summary, the research has demonstrated that a range of exercise modes have a positive effect on the physical self. In general, exercise-intervention studies report significant changes in almost all subdomains of the physical self, although the subdomains most strongly affected are perceived strength, physical condition, endurance and sport competence. By contrast, studies show that the subdomain body attractiveness has the weakest link to exercise and has consequently been targeted as the subdomain that is least susceptible to change as a function of exercise interventions (see Fox, 1997). Males and females experience similar gains in physical self-perception from participating in exercise interventions, although this finding should be interpreted carefully due to the limited number of studies in this area, small sample sizes and a reliance on university sample groups. Nevertheless, the evidence clearly shows that exercise helps people feel better about their physical abilities and personal characteristics. As a consequence, physical self constructs, which are important aspects of global self-esteem and mental well-being, should be considered target outcomes of interventions based on physical activity and exercise programmes.

4.3 Psychological Model for Physical Activity

The psychological model for physical activity (figure 5.4) was one of the first models to link

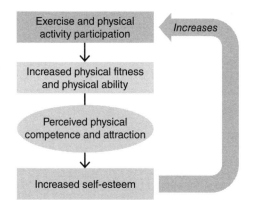

Figure 5.4 Psychological model for physical activity participation.

physical self-perception and self-esteem to physical activity (Sonstroem, 1978). It claims that participation in physical activity increases physical ability and fitness, which in turn brings about psychological benefits as reflected in positive changes in self-esteem. This change in self-esteem is mediated by perceived physical competence and body attractiveness.

Consequently, increased fitness and physical activity result in the enhancement of self-esteem in conjunction with increased perceived physical competence and attraction, which leads to increased physical activity. Moreover, the model holds that people tend to engage in modes of behaviour that will maintain their positive self-esteem and that the drive for self-enhancement

and self-development is a powerful, motivational human force that constantly affects people's lives. Hence, the model may be viewed as being based on both the skill-development and self-enhancement hypotheses (Sonstroem, 1997).

4.4 Exercise and Self-Esteem Model

The exercise and self-esteem model (EXSEM; Sonstroem & Morgan, 1989; see figure 5.5), a later model that examines the mechanisms of self-esteem change through exercise, explains how the effects of specific sessions of sport and exercise generalise to global self-esteem. It is based on the hierarchical and multidimensional model of Shavelson, Hubner and Stanton (1976) and focuses on the effects of situational experiences of competence in sport and physical activity on global self-esteem in a bottom-up fashion. The EXSEM can be seen as adopting the skill-development hypothesis.

The EXSEM consists of four key constructs: physical self-efficacy, physical competence, physical acceptance and self-esteem. Physical self-efficacy is viewed as the first cognitive link between actual behaviour and the higher-order psychological self-constructs. Physical competence refers to the broader perceptions and evaluations of one's body and its capacity for

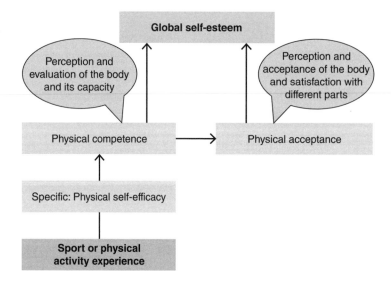

Figure 5.5 The exercise and self-esteem model.

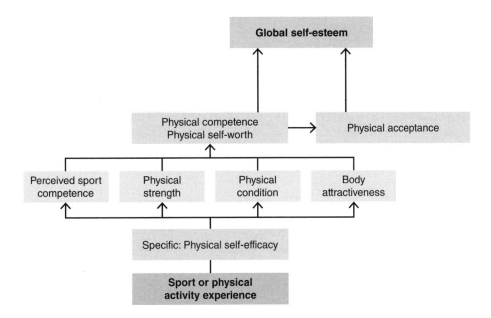

Figure 5.6   The expanded exercise and self-esteem model.

functioning and performing. Physical acceptance refers to the perceived satisfaction the individual feels about different parts of his or her body. The EXSEM is a competency-based model in which changes in physical fitness are proposed to directly lead to enhanced physical self-efficacy and indirectly affect changes in global self-esteem. Changes in physical self-efficacy influence the closely related physical competence and physical acceptance, which are also believed to affect global self-esteem (Sonstroem & Morgan, 1989).

After the development of the Physical Self-Perception Profile, the unidimensional concept of physical competence in the original EXSEM model was replaced with a multidimensional concept of physical competence (Sonstroem, Harlow & Josephs, 1994). In other words, the EXSEM was expanded to include four subdomain variables from the Physical Self-Perception Profile—perceived sport competence, physical condition, physical strength and body attractiveness—plus the general domain of physical self-worth (see figure 5.6).

Like the Psychological Model for Physical Activity, the central elements of the EXSEM have been supported. Research has confirmed the structural relationships of the EXSEM and

has validated use of the model in examining the manner in which exercise experiences influence levels of self-perception (Sonstroem et al., 1991). The EXSEM has provided researchers with a guide for examining the processes and pathways by which changes in exercise may relate to changes in self-esteem (Spence, McGannon & Poon, 2005).

4.5   Relationship Between Physical Fitness and Self-Esteem

Although sound evidence shows that exercise can produce positive self-esteem and physical self-perception, the main mechanism underpinning such changes is still not fully understood. The relationship between changes in physiological measures of physical fitness and psychological changes in self-esteem has been studied as a possible way to make this mechanism more clear.

Studies that used global measures of self-esteem report significant associations between changes in physical fitness parameters and self-esteem (Spence, McGannon & Poon, 2005). In their most recent review, Spence, McGannon and Poon (2005) analysed 113 studies. The results mainly implied that larger effect sizes were observed for those who experienced significant changes in actual physical fitness and those who participated in exercise or lifestyle programmes rather than skill training.

On the other hand, studies that measured multiple aspects of the physical self with more detailed questionnaires, such as the Physical Self-Perception Profile and the Physical Self-Description Questionnaire, indicated that underlying mechanisms were psychosocial rather than psychophysiological in nature and revealed mixed results. For example, Taylor and Fox (2005) investigated the effectiveness of a 10 wk primary care exercise-referral intervention on the physical self-perceptions of adults aged 40 to 70 yr. They reported that improvements in physiological fitness parameters, such as cardiovascular fitness and strength, were not linked to changes in physical self-perceptions. On the other hand, Schneider and colleagues (2008) reported that group participants who increased their fitness levels experienced enhanced global physical self-concept after exercise. Lindwall and Lindgren (2005) also reported significant correlation between changes in perceived physical condition and changes in physical fitness, body mass index and weight in adolescent females. However, Özdemir, Çelik and Aşçı (2010) did not find any correlation between changes in physical fitness and changes in physical self-perception of males, and Anderson and colleagues (2006) found no relationship between changes in anthropometric measures and changes in physical self-perceptions.

In accordance with current findings, the changing patterns of physical self-perception do not appear to be related to physiological changes. The nonsignificant and weak correlations could be explained by several other theoretical mechanisms for the role of exercise in physical self-perception, such as belongingness, group dynamics and feelings of self-control, competence and positive expectancies related to regular involvement in exercise. These factors, rather than psychophysiological changes, might be more important elements in the enhancement of physical self-perceptions (Fox, 2000a; Lindwall & Lindgren, 2005).

In summary, research has not clearly demonstrated the possible mechanisms of changes in physiological fitness parameters and their relationship with psychological changes. Most of the previous studies (Alfermann & Stoll, 2000; Aşçı, 2002; Aşçı, Kin & Koşar, 1998) merely investigated the effect of exercise on physical self-perceptions. As mentioned previously, only a few studies (Taylor & Fox, 2005) examined from both longitudinal and experimental perspectives the connections between physiological and psychological parameters as a consequence of regularly participating in physical activity. Moreover, nearly all of these studies (Taylor & Fox, 2005) used indirect measurement techniques to determine physiological improvements.

Several artificial, methodological factors linked to the research design may, at least partially, explain some of the effects of exercise on self-esteem (Morgan, 1997). Two such factors associated with the expectations of the experimenter are the Rosenthal effect and demand characteristics. The Rosenthal effect involves a self-fulfilling prophecy that tends to make participants improve with respect to the dependent variable due to expectations communicated by the experimenter, whereas demand characteristics involve the tendency for the participants to identify the purpose of the study in order to accord with it. In addition, the Hawthorne effect, which refers to the improvement in a variable caused by participants receiving special attention, and placebo effects (see Desharnais et al., 1993; Ojanen, 1994) may moderate any demonstrated effects.

5 Biopsychosocial Model of the Relationship Between Exercise and the Physical Self

In order to capture the complex and multilevel effects of exercise on the human psyche and develop a broad foundation for the understanding of the underlying mechanisms, it is important to simultaneously highlight psychophysiological, biological, psychological and sociocultural factors into an overarching framework. Such a framework emphasises the effects of exercise on the physical self from microlevel to macrolevel and acknowledges the roles of molecules as well as the roles of sociocultural norms and values. The biopsychosocial model presented here (Lindwall, 2004) should be perceived as a dynamic framework for future studies on the mechanisms of exercise on the physical self rather than as a complete unifying theory. Overall, the model (see figure 5.7) rests on the notion that various feedback systems linked to human functioning, occurring on different levels and through different channels, operate as active agents to make individuals feel better about themselves and their physiques when they exercise.

Starting with the psychophysiological and biological aspect, the three hypothesised mechanisms that seemingly have received the most empirical support, at least regarding effects on reducing anxiety and depression and elevating mood, are those relating to endorphin, serotonin and norepinephrine (Boecker et al., 2009; Chaouloff, 1997; Dishman, 1997; Hoffmann, 1997; Wipfli et al., 2011). In short, the endorphin hypothesis focuses on the activation of endogenous opioid systems by exercise, whereas the serotonin and norepinephrine hypotheses highlight the interaction between physical activity

and central serotonin and changes in noradrenergic activity after physical activity, respectively. The empirical support for these hypotheses rests on a combination of animal models and research in humans. However, support for the endorphin hypothesis in particular has been debated (e.g., Dishman & O'Connor, 2009).

Regarding psychological factors, research has suggested that several variables account for the positive effects of exercise on the self: increased perceived competence linked to the physical self and the body; enhanced self-acceptance and body satisfaction; increased sense of autonomy and control; and exercise as a more pertinent aspect of one's identity that affects the development of exercise-related schemas and subsequent information processing. In addition, exercise may serve as a vital token or proof of the healthy physical status of the individual in terms of bodily functions. That is, the cognitive and emotional interpretation and evaluation that occur after an exercise bout (that one can trust the body and that it will not fail in terms of functions) may contribute significantly to enhanced physical self-perception and subsequently to increased global self-esteem. This effect may be especially evident in individuals rehabilitating

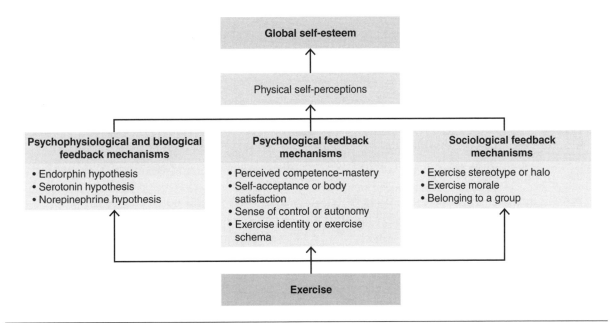

Figure 5.7 A biopsychosocial feedback model of mechanisms in the relationship between exercise and the physical self.

Reprinted from Lindwall 2004.

from various psychosomatic or stress-related health problems, in whom experiences and memories of the body losing its normal functioning may linger for a long time after the incidence and negatively affect general mental health.

Furthermore, in accordance with the work of sociologists (e.g., Featherstone, 1991; Turner, 1992), the influence of general sociocultural value systems in the modern Western world are linked to the body and its role in general health and well-being. Overall, the exercise stereotype (e.g., Hodgins, 1992 Lindwall & Martin Ginis, 2006, 2008; Martin Ginis et al., 2003) supports the notion that exercise is accompanied by other attributes that are valued highly by other people; these extend to nonphysical attributes such as self-control and being a hard worker (i.e., the halo effect; Cooper, 1981). Furthermore, given the sociocultural pressures regarding the development and maintenance of a body that is attractive, aesthetically ideal, functional, fit and, most important, healthy (e.g., Brownell, 1991a,b) and free from pandemic, modern-day, stress-related diseases, the communication to others that one subscribes to the prevalent ideals and practices regarding exercise may result in substantial positive feedback. In addition, the social support inherent in the social processes of, for example, a group exercise programme or recreational sport team provides the individual with positive feedback that reflects positively on self-evaluations. Overall, because all the factors in the model codevelop, interact and overlap and are more relevant in some situations and groups than in others, a highly relevant challenge for future researchers is to outline when, under what circumstances and for whom the various factors are most active. Another relevant task for the future is to separate the effects of the mechanisms in the model from confounding factors such as various expectancy effects.

6 Implications for Practitioners and Researchers

Positive self-esteem is widely recognised as both an important outcome in its own right and a way to facilitate other desirable outcomes in many life settings such as education, sport or exercise, health and business. Negative self-perception and low self-esteem are widely established markers of negative health and health-damaging behaviour, whereas positive self-perceptions and high self-esteem seem to accompany a wide array of positive factors linked to health, achievement and behaviour. Especially in exercise and sport settings, high self-esteem is associated with high engagement and motivation to participate in physical activity.

When translating the results of the research reviewed in this chapter to an applied setting, the main message is that exercise leads to more positive evaluations and perceptions of the physical self, especially for groups previously low in self-regard and self-esteem (e.g., those of low socioeconomic status; see chapter 4). Moreover, it seems that the frequency of the activity, rather than the duration and intensity, is the most important factor in achieving positive effects on the physical self. Although precise recommendations in terms of frequency are not available, evidence indicates that exercising regularly about 2 or 3 times/wk is enough to gain beneficial effects of exercise.

From an applied perspective, it is difficult to provide specific practical guidelines for how to build global and physical self-esteem. Coaches and teachers in physical activity, exercise and sport settings should take care to create a safe environment that highlights learning, mastery of skills and comparison with one's own progress (i.e., task involvement) rather than comparison with the progress of others (i.e., ego involvement; Roberts, 1993). Moreover, by nurturing a perspective of self-views (Dweck, 2000) in which talent and competence are viewed as a result of malleable aspects and processes such as effort rather than as fixed dispositions (e.g., "I was born a talent in sport and will therefore always be good in sport") is important for professionals. Finally, creating an environment that supports competence, autonomy and relatedness (Deci & Ryan, 2000) is likely to increase the potential for developing sound self-perceptions

EVIDENCE TO PRACTICE

- Participating in physical activity leads to more positive evaluations of the physical self and higher global self-esteem than does sedentary behaviour.

- The benefits of physical activity on self-esteem are greatest for those who initially have low levels of self-esteem.

- One must exercise at a frequency of 2 or 3 times/wk in order to gain the beneficial effects of exercise.

- Duration and intensity of exercise have less influence on whether exercise leads to increased self-esteem. Choice over exercise type and intensity is likely to lead to more self-determined motivation and adherence.

- Practitioners can maximise clients' gains in global and physical self-esteem by creating an exercise environment that highlights personal improvement in terms of physical skill and condition.

and self-esteem in the context of sport and exercise.

A vital task for exercise scientists is to spread the word and communicate their results in a meaningful way to governing health bodies and practitioners in the field (Fox, 2000b). It is, therefore, pertinent to ask what the statistical effects reported in this chapter mean in terms of relevant behavioural changes (see Kaplan, 1990; Sechrest, McKnight & McKnight, 1996). Hence, the statistical effects need to be further translated and transferred into meaningful behavioural changes. For example, what does an effect size of 0.21 for a self-esteem variable in an exercise-experiment group in a study mean in terms of changes in relevant behaviour, such as visits to the gym despite the evaluation of others? Some effects may be highly statistically significant but not practically relevant, whereas statistical trends that are nonsignificant (e.g., due to lack of power) may be highly interesting and positive from a practical or clinical perspective. Therefore, it is essential to interpret the dependent variables and the size of the effects in studies from a practical perspective (Stoové & Andersen, 2003).

7 Summary

The evidence from several meta-analyses and numerous studies suggests that exercise and self-perceptions and self-esteem do relate in a reciprocal way. That is, the way individuals perceive and evaluate themselves with regard to their bodies and their competence most likely affects how they approach exercise (i.e., motives and motivation for exercising) and their engagement patterns (i.e., type of activity, frequency of activity, exercise setting). Engaging in regular exercise also has a positive effect on individuals' self-concept, probably first on more specific domains such as self-efficacy and physical self-perception and later on broader concepts such as self-esteem. A number of moderating variables affect the exercise–self relationship; some of these have been better documented than others. For example, the effect of exercise on self-esteem will probably be larger if the individual goes into an exercise programme with lower self-esteem, lower physical fitness and a record of being sedentary. However, future research needs to further examine under what circumstances and for what groups and individuals the exercise–self relationship is strongest. The mechanisms underlying these relationships are likely a combination of biological, physiological, psychological and sociocultural factors that interrelate in a complex pattern. This notion calls for a biopsychosocial approach when trying to understand how exercise experiences influence and shape such global and important concepts as self-esteem and physical self-perceptions and, in turn, influence the motivation to start or continue to pursue a regularly active life.

8 References

Alfermann, D., & Stoll, O. (2000). Effects of physical exercise on self-concept and well-being. *International Journal of Sport Psychology*, 31, 47-65.

Anderson, A.G., Murphy, M. H., Murtagh, H., & Nevill, A. (2006). An 8 week randomized controlled trails on the effects of brisk walking and brisk walking with abdominal muscle stimulation on anthropometric, body composition and self-perception measures in sedentary adult women. *Psychology of Sport and Exercise*, 7, 437-451.

Aşçı, F.H. (2002). The effects of step dance on physical self-perception of female and male university students. *International Journal of Sport Psychology*, 33, 431-442.

Aşçı, F.H. (2004). Physical self-perception of elite athletes and non-athletes: A Turkish sample. *Perceptual and Motor Skills*, 99, 1047-1052.

Aşçı, F.H., Kin, A., & Koşar, N. (1998). Effect of participation in an 8 week aerobic dance and step aerobics program on physical self-perception and body image satisfaction. *International Journal of Sport Psychology*, 29, 366-375.

Aşçı, F.H., Koşar, ş.N., & Kin İşler, A. (2001).The relationship of self-concept and perceived athletic competence to physical activity level and gender among Turkish early adolescents. *Adolescence*, 36, 499-507.

Blackman, L., Hunter, G., Hilyer, J., & Harrison, P. (1988). The effects of dance team participation on female adolescent physical fitness and self-concept. *Adolescence*, XXIII, 90, 437-447.

Boecker H., Sprenger, T., Spilker, M.E., Henriksen, G., Koppenhoefer, M., Wagner, K.J. et al. (2008). The runner's high: opioidergic mechanisms in the human brain. *Cerebral Cortex*, 18, 2523–2531 29.

Bowker, A. (2006). The relationship between sports participation and self-esteem during early adolescence. *Canadian Journal of Behavioral Science*, 38(3), 214-229.

Brownell, K.D. (1991a). Dieting and the search for the perfect body: Where physiology and psychology collide. *Behavior Therapy, 22*, 1-12.

Brownell, K.D. (1991b). Personal responsibility and control over our bodies: When expectations exceeds reality. *Health Psychology, 10*, 303-310.

Burgess, G., Grogan, S., & Burwitz, L. (2006). Effects of 6 week aerobic dance intervention on body image and physical self-perceptions in adolescent girls. *Body Image*, 3, 57-66.

Byrne, B.M. (1996). *Measuring self-concept across the lifespan: Issues and instrumentation.* Washington, DC: American Psychological Association.

Cafri, G., Thompson, J.K., Ricciardelli, L., McCabe, M., Smolak, L. & Yesalis, C. (2005). Pursuit of the muscular ideal: Physical and psychological consequences and putative risk factors. *Clinical Psychology Review, 25(2)*, 215–239.

Campbell, R.N. (1984). *The new science: Self-esteem psychology*. Lanham, MD: University Press of America.

Chaouloff, F. (1997). The serotonin hypothesis. In W.P. Morgan (Ed.), *Physical activity and mental health* (pp. 179-198). London: Taylor & Francis.

Cooper, W.H. (1981). Ubiquitous halo. *Psychological bulletin, 90*, 218-244.

Crocker, P.R.E., Eklund, R.C., & Kowalski, K.C. (2000). Children's physical activity and physical self-perceptions. *Journal of Sports Sciences*, 18, 383-394.

Crocker, P.R.E., Sabiston, C.M., Kowalski, K.C., McDonough, M.H., & Kowalski, N. (2006). Longitudinal assessment of the relationship between physical self concept and health related behavior and emotion in adolescent girls. *Journal of Applied Sport Psychology*, 18, 185-200.

Deci, E.L., & Ryan, R.M. (2000). The "what" and "why" of goal pursuits: Human needs and the self-determination of behavior. *Psychological Inquiry*, 11, 227-268.

Desharnais, R., Jobin, J., Coté, C., Lévesque, L., & Godin, G. (1993). Aerobic exercise and the placebo effect: A controlled study. *Psychosomatic Medicine, 55*, 149-154.

Dishman, R.K. (1997). The norepinephrine hypothesis. In W.P. Morgan (Ed.), *Physical activity and mental health* (pp. 199-212). London: Taylor & Francis.

Dishman, R.K., O'Connor, P.J. (2009). Lessons in exercise neurobiology: The case of endorphins. *Mental Health and Physical Activity, 2*, 4-9.

Dweck, C.S. (2000). *Self-theories: Their role in motivation, personality, and development*. Philadelphia: Psychology Press.

Eagly, A.H., Ashmore, R.D., Makhijani, M.G., & Longo, L.C. (1991). What is beautiful is good, but...:A meta-analytic review of research on the physical attractiveness stereotype. *Psychological Bulletin, 110*, 109-128.

Ekeland, E., Heian, F., & Hagen, K.B. (2005). Can exercise improve self esteem in children and young people? A systematic review of randomised controlled trials. *British Journal of Sports Medicine*, 39(11), 792-798.

Eklund, R.C., Whitehead, J.R., & Welk, G.J. (1997). Validity of children and youth physical self-perception profile: A confirmatory factor analysis. *Research Quarterly for Exercise and Sport*, 68, 249-256.

Erol, R.Y., & Orth, U. (2011). Self-esteem development from age 14 to 30 years: A longitudinal study. *Journal of Personality and Social Psychology*, 101(3), 607-619.

Featherstone, M. (1991). The body in consumer culture. In: M. Featherstone, M. Hepworth & B.S. Turner (Eds.), The body: Social process and cultural theory. London: Sage Publications.

Feingold, A. (1992). Good looking people are not what we think. *Psychological Bulletin, 111*,304-341.

Fox, K.R. (1990). *The physical self-perception profile manual* (PRN monograph). Dekalb, IL: Northern Illinois University Office for Health Promotion.

Fox, K.R. (1997). The physical self and process in self-esteem development. In K.R. Fox (Ed.), *The physical self: From motivation to well being*. Champaign, IL: Human Kinetics.

Fox, K.R. (2000a). The effects of exercise on self-perceptions and self-esteem. In S.J.H Biddle, K.R. Fox, & S.H. Boutcher (Eds.), *Physical activity and psychological well-being* (pp. 88-118). London: Routledge.

Fox, K.R. (2000b). Self-esteem, self-perceptions and exercise. *International Journal of Sport Psychology*, 31, 228-240.

Fox, K.R., & Corbin, C.B. (1989). The physical self-perception profile: Development and preliminary validation. *Journal of Sport and Exercise Psychology*, 14, 1-12.

Gruber, J.J. (1986). Physical activity and self-esteem development and children: A meta-analysis. *American Academy of Physical Education Papers*, 30-48.

Guyot, G.W., Fairchild, L., & Hill, M. (1981). Physical fitness, sport participation, body build and self-concept of elementary school children. *International Journal of Sport Psychology*, 12, 105-116.

Harter, S. (1982). The perceived competence scale for children. *Child Development*, 53, 87-97.

Harter, S. (1993). Causes and consequences of low self-esteem in children and adolescents. In R.F. Baumeister (Ed.), *Self-esteem: The puzzle of low self-regard*, (pp.87-116). New York: Plenum Press.

Harter, S. (1999). The construction of the self: A developmental perspective. New York: Guilford Press.

Hatfield, B.D., Vaccara, P., & Benedict, G. J. (1985). Self-concept responses of children to participate in an 8 week precision jump rope program. *Perceptual and Motor Skills*, 61, 1275-1279.

Hawkins, D.B., & Gruber, J.J. (1982). Little league baseball and player's self-esteem. *Perceptual and Motor Skills*, 55, 1335-1340.

Hodgins, M (1992). A person-perception study of the "healthy body-healthy mind" stereotype. *The Irish Journal of Psychology, 13*, 161-187.

Hoffmann, P. (1997). The endorphin hypothesis. In W.P. Morgan (Ed.), *Physical activity and mental health* (pp. 163-177). London: Taylor & Francis.

Jasnoski, M.L., Holmes, D.S., Solomon, S., & Aguiar, C. (1981). Exercise, change in aerobic capacity and changes in self-perceptions: An experimental investigation. *Journal of Research in Personality*, 15, 460-466.

Kaplan, R.M. (1990). Behavior as the central outcome in health care. *American Psychologist, 45*, 1211-1220.

Knowles, A.M., Niven, A.G., Fawker, G., & Henretty, J.M. (2009). A longitudinal examination of the influence of maturation on self-perceptions and the relationship with physical activity in early adolescent girls. *Journal of Adolescence*, 32, 555-566.

Kowalski, K. C., Crocker, P. R. E., Kowalski, N. P., Chad, K. E., & Humbert, M. L. (2003). Examining the physical self in adolescent girls over time: Further evidence against the hierarchical model. *Journal of Sport and Exercise Psychology, 25*, 5–18.

Langlois, J.H., Kalakanis, L., Rubenstein, A.J., Larson, A., Hallam, M., & Smoot, M. (2000). Maxims or myths of beauty? A meta-analytic and theoretical review. *Psychological Bulletin, 3*, 390-423.

Leary, M.R. (1992). Self-presentation processes in exercise and sport. *Journal of Sport and Exercise Psychology*, 14, 339-351.

Leith, L.M. (1994). *Foundations of exercise and mental health*. Morgantown, WV: Fitness Information Technology.

Lindwall, M. (2004). *Exercising the self: On the role of exercise, gender and culture for physical self-perceptions*. Unpublished doctoral dissertation. Department of Psychology, Stockholm University: Intellecta Docusys AB.

Lindwall, M., Aşçı,, F.H., Palmeira, A., Fox, K.R., Hagger, M.S. (2011). The Importance of Importance in the Physical Self: Support for the Theoretically Appealing but Empirically Elusive Model of James. *Journal of Personality, 79, 303-333.*

Lindwall, M., & Hassmen, P. (2004). The role of exercise and gender for physical self perceptions and importance ratings in Swedish university students. *Scandinavian Journal of Medicine and Science in Sports*, 14, 373-380.

Lindwall, M., & Lindgren, E.C. (2005). The effects of a 6 month exercise intervention programme on physical self-perceptions and social physique anxiety in non-physically active adolescent Swedish girls. *Psychology of Sport and Exercise*, 6, 643-658.

Lindwall, M., & Martin Ginis, K. (2006). Moving towards a favorable image: The self-presentational benefits of exercise and physical activity. *Scandinavian Journal of Psychology. 47*, 209-217.

Lindwall, M., & Martin Ginis, K. (2008). Exercising impressive impressions: The Exercise stereotype in male targets. *Scandinavian Journal of Medicine and Science in Sports*. DOI: 10.1111/j.1600-0838.2008.00869.x.

Marsh, H.W. (1998). Age and gender effects in physical self-concepts for adolescent elite athletes and non-athletes: A multicohort-multioccasion design. *Journal of Sport and Exercise Psychology*, 20, 237-259.

Marsh, H.W., & Hattie, J. (1996). Theoretical perspectives on the structure of self-concept. In B.A. Bracken (Ed.), *Handbook of self-concept* (pp.38-90). New York: Wiley.

Marsh, H.W., Hey, R., Roche, L.A., & Perry, C. (1997). Structure of physical self-concept: Elite athletes and physical education students. *Journal of Educational Psychology*, 89, 369-380.

Marsh, H.W., & Peart, N.D. (1988). Competitive and cooperative physical fitness training programs for girls: Effects on physical fitness and multidimensional self-concept. *Journal of Sport and Exercise Psychology*, 10, 390-407.

Marsh, H.W., Richards, G.E., & Barnes, J. (1986a). Multidimensional self-concepts: A long term follow-up of the effect of participation in an Outward Bound program. *Personality and Social Psychology Bulletin*, 12, 475-492.

Marsh, H.W., Richards, G.E., & Barnes, J. (1986b). Multidimensional self-concept: The effect of participation in an Outward Bound program. *Journal of Personality and Social Psychology*, 50, 195-204.

Marsh, H.W., & Sonstroem, R.J. (1995). Importance ratings and specific components of physical self-concept: Relevance to predicting global components of self-concept and exercise. *Journal of Sport and Exercise Psychology*, 17, 84-104.

Martin Ginis, K.A., Latimer, A.E., & Jung, M.E. (2003). No pain no gain? Examining the generalizability of the exercise stereotype to moderately active and excessive active targets. *Social Behavior and Personality, 31, 283-290.*

Martin Ginis, K. A., Lindwall, M., & Prapavessis, H. (2007). Who cares what other people think? Self-presentation in sport and exercise. In G. Tenenbaum & R. Eklund (Eds.) *Handbook of Sport Psychology*, 3rd (pp. 136-157). New York: Wiley.

McAuley, E., Elavsky, S.,Motl, R.W., Konopack, J.F., Hu, L., & Marquez, D.X. (2005). Physical activity, self-efficacy, and self-esteem: Longitudinal relationships in older adults. *Journal of Gerontology, 60B*, 268-275.

McDonald, D.G., & Hodgdon, J.A. (1991). *The psychological effects of aeorobic fitness training: Research and theory*. NewYork: Springer-Verlag.

McInman, A.D., & Berger, B.G. (1993). Self-concept and mood changes associated with aerobic dance. *Australian Journal of Psychology*, 4, 134-140.

Miller, R. (1989). Effects of sports instruction on children self-concept. *Perceptual and Motor Skills*, 68, 239-242.

Morgan, W.P. (1997). Methodological considerations. In W.P. Morgan (Ed.), *Physical activity and mental health* (pp. 3-32). London: Taylor & Francis.

Morgan, C.F., Graser, S.V., & Pangrazi, R.P. (2008). A prospective study of pedometer-determined physical activity and physical self-perceptions in children. *Research Quarterly for Exercise and Sport*, 79(2), 133-140.

Murphy, G. (1947). *Personality: A biosocial approach to origins and structure*. New York: Harper & Row.

Ojanen, M. (1994). Can the true effects of exercise on psychological variables be separated from placebo effects? *International Journal of Sport Psychology*, 25, 63-80.

Olu, S.S. (1990). Effects of training in basketball and field hockey skills on self-concepts of Nigerian adolescents. *International Journal of Sport Psychology*, 21, 121-137.

Orth, U., Robins, R.W., & Widaman, K.F. (2012). Life-span development of self-esteem and its effects on important life outcomes. *Journal of Personality and Social Psychology*, 102(6), 127-1288.

Orth, U., Trzesniewski, K.H. & Robins, R.W. (2010). Self-esteem development from young adulthood to old age: A cohort-sequential longitudinal study. *Journal of Personality and Social Psychology*, 98(4), 645–658.

Özdemir, R.A., Çelik, Ö., & Aşçı, F.H. (2010). Exercise interventions and their effects on physical self perceptions of male university students. *International Journal of Psychology*, 45(3), 174-181.

Plummer, O.K., & Koh, Y.O. (1987). Effect of "aerobics" on self-concepts of college women. *Perceptual and Motor Skills*, 65, 271-275.

Raudsepp, L., Kais, K., & Hannus, A. (2004). Stability of physical self-perceptions during early adolescence. *Pediatric Exercise Science, 16*, 138-46.

Raudsepp, L., Liblik, R., & Hannus, A. (2002). Children's and adolescents' physical self-perceptions as related to moderate to vigorous physical activity and physical fitness. *Pediatric Exercise Science*, 14, 97-106.

Raustorp, A., Archer, T., Svensson, K., Perlinger, T., & Alricsson, M. (2009). Physical self-esteem, a five year follow-up study on Swedish adolescents. *International Journal of Adolescent Medicine and Health*, 21, 497-507.

Raustorp, A., Mattsson, E., Svensson, K., & Ståhle, A. (2006). Physical activity, body composition, and physical self-esteem: A three year follow-up study among adolescents in Sweden. *Scandinavian Journal of Medicine and Science in Sports, 16*, 258-66.

Roberts, G. (1993). Motivation in sport: Understanding and enhancing the motivation and achievement of children. In R.N. Singer, M. Murphey, & L.K. Tennant (Eds.), *Handbook of research in sport psychology* (pp. 517-586). New York: MacMillan.

Schneider, M., Dunton, G.F., & Cooper, D.M. (2008). Physical activity and physical self-concept among sedentary adolescent females: An intervention study. *Psychology of Sport and Exercise*, 9, 1-14.

Sechrest, L., McKnight, P., & McKnight, K. (1996). Calibration of measures for psychotherapy outcome studies. *American Psychologist, 51*, 1065-1071.

Shavelson, R.J., Hubner, J.J., & Stanton, G.C. (1976). Self-concept: Validation of construct interpretations. *Review of Educational Research*, 46, 407-441.

Sonstroem, R.J. (1978). Physical estimation and attraction scales: Rationale and research. *Medicine and Science in Sports, 10*, 97-102

Sonstroem, R.J. (1984). Exercise and self-esteem. *Exercise and Sport Sciences Reviews*, 12, 123-155.

Sonstroem, R.J. (1997). The physical self-system: A mediator of exercise and self-esteem. In K.R. Fox (Ed.), *The physical self: From motivation to well-being* (pp. 3-26). Champaign, IL: Human Kinetics.

Sonstroem, R.J. (1998). Physical self-concept: Assessment and external validity. *Exercise and Sport Sciences Reviews*, 26, 133-144.

Sonstroem, R.J., Harlow, L.L., Gemma, L.M., & Osborne, S. (1991). Test of structural relations within a proposed exercise and self-esteem model. *Journal of Personality Assessment*, 56, 348-364.

Sonstroem, R.J., Harlow, L.L., & Josephs, L. (1994). Exercise and self-esteem: Validity of model expansion and exercise associations. *Journal of Sport and Exercise Psychology*, 16, 29-41.

Sonstroem, R.J., & Morgan, W.P. (1989). Exercise and self-esteem: Rationale and model. *Medicine and Science in Sports and Exercise*, 21(3), 329-337.

Sonstroem, R.J., & Potts, S.A. (1996). Life adjustment correlates of physical self-concepts. *Medicine and Science in Sports and Exercise*, 28, 619-624.

Sonstroem, R.J., Speliotis, E.D., & Fava, J.L. (1992). Perceived physical competence in adults: An examination of the Physical Self-Perception Profile. *Journal of Sport and Exercise Psychology*, 14, 207-221.

Spence, J.C., McGannon, K.R., & Poon, P. (2005). The effect of exercise on global self-esteem: A quantitative review. *Journal of Sport and Exercise Psychology*, 27, 311-334.

Stoll, O., & Alfermann, D. (2002). Effects of physical exercise on resources evaluation, body self-concept and well-being among older adults. *Anxiety, Stress, and Coping*, 15, 311-319.

Stoové, M.A., & Andersen, M.B. (2003). What are we looking at, and how big is it? *Physical Therapy in Sport, 4*, 93-97.

Taylor, A.H., & Fox, K.R. (2005). Effectiveness of a primary care exercise referral intervention for changing physical self perceptions over 9 months. *Health Psychology*, 24, 1-11.

Trzesniewski, K.H., Donnellan, M.B., & Robins R.W. (2003). Stability of self-esteem across the life span. *Journal of Personality and Social Psychology*, 84(1), 205-220.

Tucker, L.A. (1983). Effect of weight training on self-concept: A profile of those influenced most. *Research Quarterly for Exercise and Sport*, 54(4), 389-397.

Tucker, L.A. (1987). Effect of weight training on body attitude: Who benefits most. *Journal of Sport Medicine and Physical Fitness*, 27, 70-78.

Turner, B.S. (1992). *Regulating bodies. Essays in medical sociology*. London: Routledge

Twenge, J.M., & Campbell, W.K. (2001). Age and birth cohort differences in self-esteem: A cross-temporal meta-analysis. *Personality and Social Psychology Review*, 5(4), 321-344.

Welk, G.J., Corbin, C.B., & Lewis, L.A. (1995). Physical self-perceptions of high school athletes. *Pediatric Exercise Science*, 7, 152-161.

Whitehead, J.R. (1995). A study of children's physical self-perceptions using an adapted physical self-perception profile questionnaire. *Pediatric Exercise Science*, 7, 132-151.

Wipfli, B., Landers, D., Nagoshi, C., & Ringenbach, S. (2011). An examination of serotonin and psychological variables in the relationship between exercise and mental health. *Scandinavian Journal of Medicine & Science in Sports*, 21, 474-481.

Effects of Overtraining on Well-Being and Mental Health

John S. Raglin, PhD

Indiana University, Bloomington, Indiana, United States

Gregory Wilson, PED

University of Evansville, Evansville, Indiana, United States

Goran Kenttä, PhD

The Swedish School of Sport and Health Sciences, Stockholm, Sweden

Chapter Outline

Editors' Introduction

The majority of this text explores the positive relationship between physical activity and well-being. In contrast, this chapter explores the paradox whereby very high volumes of physical activity can lead to reduced well-being and mental health as well as performance decrements. This chapter describes the signs, symptoms and stages of overtraining syndrome (OTS) and provides advice on early detection and treatment in order to reduce the impact of OTS on performance. Regular assessment using self-report psychological questionnaires is a practical and effective means of reducing the risk of developing OTS. This chapter also highlights the important role of mood disturbance in OTS.

For decades, both coaches and athletes have searched for training strategies that produce optimal sport performance. This quest has included varying the intensity, frequency, type and duration of exercise training as well as exploiting pharmaceutical agents such as androgenic anabolic steroids (Hartgens & Kuipers, 2004) or nutritional practices such as ingesting high levels of caffeine (Magkos & Kavouras, 2004). Most coaches and athletes continue to believe that the greatest improvements in sport performance are derived from training harder and more.

In the case of endurance athletes, it is widely recognised that improvements in performance depend on the physiological concept known as the principle of progressive overload, which states that the systems of the body—musculoskeletal, metabolic, cardiovascular and respiratory—must be worked at increasingly higher levels of intensity in order for optimal performance adaptations to occur (Wilmore, Costill & Kenney, 2008). As a result, a dramatic increase in both training volume and intensity by competitive athletes occurred in the latter half of the 20th century. For example, Mark Spitz, winner of 7 gold medals at the 1972 Munich Olympics, trained an average of 9,000 m/day (Counsilman & Counsilman, 1990), yet by the early 1990s some collegiate swimmers trained in excess of 36,000 m/day. Bompa (1983) estimates that the average training load for many sports increased from 10 to 22% over the period of 1975 to 1980 alone. In addition, the advent of year-round competition and training eliminated the off-season period that previously allowed athletes to recover more completely after the competitive season. Performance improvements have been significant. However, this success has been accompanied by an increase in overuse injuries. In fact, van Mechelen (1992) estimated that the yearly incidence rate for running injuries varies between 37% and 56% and that approximately 50% to 75% of these injuries are related to overuse. A further study of 1,357 Army recruits enrolled in basic training found a 17% incidence of injuries resulting from overuse (Popovich et al., 2000).

Furthermore, at the 2009 world championships in athletics held in Berlin, 236 injury incidents due to overuse (44.1% of reported injuries) were reported (Alonso et al., 2012. Moreover, researchers have suggested that the incidence of overuse injuries may actually be underestimated when a traditional time-loss definition is used to record injuries because many athletes continue to train using nonsteroidal anti-inflammatory agents despite pain (Tschol, Junge & Dvorak, 2008).

1 Paradox of Increased Training and Decreased Performance

Some athletes experience a prolonged decline in performance as a direct consequence of excessive training. This paradoxical consequence of physical training is not a recent phenomenon; it was described in the medical literature over a century ago as well as in the personal accounts of athletes. Gunter Hägg, who established several world records at distances between 1,500 and 5,000 m during the period from 1939 and 1945, also experienced persistent slumps. After a hard training period leading up to the 1943 season, Hägg (1952) wrote, "I never thought one could be training this hard day in and day out, but it is possible and I grow stronger and stronger. But I can't imagine training any harder without losing my motivation and interest for the upcoming race season" (p. 51). Despite this declaration, Hägg proved not to be immune to the stress of hard training. In the summer of 1942 he experienced a serious decrease in performance, which a newspaper described as a condition of "burnout"; this was perhaps the first public use of the term in the context of sport. Hägg (1952), however, felt differently and responded by stating, "I am not burned out, but I am ill" (p. 47). Given that he ran 13 races and broke 3 world records between July 1 and July 23, his self-diagnosis was likely correct. The few days of rest between races were spent traveling to race sites. He refrained from training between July 24 and July 28 and nearly broke another world record on July 29, perhaps as a consequence of allowing himself some necessary recovery.

This phenomenon, initially labelled as staleness (Griffith, 1926), is now more commonly depicted as OTS (Meeusen et al., 2006), but it has also been called inadequate recovery syndrome and unexplained underperformance syndrome. The defining symptom of OTS is a serious reduction in the capacity to train and compete at customary levels that persists for several weeks or months and is a direct consequence of the stress of training paired with insufficient recovery (Kreider, Fry & O'Toole, 1998; Kuipers & Keizer, 1988; Meeusen et al., 2006; Morgan et al., 1987). Other potential causes, such as injury and illness, must be ruled out. Researchers generally believe that nonsport sources of stress (e.g., psychosocial stressors) also contribute to the development of OTS, but direct evidence of the magnitude of impact of these stressors is lacking.

One must distinguish OTS from what has been called exercise addiction or dependence (see chapter 13). The latter phenomenon is largely confined to the recreational exerciser who, although preoccupied with increasing the amount of time devoted to physical activity, typically has little or no interest in athletic achievement or even improved performance (Raglin, 2012). OTS is also distinct from burnout, although sport psychologists and practitioners in the field commonly and mistakenly use the terms synonymously. Burnout was originally linked to occupational stressors (Maslach et al, 2001), and far less empirical research has been conducted on athletes (Goodger et al., 2007; Gustafsson, Kenttä & Hassmén, 2011). Although chronic imbalance is a key element in both concepts, the predominant stressors associated with each condition are distinct: physical training in the case of OTS and occupational stress in most research on burnout. In the sport psychology literature, burnout has typically been regarded as a consequence of excessive stress demands placed on the individual, although some researchers have emphasised that the influence of the social organisation in sport can potentially result in feelings of entrapment (Brewer, 1993; Brustad & Ritter-Taylor, 1997). More recently, a stress-recovery perspective on burnout in sport (Kellmann & Kallus, 2001; Kenttä et al., 2001), which argues that poor recovery is a major risk factor, has emerged. Consequently, both enhancing and monitoring effective strategies of recovery are essential in preventing burnout. Research

KEY CONCEPTS

- The role of stress in an athletic context is complex. Stress is necessary for improving performance but can be a potential problem that may result in performance decrements.

- Exercise at mild to moderate levels has proven beneficial for mental health. However, this beneficial relationship breaks down when training load is increased beyond a certain point.

- Based on the physiological concept known as the overtraining principle, athletes must stress the body above what is normally required for general fitness in order to maximise performance gains. However, some athletes respond in a negative manner to this increase in training volume and instead suffer from OTS.

- Physiological markers for monitoring how an athlete is responding to training have been proposed. However, these markers have proven inconclusive.

- Various forms of psychological assessments have proven effective in monitoring the response of individual athletes to training (Raglin & Wilson, 2000). Specifically, psychological instruments such as the Profile of Mood States and other newly developed questionnaires that specifically assess overload training and recovery have shown promise in predicting cases of OTS in athletes.

into burnout has been hampered by the lack of a single definition of burnout, but an emerging consensus around Raedeke, Lunney and Venables' (2002) athlete-specific definition of burnout as "a withdrawal from [sport] noted by a reduced sense of accomplishment, devaluation/resentment of sport and physical/psychological exhaustion" (p. 181) is allowing research in this area to move forward (Goodger et al., 2007).

2   Signs and Symptoms of Overtraining Syndrome

OTS is associated with a broad range of signs and symptoms not found in burnout. Those most frequently reported include medical illnesses such as upper-respiratory infections, sleep disturbances (longer sleep onset, frequent waking, poor sleep quality), loss of appetite, muscle soreness, feelings of heaviness in the arms and legs and an increase in the perception of effort associated with training (Fry, Morton & Keast, 1991; Kuipers & Keizer, 1988). Psychological symptoms such as mood disturbances, irritability and depression are among the most frequently reported symptoms in overtrained athletes. Research indicates that as many as 80% of overtrained athletes exhibit depression of clinical significance (Armstrong & VanHeest, 2002; Morgan et al., 1987). This is in sharp contrast to individuals who train at low and moderate volumes (e.g., 20-60 min/day of exercise), which have been found to effectively enhance mood in healthy individuals (Martinsen & Raglin, 2007; Morgan, 1997). Low-intensity exercise has also been found to be effective in treating mild to moderate depression and anxiety disorders and to rival the benefits of traditional forms of medication (Blumenthal et al., 2007) (see chapter 8). However, at the training duration and intensity routinely used by competitive athletes, OTS is more often associated with worsened emotional states and, in the most severe cases, clinical depression. Hence, these findings illustrate the complex and paradoxical effect that physical activity has on mental health.

Because OTS is a syndrome, it is associated with a broad range of symptoms that occur with varying degrees of frequency and intensity. However, because these symptoms are also common to other illnesses or conditions (e.g., chronic fatigue syndrome), the diagnosis of OTS is necessarily based on exclusion. Pre-existing conditions such as an illness, injury or medical conditions that share common symptoms with OTS must first be ruled out. Thus, making a definitive diagnosis is often difficult (Meeusen et al., 2006).

The initial stage of OTS during which performance has stagnated or is just beginning to worsen is often referred to as nonfunctional overreaching (NFOR; Meeusen et al., 2006). Unlike fully developed cases of OTS, NFOR can be effectively treated by simply reducing or ceasing training for several days. Although NFOR is regarded as an undesirable outcome, Kenttä and Hassmén (1998) propose that overreaching that is appropriately managed actually stimulates physiological training adaptations derived from the overload principle. As a result, researchers now differentiate NFOR from functional overreaching. In practice, however, it is difficult if not impossible to determine whether training regimens that incorporate periods of intensive overload training will ultimately benefit or harm the athlete until the actual consequences become evident.

Reducing the rigour of training programmes can reduce or even eliminate the risk of NFOR and OTS. However, the resulting subpar performance would clearly be unacceptable to any serious coach or athlete. Consequently, there has been considerable interest in identifying symptoms that are reliable precursors to OTS.

3   Treatment of Overtraining Syndrome

Treatment requires the athlete to refrain from training for a period that may last from days to months, although participation in recreational activities, even those involving moderate physical exertion, is encouraged. Medical evaluation is necessary both to rule out more serious medical conditions and to treat the athlete for infections common to OTS. Proper nutrition and hydration are crucial because some evidence suggests that overtrained athletes may consume calories that are insufficient to meet their energy demands (Costill et al., 1988). Although use of nutritional supplements has been proposed, the effectiveness of these agents has not been systematically evaluated. The severity of the depression and mood disturbances of the overtrained athlete warrants professional intervention such as counselling, psychotherapy or pharmacological treatment (Morgan et al., 1987). Morgan and colleagues (1987) cite an example of a male swimmer who during a season experienced overtraining that resulted in chronic fatigue and a diagnosis of depression by a clinical psychologist. After short-term psychotherapy, a rest period of 1 wk and a reduced training load, the swimmer recovered and was swimming competitively again by the end of the season. However, the psychological support and treatment required by athletes with OTS depend on the needs of each athlete and the context in which they are training. Most athletes do successfully recover from OTS and resume training and competing, but evidence suggests that these athletes are at an increased risk of relapse (Raglin, 1993). Unfortunately, a small minority of athletes never regain their previous level of performance, potentially as a consequence of a gradual transition from OTS to burnout syndrome (Gustafsson et al., 2011; Meeusen et al., 2006).

4   Prevalence and Susceptibility in Athlete Samples

Retrospective and prospective research with collegiate swimmers and other endurance athletes who undergo an extended period of intensive overload training indicates that approximately 10% of athletes experience at least some signs of OTS (Raglin & Wilson, 2000). This risk is compounded over time. Studies of adults found that 64% of elite American male and 60% of female distance runners reported experiencing OTS one or more times during their athlete career. Female nonelite distance runners reported a lifetime rate

of only 33%; the difference was attributed to the significantly lower weekly training distance in this group (Morgan et al., 1987b, 1988b). Moreover, the push to train young athletes harder across longer competitive seasons has resulted in rates of OTS that rival those for adult athletes. In a study of 231 competitive swimmers aged 13 to 17 yr from 4 countries, 34.6% reported experiencing OTS at least once (Raglin et al., 2000). Of particular interest is that the rate of OTS was higher for swimmers who had been involved in the sport longer and who were faster as reported by their personal best times. A related study of 272 elite Swedish high school athletes in 13 sports found an overall OTS rate of 37% (Kenttä, Hassmén & Raglin, 2001). These retrospective findings have been corroborated by a recent prospective study involving British age-group swimmers (Matos et al., 2011). This study found that 29% developed NFOR or OTS, with the highest rates found among swimmers in the top performance category. Comparable rates have been found in athletes in nonendurance sports (e.g., basketball) that place a premium on top physical conditioning (Raglin & Wilson, 2000).

It also appears that some athletes are inherently prone to this disorder. For example, research involving collegiate varsity swimmers found that 91% of athletes who developed OTS during their first year of collegiate competition became overtrained again at least once over the following three seasons, whereas the rate decreased to 34% among swimmers who did not become overtrained during their first year of college (Raglin, 1993). Other controlled research with a sample of 10 competitive swimmers who completed 10 days of intensified training at the same volume and relative intensity (8970 m/day at 94% $\dot{V}O_2$max) found that 3 of the 10 swimmers had difficultly completing the training requirements and exhibited signs of NFOR. These athletes possessed greater total mood-disturbance scores on the Profile of Mood States (POMS) (Morgan et al., 1988) and had lower levels of muscle glycogen (Kirwan et al., 1988) at the end of training compared with the rest of the sample. Research has not yet revealed whether some athletes are inherently predisposed to OTS when exposed to overload training or whether succumbing to OTS increases the risk of subsequent relapse. Research on potential psychological mediators has been conducted, but the risk of OTS has not been found to be mediated by intrinsic motivation (Raglin, Morgan & Luchsinger, 1990), hardiness, or optimism (Wilson & Raglin, 2004).

5 Early Detection Using Physiological Measures

Given the considerable variability in the responses of athletes to standardised training regimens as well as the previously described individual differences in susceptibility to OTS, it remains a difficult if not impossible task to prescribe training regimens that minimise or obviate OTS while at the same time maximise training adaptation according to the overload principle. As a consequence, considerable efforts have been made to identify reliable signs or symptoms that occur early enough that brief training breaks or reductions would effectively forestall OTS. Studies initiated several decades ago have yielded more than 80 putative measures involving cardiovascular, metabolic and hormonal variables (Fry, Morton & Keast, 1991; Kuipers & Keizer, 1988; Urhausen & Kindermann, 2002) that have been tested in this capacity. Unfortunately, despite this extensive work, the view expressed by Urhausen and Kindermann (2002) that "there has been little improvement in recent years in the tools available for the diagnosis of OTS" (p. 95) remains unchallenged (Meeusen et al., 2006). A small number of hormonal measures appear to provide some sensitivity for identifying overtrained athletes, but their practical utility is limited by expense, technical requirements and the invasiveness that many physiological variables (e.g., blood draws) entail. Performance measures are also of limited utility because many coaches are reluctant to subject athletes to all-out physical tests during periods of heavy training or during an intensive competitive schedule.

6 Early Detection Using Psychological Measures

To address the concerns over physiological markers of OTS and the fact that psychological changes have long been noted anecdotally in the overtraining literature, research turned to the examination of psychological variables. The primary instrument used for this research was the POMS (McNair, Lorr & Dropplemann, 1971), a Likert-format questionnaire that measures tension, depression, anger, vigor, fatigue and confusion. Summing the negative POMS factors (tension, depression, anger, fatigue and confusion), subtracting the positive POMS factor (vigor) and adding a constant of 100 to prevent negative scores yield a global measure of mood disturbance. Individuals answer POMS items according to how they have been feeling "last week, including today"; this yields a moderately stable measure of mood that falls between true psychological states and more stable traits and exhibits an appropriate degree of responsiveness to the stressors associated with athletic training.

Research with POMS has revealed that intensive athletic training is consistently associated with significant elevations in negative POMS factors and reduced vigor in athletes who exhibit positive scores on all the POMS factors during the off-season or periods of easy training. Morgan (1985) labelled this distinctive pattern of positive scores on all POMS factors the iceberg profile. It is so named because research comparing athletes with the population norm found that athletes' scores for negative mood factors each fall significantly below that of the population norm, whereas athletes' scores for the positive mood factor vigor are typically one to two standard deviations above the norm. When the standardised POMS scores of athletes are plotted as in figure 6.1, the horizontal line representing the population norm can be imagined as the surface of the sea and the plot of the athlete's POMS scores as an iceberg. Only the vigor score rises above the sea's surface, just like only a small proportion of the ice in an iceberg is visible above the sea's surface.

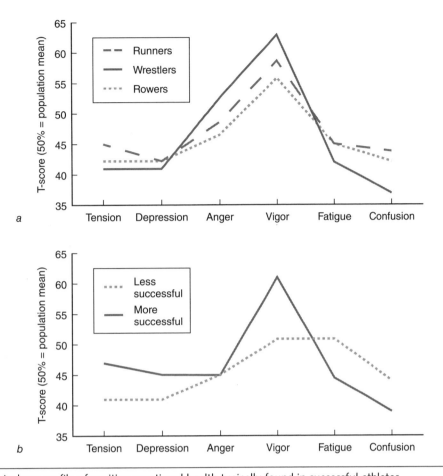

Figure 6.1   The iceberg profile of positive emotional health typically found in successful athletes.

Adapted from W. Morgan, 1979, *Coach, athlete and the sport psychologist* (Toronto: University of Toronto School of Physical Health and Education), 185. By permission of W. Morgan.

Subsequent studies that have examined the relationship between training load and mood state on a monthly or weekly basis have found that a predictable relationship exists between training load and mood disturbance. When training volume or intensity increase, there is a corresponding increase in mood disturbances and decrease in vigor, the lone positive factor assessed by the POMS. Mood disturbances are typically highest during the most intense training period. Mood disturbances decrease as training load is reduced or tapered, and mood profiles return to baseline values by the end of the season for the majority of athletes. The mood-state responses were found to be similar in male and female swimmers except in cases in which their training regimens differed significantly (Morgan et al., 1987; Raglin, Morgan & O'Connor, 1991). Subsequent research has shown that this

dose–response relationship between training load and mood state occurs in a wide variety of endurance and nonendurance sports (Raglin & Wilson, 2000) where the changes in training load are sufficiently intense (i.e., >2 h/day of training) and efforts have been made to control or minimise the potential for response distortion.

These findings involved regimens in which training volumes slowly changed over a period of weeks or months. Many sports utilise conditioning programmes that rapidly increase training loads over the course of a few days, and research has shown that this form of training can result in NFOR or OTS (Costill et al., 1988; Kenttä, Hassmén & Raglin, 2006). To assess mood in this context, the instructions of the POMS are amended so that the athlete responds according to how he or she feels "today" or "right now" in order to yield a true state measure of mood that is sensitive to acute stressors. It has been found that as few as 2 days of intensified training can result in significant elevations in mood disturbance (e.g., O'Connor et al., 1989); these elevations are greatest in athletes showing signs of NFOR (Kenttä, Hassmén & Raglin, 2006; Morgan et al., 1988; O'Connor et al., 1989). In research that has contrasted psychological responses with commonly used physiological markers of training stress such as cortisol secretion or heart rate, elevations in mood disturbances precede changes in physiological variables (O'Connor et al., 1989). This provides further evidence in support of using psychological measures in this context. The elevations in mood disturbances that occur with training often coincide with other perceptual and behavioural symptoms (e.g., perceived exertion, muscle soreness and feelings of heaviness) that are assessed using simple self-report questionnaires (Morgan et al., 1988), although the magnitude by which these variables change in response to training differs.

6.1   Mood-State Responses to Training

In the initial stages of the training season when the workload is light, the mood-state scores of athletes who later develop signs of NFOR or OTS are indistinguishable from scores of those who successfully adapt to the training regimen (O'Connor et al., 1989; Raglin & Morgan, 1994; Verde, Thomas & Shephard, 1992). However, as training loads reach more intense levels, athletes showing signs of NFOR or OTS have greater increases in total mood disturbance and exhibit a unique configuration of changes in the specific POMS variables. Several studies involving long-term training paradigms (O'Connor et al., 1989; Raglin & Morgan, 1994; Raglin et al., 1991) have shown that the POMS factors of fatigue and vigor are the most responsive to increased training and that the POMS factor of depression is often the least affected in healthy athletes. However, in athletes with OTS, there is a greater elevation in total mood disturbance; more important, depression increases the most

of all POMS variables. Other research (O'Connor et al., 1989) has found that POMS depression scores are significantly correlated with salivary cortisol levels in overtrained swimmers, suggesting that the depression commonly seen in overtrained athletes has a biological basis and is not merely the reaction of athletes to poor performance as some have contended (Martin et al., 2000). This finding reinforces the need for intervention by appropriately trained clinicians rather than traditional applied sport psychology techniques such as arousal regulation, goal setting, self-talk and psychological skills training.

Based on salient research findings, one can conclude that mood state will predictably fluctuate in accordance with changes in the volume and intensity of training (i.e., respond to the total workload) when mood state is appropriately monitored in competitive athletes who are undergoing significant periodisation cycles involving periods of heavy training. In many cases both a greater elevation in total mood disturbance and a unique pattern of specific mood disturbances are observed in individuals who are at an increased risk of developing OTS.

6.2   Using Mood-State Responses to Reduce the Risk of Overtraining Syndrome

The finding that disturbed mood is the symptom that perhaps occurs most consistently in OTS has led to some attempts to prevent these symptoms by regularly monitoring athletes during intense training and altering training in cases of extreme mood scores. In one study the mood state of members of a collegiate men's and women's swimming team undergoing a period of intense training was assessed daily using the "today" version of the POMS (Raglin, 1993). The total mood-disturbance score of each swimmer was contrasted with the mean of the entire team for the same day. When the total mood-state score of a swimmer was elevated by 1 standard deviation or more above the team average, training loads for the individual swimmer were reduced until the score fell below this threshold.

Conversely, when the total mood-state score of a swimmer fell 1 standard deviation or more below the team average, it was assumed that the swimmer was insufficiently stressed by the training load and the volume of subsequent workouts was increased until the swimmer's total mood-disturbance score increased to within 1 standard deviation. The researchers concluded that the intervention was successful because, for the first time in a decade, the coaches reported no cases of OTS in the swimmers.

In a study using an intraindividual intervention paradigm, Berglund and Säfström (1994) used off-season baseline scores of Swedish male and female race canoeists to modulate training loads as the athletes prepared for Olympic competition. The athletes were assessed weekly using the Swedish-language version of the POMS, and training load was adjusted on the basis of total mood-state scores. Training load was reduced when the athlete's total mood-disturbance score exceeded the athlete's baseline score by at least 50%, and loads were increased when scores decreased to within 10% of the baseline. Both interventions were frequently employed. Training was reduced in 64% of the athletes sampled and increased in 57%, indicating some athletes required each intervention at some point during training. No cases of OTS occurred, and the authors concluded the intervention programme was successful. Although these findings are promising, replications with a larger sample and appropriate control conditions are needed.

6.3 Specialised Overtraining Syndrome Scales

Some researchers have attempted to create novel scales based on the POMS for use in basic and applied research on athletes at risk of OTS. Raglin and Morgan (1994) used statistical techniques to identify POMS items that most reliably distinguished healthy from overtrained athletes in a sample of 186 college varsity swimmers who completed the POMS on a monthly basis throughout training. The resulting seven-item scale, labelled the Training Distress Scale (TDS),

consisted of five depression and two anger items derived from the POMS. Interestingly, the TDS was found to be more accurate than predictions based on either POMS total mood disturbance or POMS depression in identifying overtrained college track athletes. Subsequent research involving translations of the TDS (Kenttä, Hassmén & Raglin, 2001; Raglin et al., 2000) indicates that athletes with symptoms of OTS had significantly higher TDS scores than did healthy athletes.

A different approach was used by Kenttä, Hassmén and Raglin (2006), who created a POMS energy index scale by subtracting fatigue from vigor. The purpose of this measurement tool was to develop a brief measure sensitive enough to monitor mood responses to training load as well as recovery on a daily basis. Consequently, a composite score was based on fatigue and vigor because previous research shows that these factors are the most sensitive to increased training. In an examination of the test's sensitivity, elite kayakers completed the POMS twice daily (i.e., before and after practices) throughout an intensive 3 wk training camp. The POMS energy index scores responded significantly to training stress and recovery, whereas POMS depression scores and other variables remained unchanged throughout the training intervention. The authors concluded that the energy index appeared to be a sensitive measure for assessing the ability of athletes to adapt to brief but intense training cycles.

Other overtraining scales have been developed under the presumption that measures specifically devised to assess overtraining and recovery should provide even greater efficacy than general instruments such as the POMS. The most popular among these is the Recovery Stress Questionnaire for athletes (RESTQ; Kellman & Kallus, 2001), a 77-item questionnaire that assesses 19 factors based on stressful and restful events that occur over a period of 3 days. Initial work indicates that the RESTQ can identify athletes with signs of OTS, but its accuracy has yet to be compared with that of the POMS and other scales. In addition, Kenttä and Hassmén (1998), who emphasised monitoring recovery as a means for preventing overtraining, published a

EVIDENCE TO PRACTICE

- Intensive overload training is common among both young and adult competitive athletes in endurance and nonendurance sports.
- Intensive overload training is typically associated with disturbances in mood state, but physiological responses have been found to be less consistent.
- For most athletes, tapers or breaks after intensive training are associated with small but meaningful improvements in performance and a return to positive mood-state profiles.
- Approximately 10% of athletes who undergo intensive training schedules do not adapt or respond favorably and exhibit signs of OTS.
- OTS is associated with a chronic loss of physical capacity and significant mood disturbances, including clinical depression.
- OTS treatment requires that athletes discontinue training for a period of weeks or months. Medical and psychological attention is generally necessary as well.
- Tests of a variety of biological and psychological training markers have revealed that assessments of mood state and perceptions related to fatigue have potential in monitoring and preventing OTS.

conceptual model on overtraining and recovery that includes the Total Quality Recovery Scale (TQR). The scale assesses both the athletes' self-perception of recovery and recovery actions in four essential categories: nutrition and fluid, sleep and rest, relaxation and emotional support and, finally, active recovery. Most recently, Lundqvist and Kenttä (2010) developed the Emotional Recovery Questionnaire (EmRecQ). The purpose of this instrument is to account for the comprehensive variables associated with the process of recovery in order to prevent OTS by effectively monitoring training and enhancing the periods of recovery in a training cycle.

7　Summary

Compelling evidence shows that physical exercise and participation in physical activity are associated with improved mood and can be an effective means of alleviating symptoms of mild to moderate anxiety and depression (Blumenthal et al., 2007; Martinsen & Raglin, 2007; Morgan, 1997). However, studies of competitive athletes indicate that regimens of physical training that involve high volumes or intensities routinely result in worsened mood state and, in the extreme case of athletes suffering from OTS, and

clinical depression. Athletes suffering from fully developed OTS generally must cease training and competing for a period of weeks or months and, in rare cases, perhaps years (Meeusen et al., 2006). OTS is a multifactorial phenomenon that has continually defied the concerted efforts of scientists to identify its root causes and establish reliable diagnostic markers that could help reduce its incidence. However, promising evidence shows that athletes undergoing intensive periods of training may be reliably assessed and monitored using psychological instruments such as the POMS or newly developed questionnaires that assess overload training and recovery. Hence, these tools may provide an effective means of reducing, if not eliminating, the risk of OTS in susceptible athletes (Berglund & Säfström, 1994; Kellman & Kallus, 2001; Kenttä, Hassmén & Raglin, 2006; Raglin, 1993). Any psychological or behavioural monitoring tool must be integrated into a comprehensive monitoring strategy in which relevant physiological, performance and nutritional factors are regularly assessed and a clear plan for intervention and treatment involving appropriately trained professionals has been established.

The finding that athletes who undergo increases in training volume experience elevations in mood disturbances that are closely associated with training volume reveals that physical exercise is a complex stressor that can result in both beneficial and detrimental outcomes. The literature supporting this relationship involves samples totaling more than 2,000 athletes involved in a wide range of sports. However, these findings are rarely described in overviews of the literature (e.g., Weir, 2011). This is unfortunate because the findings from this literature have implications in relation to the relationship between exercise and mental health. The findings also have implications for sports medicine because this field has long been dominated by a purely biological approach. The value of an enlarged psychobiological perspective has only recently come to the fore but was recognised long ago by the early American psychologist Coleman Roberts Griffith (1926), who said "The athlete, at work and at play, constitutes a fine laboratory for the study of vexing physiological and psychological problems, many of which are distorted by the attempt to reduce them to simpler terms" (p. vii).

8 References

Alonso, J.M., Edouard, P., Fischetto, G., Adams, B., Depiesse, F., Mountjoy, M. (2012). Determination of future prevention strategies in elite track and field: Analysis of Daegu IAAF Championships injuries and illnesses surveillance. *British Journal of Sports Medicine*. 2012 Jun;46(7):505-14.

Armstrong, L.E., & VanHeest, J.L. (2002). The unknown mechanism of the overtraining syndrome: Clues from depression and psychoneuroimmunology. *Sports Medicine*, 32, 185-209.

Berglund, B., & Säfström, H. (1994). Psychological monitoring and modulation of training load of world-class canoeists. *Medicine and Science in Sports and Exercise*, 26, 1036-1040.

Blumenthal, J.A., Babyak, M.A., Murali Doraiswamy, P., Watkins, L., Hoffman, B.M., Barbour, K.A., et al. (2007). Exercise and pharmacotherapy in the treatment of major depressive disorder. *Psychosomatic Medicine*, 69, 587-596.

Bompa, T.O. (1983). *Theory and methodology of training: The key to athletic performance*. Dubuque, IA: Kendall-Hunt.

Brewer, B.W. (1993). Self-identity and specific vulnerability to depressed mood. *Journal of Personality* 61(3) , 343-364

Brustad, R.J., Ritter-Taylor, M. (1997). Applying social psychological perspectives to the sport psychology consulting process *Sport Psychologist* 11, 107-119

Costill, D.L., Flynn, M.G., Kirwan, J.P. Houmard, J.A., Mitchell, J.B., Thomas, R. et al. (1988). Effects of repeated days of intensified training on muscle glycogen and swimming performance. *Medicine and Science in Sports and Exercise*, 20, 249-254.

Counsilman, J.E., & Counsilman, B.E. (1990). No simple answers. *Swimming Technique*, 26, 22-29.

Fry, R.W., Morton, A.R., & Keast, D. (1991). Overtraining in athletes: An update. *Sports Medicine*, 12, 32-65.

Goodger, K., Gorely, T., Lavallee, D., & Harwood, C. (2007). Burnout in sport: A systematic review. *The Sport Psychologist*, 21, 127-151.

Griffith, C.R. (1926). *Psychology of coaching*. New York: Scribner.

Gustafsson, H., Kenttä, G., & Hassmén, P. (2011). Athlete burnout: An integrated model and future research directions. *International Review of Sport and Exercise Psychology*, 4(1), 3-24.

Hägg, G. (1952). Gunder Häggs dagbok, en världsmästares erfarenheter och träningsråd [Gunder Häggs diary, a world champions experiences and training advises]. Stockholm, Sweden: Tryckeriaktiebolaget Tiden.

Hartgens, F., & Kuipers, H. (2004). Effects of androgenic-anabolic steroids in athletes. *Sports Medicine*, 34, 513-554.

Kellmann, M., & Kallus, K.W. (2001). *Recovery-stress questionnaire for athletes*. Champaign, IL: Human Kinetics.

Kenttä, G., & Hassmén, P. (1998). Overtraining and recovery: A conceptual model. *Sports Medicine*, 26, 1-16.

Kenttä, G., Hassmén, P., & Raglin, J. (2001). Overtraining and staleness in Swedish age-group athletes: Association with training behavior and psychosocial stressors. *International Journal of Sports Medicine*, 22, 460-465.

Kenttä, G., Hassmén, P., & Raglin, J.S. (2006). Mood state monitoring of training and recovery in elite kayakers. *European Journal of Sport Science*, 4, 245-253.

Kirwan, J.P., Costill, D.L., Mitchell, J.B., Houmard, J.A., Flynn, M.G., Fink, W.J., Beltz, J.D. (1988) Carbohydrate balance in competitive runners during successive days of intense training *Journal of Applied Physiology* 65, 2601-2606

Kreider, R.B., Fry, A.C., & O'Toole, M.L. (1998). *Overtraining in sport.* Champaign, IL: Human Kinetics.

Kuipers, H., & Keizer, H.A. (1988). Overtraining in elite athletes: Review and directions for the future. *Sports Medicine*, 6, 79-92.

Lundqvist, C., & Kenttä, G. (2010). Positive emotions are not simply the absence of the negative ones: Development and validation of the Emotional Recovery Questionnaire (EmRecQ). *Sport Psychologist*, 24(4), 468-488.

Magkos, F., & Kavouras, S.A. (2004). Caffeine and ephedrine: Physiological, metabolic and performance-enhancing effects. *Sports Medicine*, 34, 871-889.

Martin, D.T., Andersen, M.B., & Gates, W. (2000). Using Profile of Mood States (POMS) to monitor high-intensity training in cyclists: Group versus case studies. *The Sport Psychologist*, 14, 138-156.

Martinsen, E., & Raglin, J. (2007). Themed review: Anxiety/depression. *American Journal of Lifestyle Medicine*, 1, 159-166.

Maslach C, Schaufeli WB, Leiter MP. (2001) Job burnout. *Annual Reviews of Psychology.* 2001;52:397-422.Matos, N., Winsley, R., & Williams, C. (2011). Prevalence of nonfunctional overreaching/overtraining in young English athletes. *Medicine and Science in Sports and Exercise*, 43, 1287-1294.

McNair, D.M., Lorr, M., & Dropplemann, L.F. (1971). *Profile of Mood States manual.* San Diego: Educational and Testing Service.

Meeusen R., Duclos, M., Gleeson, M., Rietjens, G., Steinacker, J., & Urhausen, A. (2006). Prevention, diagnosis and treatment of the overtraining syndrome. ECSS Position Statement "Task Force." *European Journal of Sport Science*, 6(1), 1-14.

Morgan, W.P. (1985). Selected psychological factors limiting performance: A mental health model. In D.H. Clarke & H.M. Eckert (Eds.), *Limits of human performance* (pp. 70-80). Champaign, IL: Human Kinetics.

Morgan, W.P. (Ed.). (1997). *Physical activity and mental health.* Washington, D.C.: Taylor & Francis.

Morgan, W.P., Brown, D.R., Raglin, J.S., O'Connor, P.J., & Ellickson, K.A. (1987a). Psychological monitoring of overtraining and staleness. *British Journal of Sports Medicine*, 21, 107-114.

Morgan, W.P., Costill, D.L., Flynn, M.G., Raglin, J.S., & O'Connor, P.J. (1988a). Mood disturbances following increased training in swimmers. *Medicine and Science in Sports and Exercise*, 23, 408-414.

Morgan, W.P., O'Connor, P.J., Ellickson, K.A., & Bradley, P.W. (1988b). Personality structure, mood states, and performance in elite male distance runners. *International Journal of Sport Psychology*, 19, 247-263.

Morgan, W.P., O'Connor, P.J., Sparling, P.B., & Pate, R.R. (1987b). Psychological characterization of the elite female distance runner. *International Journal of Sports Medicine*, 8(Suppl.), 124-131.

O'Connor, P.J., Morgan, W.P., Raglin, J.S., Barksdale, C.N., & Kalin, N.H. (1989). Mood state and salivary cortisol levels following overtraining in female swimmers. *Psychoneuroendocrinology*, 14, 303-310.

Popovich, R.M., Gardner, J.W., Potter, R., Knapik, J.J., & Jones, B.H. (2000). Effect of rest from running overuse injuries in Army basic training. *American Journal of Preventive Medicine*, 18(3), 147-155.

Raedeke, T.D., Lunney, K., & Venables, K. (2002). Understanding athlete burnout: Coach perspectives. *Journal of Sport Behavior*, 25(2), 181-206.

Raglin, J.S. (1993). Overtraining and staleness: Psychometric monitoring of endurance athletes. In R.N. Singer, M. Murphey, & L.K. Tennet (Eds.), *Handbook of research in sport psychology* (pp. 840-850). New York: MacMillan.

Raglin, J.S. (2012). Addiction to physical activity. In J. Rippe (Ed.), *Encyclopedia of lifestyle medicine and health*. Thousand Oaks, CA: Sage.

Raglin, J.S., & Morgan, W.P. (1994). Development of a scale for use in monitoring training-induced distress in athletes. *International Journal of Sports Medicine*, 15, 84-88.

Raglin, J.S., Morgan, W.P., & Luchsinger, A.E. (1990). Mood and self-motivation in successful and unsuccessful female rowers. *Medicine and Science in Sports and Exercise*, 22, 849-853.

Raglin, J.S., Morgan, W.P., & O'Connor, P.J. (1991). Changes in mood states during training in female and male college swimmers. *International Journal of Sports Medicine*, 12, 585-589.

Raglin, J.S., Sawamura, S., Alexiou, S., Hassmén, P., & Kenttä, G. (2000). Training practices and staleness in 13-18 year old swimmers: A cross-cultural study. *Pediatric Sports Medicine*, 12, 61-70.

Raglin, J.S., & Wilson, G. (2000). Overtraining and staleness in athletes. In Y.L. Hanin (Ed.), *Emotions in sports* (pp. 191-207). Champaign, IL: Human Kinetics.

Tschol, P., Junge, A., & Dvorak, J. (2008). The use of medication and nutritional supplements during FIFA World Cups 2002 and 2006. *British Journal of Sports Medicine*, 42, 725-730.

Urhausen, A., Kindermann, W. (2002) Diagnosis of overtraining: What tools do we have? *Sports Medicine* 32, 95-102.

van Mechelen, W. (1992). Running injuries: A review of epidemiological literature. *Sports Medicine*, 14(5), 320-335.

Verde, T., Thomas, S., & Shephard, R. (1992). Potential markers of heavy training in highly trained distance runners. *British Journal of Sports Medicine*, 26, 167-175.

Weir, K. (2011). The exercise effect. *APA Monitor*, 42(11), 49-52.

Wilmore, J.H., Costill, D.L., & Kenney, W.L. (2008). *Physiology of sport and exercise* (4th ed.). Champaign, IL: Human Kinetics.

Physical Functioning and Mental Health in Older Adults

Donald H. Paterson, PhD
University of Western Ontario, London, Ontario, Canada

Juan M. Murias, PhD
University of Western Ontario, London, Ontario, Canada

Chapter Outline

Editors' Introduction

This chapter provides an overview of the evidence that level of physical activity affects the mental health and physical functioning of older adults. It makes the case that routine activities of daily life in this age group are not adequate to alleviate the negative impact of aging and that more is better in terms of both intensity and amount of physical activity performed. Given the challenges presented by caring for aging populations, this timely chapter is essential reading for students, researchers, exercise professionals and those working in primary care and public health settings. This chapter provides practical, age-appropriate advice and guidelines for policy makers and professionals who seek to promote enhanced mental health as well as sustained physical functioning into older age via exercise programmes. The chapter has a very important message for everyone experiencing the aging process.

The baby boomer generation is now reaching 65 and life expectancy is increasing, leading to a rapidly increasing number of older adults. The expanding number of older adults combined with a relative birth dearth results in a staggering proportion of older adults. By 2050, older adults will make up an estimated 15% to 20% of the global population. Aging is characterised by loss of function, chronic diseases of aging and sedentary lifestyles. More than 50% of older adults do not meet the minimal guidelines for physical activity. Given these factors, for many, life expectancy now exceeds the ability to maintain function. For example, loss of aerobic cardiorespiratory fitness impinges on the available energy for daily activities and results in fatigue and further loss of function. Thus, with older age can come reduced health and quality of life, increased reliance on long-term care and greatly increased health care costs.

In developed countries health care for the older adult costs an estimated four times more than health care for the adult under age 65 yr. Many have warned that the increasing number and proportion of older adults challenge the sustainability of the health care system. Yet substantial research evidence shows that a relationship exists between greater levels of physical activity or exercise and disease prevention, compression of the period of morbidity, reduced risk of functional losses and maintenance of independence. In fact, among various factors related to population health, increased physical activity in the older population is estimated to have the greatest impact on public health. Evidence shows that a relationship exists between physical activity and mental health, physical health and independence (all of which are intertwined). This chapter reviews this evidence as well as the theory of the pathways or mechanisms through which exercise leads to benefits in the older adult. Practitioners need to promote physical activity to their patients and clients. The evidence in this chapter will help health professionals and those in the fitness industry enhance the mental health and functioning of older adults with whom they work. The analyses include applied examples of interventions that are relevant to older adults along with notes on some popular interventions that may be of little effect.

Although the first studies of exercise-training interventions were published in the early 1940s, the earliest studies of exercise training in older adults were not published until some 20 yr later. In fact, even as the early studies proceeded, concerns about the safety of older adults exercising as well as scepticism about the effectiveness and the trainability of exercise training in older adults. Bassey (1978) stated, "Vague fears that too much exercise will precipitate injury, catastrophic exhaustion, or overt illness bedevil the situation and have fostered disapproval of all but the mildest exertion" (p. 67). Thus, the earliest exercise trials used mild exercise and very slow progression. This resulted in little gain and led to the suggestion that older adults lose the ability to adapt to the stress of physical exercise. Just before 1980, studies showed that exercise-training programmes for older adults were effective in terms of physiological adaptations and health benefits. These studies included laboratory-based prescribed-exercise regimens that carefully measured physiological outcomes (e.g., Seals et al., 1984) as well as clinical trials or randomised controlled trials of exercise interventions in larger subject groups (e.g., Blumenthal et al., 1989; Cunningham et al., 1987).

Epidemiological studies have also contributed a great deal of the evidence of the relationship between physical activity and disease prevention (and loss of function). The pioneering work in leisure-time physical activity epidemiology was conducted by Morris and colleagues (1973) in the United Kingdom and Paffenbarger, Wing and Hyde (1978) in the United States. Their data showed that participation in moderate- to vigorous-intensity sport or fairly brisk walking are necessary in order to lower the risk of heart disease or death in older adults.

This chapter assesses the epidemiological and experimental (exercise-training interventions) research literature in order to provide evidence for the recommendations of the dose (amounts and types) of physical activity that healthy, community-dwelling older adults need to prevent disease, promote health and maintain function, well-being and independence into older age. For more in-depth reviews of the cited studies about physical activity for older adults, see reviews by Paterson, Jones and Rice (2007) and Paterson and Warburton (2010).

1   Physical Activity and Mortality

As reviewed in chapter 1, a large number of epidemiological studies unequivocally support that physical inactivity is a major risk factor and that physical activity or fitness is associated with a decreased risk of morbidity (e.g., cardiovascular disease, diabetes, colon cancer) and all-cause mortality. These studies have been influential in informing the physical activity guidelines for adults. This chapter analyzes these studies because they inform levels of physical activity

older adults need to prevent morbidity and early mortality. A number of studies by Morris and colleagues (published between 1973 and 1990) concluded that to achieve strikingly lower rates of heart disease or death for the older age group, the exercise dose needed to include occasional sport and fairly brisk walking (referred to as moderately vigorous activity). More leisurely walking (ordinary walking, walking to work) and activities such as yard work, gardening and household repairs were not associated with reduced risk of disease or death. A number of studies by Paffenbarger and colleagues (between 1978 and 1994) and Lee and colleagues (between 1995 and 2000) concluded that participating in moderately vigorous sport or a high volume of physical activity that included walking, stair climbing and sport was associated with a 30% lower risk of disease incidence or death, whereas participating in light sport or light activities such as walking, golfing and gardening did not reduce risk. These

KEY CONCEPTS

Prospective cohort epidemiological studies have provided overwhelming evidence of the effectiveness of physical activity in increasing active life expectancy and in preventing

- functional losses leading to loss of independence and well-being and, potentially, some aspects of cognitive losses and depression and
- disease (cardiovascular diseases, diabetes, some cancers) and all-cause mortality.

The dose of physical activity that is needed to achieve these benefits has been assessed and used to derive guidelines for physical activity for older adults. The consensus recommendations are as follows:

- Perform moderate- to vigorous-intensity aerobic activities (e.g., brisk walking or walking for exercise, some uphill walking or participation in aerobic sport) to enhance cardiorespiratory fitness.

- Perform a minimum of 150 min/wk of moderate-intensity activity that amounts to an energy expenditure of approximately 1000 kcal/wk (or ~90 min/wk of vigorous exercise).
- Gain additional benefits from adding 2 sessions/wk of muscle-strengthening activities (e.g., callisthenic exercises, resistance training).
- If balance and mobility are limitations, include balance-related activities (e.g., walking on uneven surfaces such as trails).
- Structured exercise-training programmes, usually consisting of 30 min/session of moderate- and vigorous-intensity exercise, have been shown to be effective and safe.
- It is possible that lower levels of activity may yield some health benefits. However, the guidelines all report that more is better.

studies suggested that at least 4200 kJ/wk (1000 kcal/wk; see "$\dot{V}O_2$max, Metabolic Equivalent and Units of Energy Expenditure $\dot{V}O_2$max") of moderately vigorous activity is needed to lower mortality. Paffenbarger and colleagues (1994) also commented that "it seems not too late to adopt favourable lifeway habits" (p. 864). Data showed that those who changed their physical activity habits by taking up moderately vigorous sport or substantial increases in energy expenditure showed a 30% reduction in risk compared with those who remained sedentary.

Lee, Hsieh and Paffenbarger (1995) concluded that "the inverse association between physical activity and mortality is related not so much to the exercise itself, but to the improved cardiorespiratory fitness that it induced" (p. 1184). When relative cardiorespiratory fitness increases, risk of both mortality and morbidity linearly decreases. Risk is reduced 25% in those who are moderately fit and 40% to 50% in those who are most fit (see figure 7.1, which shows average relative risk versus fitness percentile). Improvement in fitness is inversely related with mortality irrespective of the initial fitness of the individual. A change from unfit to fit (or an increase in fitness of 2 MET or $\dot{V}O_2$max of 7 ml·kg^{-1}·min^{-1}; see "$\dot{V}O_2$max, Metabolic Equivalent and Units of Energy Expenditure") was associated with 50% lower risk of morbidity and a 30% lower all-cause mortality (Blair et al., 1995).

A number of studies have focussed on older groups beyond age 70 yr. A 12 yr follow-up

study of men with a mean age of 68 yr noted that those who walked 1.6 to 3.2 km/day showed a lower all-cause mortality than did those who walked less than 1.6 km/day, and those who walked more than 3.2 km/day showed a 50% lower mortality rate (Hakim et al., 1998). Another study monitored 5 yr changes in physical activity of men with a mean age of 75 yr. Those who walked or cycled for 20 min more than 3 times/wk had an almost 50% lower risk of all-cause mortality, and those who moved from being sedentary to active, even at this older age, showed a nearly 25% reduction in risk (Bijnen et al., 1999).

In summary, the epidemiology of cardiorespiratory fitness shows that risk of morbidity and mortality has a strong inverse relationship with a midlife change in fitness. Taking up a more active lifestyle in older age also reduces risk of morbidity and mortality. The physical activity dose for these outcomes appears to be that which also enhances cardiorespiratory fitness. Moderate to moderately vigorous activity translates to approximately 50% to 60% of the maximal oxygen uptake (see "$\dot{V}O_2$max, Metabolic Equivalent and Units of Energy Expenditure") of average older adults, and a total energy expenditure of 4200 kJ/wk (1000 kcal/wk) translates to just over 3 h/wk of brisk walking. A number of studies indicate that intensity and duration of physical activity must exceed a threshold in order to reduce risk and note that ordinary walking, gardening and general housework were not associated with reduced risk of disease or death.

Some controversy exists regarding the dose of physical activity that results in benefit. In a large prospective cohort study of Taiwanese men and women, Wen et al. (2011) analysed data for the minimum amount of physical activity required for reduced mortality. Their data showed that 15 min/day (90 min/wk) of physical activity reduced the risk of all-cause mortality by 14%. Therefore, compared with the very inactive totally sedentary group, 90 min/wk (rather than the usual recommendation of 150-180 min/wk) was of health benefit. Nevertheless, even in that study more was better. Vigorous-intensity exercise yielded greater health benefits

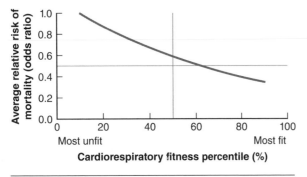

Figure 7.1 Cardiorespiratory fitness dose–response relationship with coronary heart disease and all-cause mortality from the consensus of a number of studies as reviewed in Paterson, Jones and Rice (2007).

Adapted from Paterson et al. 2007.

than did moderate-intensity exercise in terms of reducing all-cause mortality: 30 min/day of vigorous-intensity exercise yielded an almost 40% reduction in risk, whereas 30 min/day of moderate-intensity activity yielded somewhat less than a 20% reduction. Despite the debate about a threshold and the concept that accumulating small bouts of physical activity throughout the day does have some health benefit, studies show that moderate-intensity aerobic activity and a volume of 1000 kcal/wk reduce risk of morbidity and mortality by approximately 30% and that more is better.

2 Physical Activity, Functional Abilities, Independence and Well-Being Into Older Age

With age-related losses of cardiorespiratory fitness, muscle mass and strength, the average

---

$\dot{V}O_2$max, Metabolic Equivalent and Units of Energy Expenditure $\dot{V}O_2$max

$\dot{V}O_2$max (also maximal oxygen uptake or aerobic power) is the maximum capacity to transport and use oxygen during incremental exercise that progresses to volitional fatigue. This exercise is usually performed on a treadmill or cycle ergometer. $\dot{V}O_2$max is the standard measure of cardiorespiratory or cardiovascular fitness. $\dot{V}$ = volume per time (ventilation), O_2 = oxygen, max = maximum.

$\dot{V}O_2$max is expressed either as an absolute rate in litres of oxygen per minute (L/min) or as a relative rate in millilitres of oxygen per kilogram of body weight per minute ($ml \cdot kg^{-1} \cdot min^{-1}$). The latter expression is used to assess an individual's ability to perform exercises carrying his or her own body weight (e.g., walking, jogging, running). Average values for young males and females are approximately 45 and 38 $ml \cdot kg^{-1} \cdot min^{-1}$, respectively. $\dot{V}O_2$max declines by approximately 10% per decade such that by age 70 yr the $\dot{V}O_2$max of average men and women declines to 20 to 25 $ml \cdot kg^{-1} \cdot min^{-1}$.

METABOLIC EQUIVALENT

The metabolic equivalent (MET) is an expression of the energy cost of physical activities as multiples of resting metabolic rate. The reference resting metabolic rate (i.e., 1 MET; sitting quietly) is set by convention as 3.5 ml of $O_2 \cdot kg^{-1} \cdot min^{-1}$ (or 1 $kcal \cdot kg^{-1} \cdot h^{-1}$, or 4.184 $kJ \cdot kg^{-1} \cdot h^{-1}$). MET values are an index or ratio of the exercise metabolic rate relative to the resting 1 MET. Intensity values of various activities range from 0.9 (sleeping) to 18 (running at 17.5 km/h or a 5:31 min mile pace).

The term *MET* has been used in epidemiology and public health to provide general exercise thresholds and guidelines. Activities of less than 3 METs are classified as light intensity [e.g., walking at 4 km/h (2.5 miles/h) is 2.9 METs]. Activities of 3 to 6 METs are classified as moderate intensity [e.g., walking at 4.8 km/h (3 miles/h) is 3.3 METs and at 5.5 km/h (3.4 miles/h) is 3.6 METs; leisure cycling at (~10 miles/h) is ~4 METs]. Activities of greater than 6 METs are classified as vigorous (e.g., jogging is ~7 METs).

The concept of the MET minute can be used to quantify the total amount of physical activity in a way that is comparable across persons and types of activities. Thus, briskly walking at 5 km/h for 30 min (a moderate-intensity activity of 3.3 METs) accounts for about 100 MET minutes and is in this aspect equivalent to running at 10 km/h for 10 min (a vigorous-intensity activity of 10 MET). This way, the total accumulated effort expended in different activities over a period of time can be calculated. Health benefits of physical activity increase with increasing levels of activity and do not plateau until levels that are quite high.

KILOCALORIES PER MINUTE

An oxygen uptake ($\dot{V}O_2$) of 1 L/min is equivalent to an energy expenditure of approximately 5 kcal/min. This energy expenditure is also expressed as kilojoules per minute (1 kcal = 4.2 kJ).

older adult loses functional abilities to the point where activities of daily living (see "Activities of Daily Living and Instrumental Activities of Daily Living to Assess Functional Abilities in Older Adults") become too difficult. Mobility (walking) is a challenge, which can lead to loss of independence and reduced quality of life. Such reductions in health-related quality of life are associated with reduced general well-being (e.g., Muldoon et al., 1998; also see chapter 1 in this text). It appears that a $\dot{V}O_2$max of 15 ml·kg^{-1}·min^{-1} is the minimum level of cardiorespiratory fitness in those who remain independent and above some minimal level of functioning into old age (see Paterson, Jones & Rice, 2007). The decline in $\dot{V}O_2$max with age suggests that routine physical activity in that age group is not enough to prevent the loss of cardiorespiratory fitness. This section describes the relationship between fitness levels and the maintenance of functional abilities, independence and well-being into older age.

Fries (1980) stated that "insofar as frailty and dependence may be the result of loss of physical function, physical activity (or improved 'fitness') is one intervention which may reduce the years of dependent living and improve quality of life of older adults." As reviewed in Paterson, Jones and Rice (2007), a few cross-sectional studies in the late 1990s attested to this hypothesis. Reduced cardiorespiratory fitness and muscle strength were found to be associated with loss of function. Performance tests (e.g., time to rise from a lying to standing position or self-reported abilities in various activities such as walking or lifting objects) showed that cardiorespiratory fitness is directly related to disease outcomes and independently related to functional limitations. Relative to the low-fitness group, risk of functional limitations was reduced by 50% to 60% in the moderately fit group and by 70% in the very fit group. Ferrucci and colleagues (1999) performed annual follow-ups in a group with a mean age of 65 yr. The life expectancy of those involved in moderate and vigorous activities was increased by 3 to 6 yr compared with those involved in low levels of activity, and the delay in the onset of disability increased disability-free

Activities of Daily Living and Instrumental Activities of Daily Living to Assess Functional Abilities in Older Adults

Activities of daily living (ADL) are the daily self-care activities that individuals routinely need to perform in order to care for themselves and maintain functional independence. A person's ability or inability to perform ADL provides a measure of the functional status of the person and of whether they have limitations or disabilities. Basic ADL consist of the following self-care tasks:

- Personal hygiene and grooming
- Dressing and undressing
- Self-feeding
- Functional transfers (e.g., getting out of bed, getting on or off the toilet)
- Bowel and bladder management

- Ambulation (i.e., walking without use of an assistive device such as a walker, cane, or crutches)

Instrumental ADL are not necessary for fundamental functioning but they allow an individual to live independently in a community. Instrumental ADL include the following:

- Performing housework
- Taking medications as prescribed
- Managing money
- Shopping for groceries or clothing
- Using a telephone or other form of communication
- Using technology (as applicable)
- Using transportation in the community

years by 2 yr in those in the more active quartile compared with those in the lower activity quartile. Their data confirmed a compression of morbidity, as originally proposed by Fries (1980).

Paterson and colleagues (2004) recognised that loss of independence is a major concern of older adults and a major health care cost and thus designed a prospective study to determine factors related to loss of independence. The cohort studied was initially healthy community-dwelling men and women of mean age 70 yr. In an 8 yr follow-up, initial cardiorespiratory fitness ($\dot{V}O_2$max) was a significant variable in those who became dependent compared with those who remained independent. Those who were initially in the moderately and highly fit groups showed a 30% and 50% lower risk of becoming dependent, respectively, compared with the low-fit group. Thus, cardiorespiratory fitness was an independent determinant of becoming dependent in older age. Further, data did not show a relationship between the habitual levels of leisure-time physical activity of this study group and independence or dependence. This finding was consistent with the data of others that habitual activity or general leisure activities did not alter the odds of dependent living in older adults, although routine exercise and consistent walking did (see Paterson, Jones & Rice, 2007). Thus, only activities of higher intensity and sustained duration—activities that would increase cardiorespiratory fitness—were effective in maintaining functional abilities for independent living and resultant well-being.

In a systematic review of the literature on the relationship between physical activity and functional outcomes in older community-dwelling adults, Paterson and Warburton (2010) summarised 35 prospective cohort (epidemiological) studies representing data from approximately 84,000 participants. In these studies, physical activity levels (usually assessed by questionnaire) were related to outcomes (also assessed by self-report but in some cases by batteries of physical performance tests) of impairment or functional limitations, disability or loss of independence. With regard to the outcomes of disability in activ-

ities of daily living (ADL) or instrumental ADL (see "Activities of Daily Living and Instrumental Activities of Daily Living to Assess Functional Abilities in Older Adults"), the consensus was that higher levels of physical activity reduced the risk of an outcome related to functional limitation or disability by 50% (figure 7.2). Although it is difficult to quantify the effective dose of physical activity, these studies indicated moderate to high levels were necessary to induce benefit, and that an effective activity is walking at a speed described as an intention to exercise for more than 1.6 km (1 mile)/session, walking 1 h/day or walking for exercise 20 min/day 3 days/wk.

From the review of Paterson and Warburton (2010) it appears that moderate activity was effective in preventing declines or limitations in performance and reduced well-being. However, many of the studies the physical activities that substantially reduced risk of functional limitations were described as vigorous or as exercise (figure 7.2). Only one study showed similar substantial reductions in functional limitations in those who had been inactive but had taken up moderately vigorous activity. From the review of Paterson and Warburton (2010) an example of an effective dose was described as

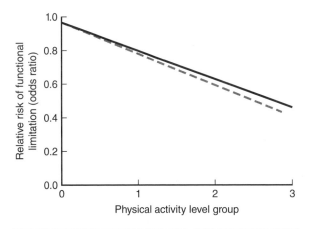

Figure 7.2   Relative risk (odds ratio) of functional limitation in relation to physical activity level in older adults. Dashed line represents data from prospective cohort studies with an outcome of disability in activities of daily living and instrumental activities of daily living. Solid line represents data from prospective cohort studies with an outcome of functional limitations.

Adapted from Paterson and Warburton 2010.

vigorous exercise of greater than 30 min 3 times/ wk, exercise at high aerobic levels, exercising 3 times/wk or more or often walking for exercise. Overall, these prospective studies showed that regular participation in aerobic physical activities reduced risk of functional limitations and disability in older age by 30% to 50%. It appears that reduction in functional limitations and disability in older groups is achieved through physical activity (including walking and other moderate-intensity aerobic activities) totalling 150 min/ wk or moderately vigorous exercise of 30 min 3 times/wk. In an intervention study of sedentary 70- to 89-yr-olds, Pahor and colleagues (2006) showed that an exercise programme of 150 min/ wk of moderate-intensity walking plus strength and balance exercises reduced major mobility disability by 30% and, thus, helped participants maintain independent living.

3   Physical Activity, Cognitive Function and Mental Health in Older Adults

Also of major concern to older adults is declining cognitive function. Does a physically active lifestyle preserve cognitive function into older age, and in older age can a fitness programme result in enhanced cognitive function? Paterson and Warburton (2010) conducted a systematic review of associations between physical activity and cognitive function outcome measures in studies up to 2008. Results convincingly showed that the risk of dementia and Alzheimer's disease was reduced in the physically active groups (see also chapter 10). A review by Voss and colleagues (2011) showed that epidemiological and prospective studies generally support the position that physical activity and perhaps aerobic fitness prevent the onset of various types of dementia and likely have a role in preserving a healthy brain and optimal cognitive functioning.

Extensive literature espouses the cognitive and mental health and benefits of physical activity (see chapter 1), particularly the positive outcomes of exercise interventions in the treat-

ment of depression (see chapter 9). A recent study by Pasco and colleagues (2011) examined the relationship between habitual physical activity and the incidence of depressive and anxiety disorders in older men and women in the general population. The results provided further evidence that higher levels of physical activity are protective against the risk of developing depressive and anxiety disorders. Proposed physiological mechanisms include increases in neurotransmitters (specifically serotonin and noradrenaline) or psychosocial advantages of physical activity as a scheduled productive activity, social activity and benefit to self-efficacy. Nevertheless, to date studies of physical activity and the reduction of risk of depression and anxiety in older people have not established a body of evidence regarding the types or dose (i.e., intensity or volume) of physical activity needed.

The key concepts of the scientific evidence of the benefits of physical activity for older adults are summarised in the following Physical Activity Guidelines for Older Adults box.

4   Physical Activity Guidelines for Older Adults

The United States, United Kingdom and Canada as well as other countries and the World Health Organisation (WHO) have published physical activity guidelines for older adults. Although the messages accompanying these guidelines do not usually mention increased well-being and mental health, improvement in these elements is typically consequential to improvements in physical health and functioning (see chapter 2). The content of the various guideline statements is similar, although the degree of detail in the messages that accompany each guideline varies. Canada's Physical Activity Guidelines for Older Adults are displayed in the following highlight box.

It is necessary to translate what moderate and vigorous intensity may mean for older adults (see "Evidence to Practice"). In the epidemiological studies from which the recommendations were derived and in which the average age of the study population was approximately 45 yr,

Canadian Physical Activity Guidelines

- To achieve health benefits and improve functional abilities adults aged 65 years and older should accumulate at least 150 minutes of moderate to vigorous-intensity aerobic physical activity per week, in bouts of 10 minutes or more.

- It is beneficial to add muscle and bone strengthening activities using major muscle groups, at least 2 days per week.

- Those with poor mobility should perform physical activities to enhance balance and prevent falls.

- More physical activity provides greater health benefits.

The new guidelines emphasise the following:

- Perform 150 min/wk (more is better) of moderate- to vigorous-intensity aerobic activities in bouts of at least 10 min. WHO, U.S. and U.K. guidelines also suggest an alternative of 75 min/wk of vigorous-intensity activity. WHO, U.S. and U.K. guidelines suggest increasing moderate-intensity aerobic activity to 300 min/wk or engaging in 150 min/wk of vigorous-intensity activity or a combination of both types of activity (preferably spread throughout the week; U.K. example: 30 min on ≥5 days/wk) for additional health benefits.

- Add muscle- and bone-strengthening activities at least 2 times/wk. WHO, U.S. and U.K. guidelines agree and suggest per-

forming muscle-strengthening activities (major muscle groups, moderate to high intensity) at least 2 days/wk for additional health benefits.

- Those with poor mobility should perform physical activities that enhance balance and prevent falls. WHO, U.S. and UK guidelines suggest performing these activities at least 2 days/wk.

- Flexibility or stretching exercises offer no known health benefits. Individuals should devote time and energy to the other aspects of fitness.

The full guidelines and notes on their development are available at the following websites:

Canada: www.phac-aspc.gc.ca/hp-ps/hl-mvs/pag-gap/index-home-accueil-eng.php

United Kingdom: www.bhfactive.org.uk/home/index.html

United States: www.cdc.gov/physicalactivity/everyone/guidelines/index.html

Australia: www.health.gov.au/internet/main/publishing.nsf/Content/health-pubhlth-strateg-phys-act-guidelines

New Zealand: www.moh.govt.nz/moh.nsf/indexmh/activity-guidelines

WHO: www.who.int/dietphysicalactivity/factsheet_recommendations/en/index.html

Reprinted, by permission, from Canadian Society for Exercise Physiology, 2011, *Physical activity guidelines for older adults* (Ottawa, Canada: Canadian Society of Exercise Physiology).

activities that met the criteria for being moderate intensity ranged from 4 to 4.5 METs and vigorous-intensity activities were near 6 METs (refer to "$\dot{V}O_2$max", Metabolic Equivalent and Units of Energy Expenditure" for a definition and explanation of MET). An MET is an absolute intensity (a standard energy cost per kilogram of body mass); this intensity needs to be translated to a relative intensity to express the energy cost as a

proportion of an individual's maximum capacity. Given the age-related decline in cardiorespiratory fitness, a 20% to 25% decline in $\dot{V}O_2$max) might be expected between age 45 and 70 yr. Thus, 4 to 4.5 METs in a 45-yr-old would translate to 3.2 to 3.6 METs for moderate intensity in older adults and 6 METs would translate to approximately 4.0 to 4.5 METs for vigorous intensity. Thus, older adults of average fitness at ages

Table 7.1 Energy Cost Equivalents and Relative Intensity of Moderate- and Vigorous-Intensity Walking Speeds for Older Adults

Physical activity description	Moderate-intensity walking	Vigorous-intensity walking
Speed	4.8 km/h (3 miles/h)	6.4 km/h (4 miles/h)
Energy cost in metabolic equivalent	3.3	4.2
Energy cost in $\dot{V}O_2$ units (ml·kg−1·min−1)	11.6	14.7
Energy cost in $\dot{V}O_2$ units for 60 or 80 kg individual (ml/min)	700-900	880-1,180
Energy cost in kcal/min	3.5-4.5	4.4-5.9
Relative intensity* (%$\dot{V}O_2$max)	46-58	59-74
Total energy expenditure with 150 min of activity (kcal)	525-625	660-885

*Percentage $\dot{V}O_2$max for older adults with a $\dot{V}O_2$max of 20 to 25 ml·kg^{-1}·min^{-1}.

65 to 70 can achieve moderate and vigorous intensities with walking paces (described in the literature as brisk walking, fast walking or walking for exercise). Table 7.1 shows the MET cost of different walking speeds for typical older adults and the relative intensity of these walking speeds. Note that in the case of older adults the scale of what is considered moderate and what is vigorous is narrow; vigorous does not equal twice the intensity of moderate. In younger adults 75 min of vigorous exercise may equal the energy expenditure of 150 min of moderate exercise, whereas in older adults more than one half of the volume of moderate exercise is needed (e.g., 90 min of vigorous exercise may approximate 150 min of moderate exercise).

5 Aerobic Exercise-Training Interventions

Reductions in aerobic performance throughout the life span have been well documented and have been associated with age-related decreases in physical functional capacity, loss of independence and detriment of cognitive function (Paterson, Jones & Rice, 2007). As noted earlier, Paterson and colleagues (2004) showed in an 8 yr follow-up study that a higher initial $\dot{V}O_2$max) in independently living older men and women reduced the odds ratio of becoming dependent by 14% for each millilitre of oxygen per kilo-gram of body weight per minute (~50%/MET). As such, these data suggest that maintaining or gaining a high maximal aerobic power is an important component in healthy aging.

Although an early training study in older adults failed to show significant changes in fitness, subsequent studies including exercise-training programmes of higher relative intensity have consistently shown successful responses in older adults. Longer-term (~6-12 mo duration) training studies in older adults have yielded improvements in $\dot{V}O_2$max) ranging from 15% to 29%, and even shorter-term (~9-12 wk duration) exercise-training interventions have produced increases in $\dot{V}O_2$max) ranging from approximately 6% to 30% (see Paterson, Jones & Rice, 2007, for a review). Importantly, the percentage increase in $\dot{V}O_2$max) in older adults has been reported to be similar to that observed in young individuals even when older and young adults are directly compared.

5.1 Duration and Intensity of the Training Programme

Several studies have shown the importance of higher exercise intensities in the improvement of fitness. For example, Seals and colleagues (1984) demonstrated that a 12 mo training programme produced an increase in $\dot{V}O_2$max) of approximately 30% in men and women between

60 and 70 yr of age. Interestingly, a programme of relatively low intensity during the first 6 mo induced a 12% increase in $\dot{V}O_2$max), whereas an intervention of higher relative intensity (~75% of $\dot{V}O_2$max)) during the following 6 mo resulted in a further 18% improvement. The authors attributed the success to first the volume (at least 3 times/wk) and then the intensity of the programme.

Kohrt and colleagues (1991) also showed that older men and women (aged 60-71 yr) had similar average improvements in $\dot{V}O_2$max) (~20%) in response to 9 to 12 mo of training performed 3 times/wk at 70% to 80% of heart rate reserve. The improvements were similar in those with the lowest and the highest initial $\dot{V}O_2$max) as well as in the youngest and oldest participants. This means that neither initial fitness level nor age (at least within this age range) determined the rate of adaptation. Importantly, improvements in $\dot{V}O_2$max) brought measures of cardiovascular function in this group to a level equivalent to a person 20 yr younger.

Hagberg and colleagues (1989) conducted another successful endurance-training programme in older men and women aged 70 to 79 yr. Participants demonstrated a 22% increase in $\dot{V}O_2$max) after 6 mo of training 3 times/wk at approximately 70% of $\dot{V}O_2$max). Subjects in this study mostly walked fast in order to achieve the target training intensity, which led the authors to speculate that fast walking can substantially improve $\dot{V}O_2$max). However, in the younger old, this type of activity may not be enough to reach the level of stress required for $\dot{V}O_2$max) to increase. Using a similar training protocol, Spina and colleagues (1993) confirmed that both older men and women undergo a similar increase in $\dot{V}O_2$max) after endurance exercise training (19% in men and 22% in women).

Short-term endurance-training interventions have also been shown to be effective in improving cardiovascular fitness in older populations. Although Gass and colleagues (2004) reported significant but rather modest improvements (6%-8%) in $\dot{V}O_2$max) in response to a 12 wk endurance-training programme consisting of 30 min sessions 3 times/wk at either 50% or 70% $\dot{V}O_2$max), larger increases in $\dot{V}O_2$max) ranging from 6% to 30% have been shown in response to short-term endurance-training programmes. For example, studies have shown increments in $\dot{V}O_2$max) of approximately 20% after 12 wk of training performed 3 times/wk at an intensity that would elicit approximately 75% of maximum heart rate (Beere et al., 1999) or 100% of heart rate at the anaerobic threshold (Pogliaghi et al., 2006). More recently, Murias, Kowalchuk and Paterson reported similar increases in $\dot{V}O_2$max) of approximately 20% in older women (2010a) and approximately 30% in older men (2010b) in response to a 12 wk endurance-training programme performed 3 times/wk at approximately 70% of $\dot{V}O_2$max) and during which training intensity was adjusted every third week to account for improvements in $\dot{V}O_2$max).

An important aspect to consider is that the studies that show the largest increases in $\dot{V}O_2$max) in response to endurance training were conducted using training intensities that could be considered at least moderately high for this type of training (~50%-70% $\dot{V}O_2$max)). Studies in which the training intensity was lower have found more modest changes in $\dot{V}O_2$max) that range from approximately 0% to 7%. Overall, these investigations show that training at relatively light intensity results in small improvements in cardiorespiratory fitness, mainly in those with low initial levels of fitness and only over the initial period of the programme, whilst they have low levels of fitness.

Collectively, these studies demonstrate that older adults, at least up to the age of approximately 75 yr, respond to endurance-training programmes in a way that is similar to that of their younger counterparts and that both long-term and short-term programmes can result in large increases in $\dot{V}O_2$max) that would decrease the likelihood of becoming dependent. Additionally, the available data suggest that higher-intensity training programmes are more likely than lower-intensity programmes to produce improvements in cardiorespiratory fitness.

5.2   Mechanisms of Adaptation

Some studies exploring the physiological mechanisms underlying adaptations to endurance training in older adults noted peripheral (i.e., muscle increases in the activity of aerobic enzymes) (Meredith et al., 1989; Suominen, Heikkinen & Parkatti, 1977) or central (i.e., cardiac function) changes (Ehsani et al., 1991). Makrides, Heigenhauser and Jones (1990) showed that after 12 wk of training the majority of the gain in $\dot{V}O_2$max) in a group of older men was explained by increases in central factors of cardiac output and stroke volume. A small portion of the change was attributed to peripheral factors indicated by a widened arterial–venous O_2 difference (a-vO_2diff), indicating extraction of the available oxygen at the muscle. Ehsani and colleagues (1991) also reported left ventricular heart enlargement with increases in stroke volume and cardiac ejection fraction in older men after 1 yr of endurance training.

Classic studies by Spina and colleagues (1993, 1996) attributed two thirds of the increase in $\dot{V}O_2$max) in older men after 12 mo of endurance training to larger cardiac output. However, only changes in a-vO_2diff (likely due to peripheral adaptations) with no increments in cardiac output explained the similar percentage increase in $\dot{V}O_2$max) observed in older women. Murias and colleagues (2010a,b) further demonstrated this sex-dependent type of adaptation to increases in $\dot{V}O_2$max) in the older population. These short-term (12 wk) endurance-training programmes confirmed that the majority of the increase in $\dot{V}O_2$max) in older men is explained by central adaptations (approximately two thirds of an approximately 30% increase in $\dot{V}O_2$max) was explained by a larger maximal cardiac output and stroke volume), that this adaptation occurs very quickly (~3 wk) and that it progressively continues throughout the duration of the programme (Murias et al., 2010b). Additionally, the training-induced increase (~20%) in $\dot{V}O_2$max in the older women was explained by a widened a-vO_2diff (Murias et al., 2010a). An interesting aspect of this study is that although a widened maximal a-vO_2diff increased $\dot{V}O_2$max) in the older women, the absolute level of a-vO_2diff in the older women was lower than that observed in the older men. The lack of central adaptations in older women together with a levelling off of benefit or ceiling effect for peripheral adaptations could explain the plateau-like response in the increase of $\dot{V}O_2$max) after 9 wk of training that was not present in the older men. Interestingly, in a cross-sectional study of men and women with a mean age of 69 yr, age-related decline of left ventricular compliance, or the increased stiffness of the cardiac muscle, was found in the sedentary group but not in endurance-trained masters athletes (Arbab-Zadeh et al., 2004). This could indicate that chronic adaptations to prolonged exercise training may prevent the decline in fitness even in older women.

Overall, despite the evidence of increases in $\dot{V}O_2$max) in response to training in older men and women, evidence strongly supports that cardiac adaptations (predominantly central, although peripheral as well) are a determinant for increasing $\dot{V}O_2$max) in older men. However, peripheral muscle adaptations seem more important in older women. As such, exercise-training programmes should consider these differential mechanisms of adaptation and thus include activities specific to the muscle groups used in ADL in older women (e.g., emphasis on walking or jogging exercise). However, older men may benefit from more generalised exercise protocols (e.g., cycling, swimming, rowing).

Positive exercise-training adaptations have also been observed in groups of octogenarians. However, the magnitude of the adaptations is suggested to be smaller compared with that of older individuals in their 60s and 70s. $\dot{V}O_2$max) increased between 12% and 15%. Evans and colleagues (2005) showed that a 10 to 12 mo programme in which a group (mean age 80 yr) performed various modes of aerobic activity at 60% to 75% $\dot{V}O_2$max) with progressive increases of intensity increased $\dot{V}O_2$max by 15%. Ehsani and colleagues (2003) showed in octogenarians (men and women; mean age 83 yr) a 14% increase in $\dot{V}O_2$max) that was explained by gains in stroke volume and cardiac output and no widening of a-vO$_2$diff after 1 yr of training. Spina and colleagues (2004) reported no changes in the volume of blood filling the ventricle of the heart during diastole (diastolic filling) or the ability of the ventricule to eject the blood (left ventricular function) related to the larger (12%) $\dot{V}O_2$max) in a group of frail older men and women (mean age 78 yr). In this study, the control group had a 7% reduction in $\dot{V}O_2$max). Although the results from studies in the older old suggest that an age limit might exist for cardiovascular adaptations—considering the more pronounced reductions in $\dot{V}O_2$max) that occur after the fifth decade of life and the need for older adults to keep a minimum functional fitness—avoiding further decreases in $\dot{V}O_2$max) may be critical even if the improvements are not as pronounced as those noted in groups of younger old individuals.

6   Strength-Training Interventions

Starting at approximately 30 yr of age, strength declines at a rate of approximately 10% to 15% per decade. As with cardiovascular fitness, this decline is more pronounced after the fifth decade of life and appears to increase with severity after age 65 yr (Paterson, Jones & Rice, 2007). This reduction in strength is mainly caused by the loss of muscle mass (sarcopenia). Another detrimental change observed with age is a reduction in contractile speed. The combined reductions in strength and speed may severely affect functional capacity in older adults. Thus, the reduction in power (strength × velocity of movement) in the elderly may be double that of the strength loss alone (Macaluso & De Vito, 2004). The loss of power (rather than the loss of strength alone) is more closely related to ADL and loss of independence (Bassey et al., 1992; Miszko et al., 2003).

Importantly, the skeletal muscles of older adults do not seem to lose the ability to adapt in response to resistance-training programmes. In fact, the responses to these programmes are similar or even superior to those observed in young adults (Macaluso & De Vito, 2004). As pointed out in the meta-analysis by Peterson and colleagues (2010), evidence clearly indicates that muscle weakness is a reversible cause of disability and that older adults are probably likely to benefit the most from resistance-training programmes.

Early studies on the effect of resistance training in older adults were conservative in terms of intensity and exercise prescription (Granacher et al., 2011). Research starting in the late 1980s showed that higher-intensity [~80% of 1 maximal repetition (RM)] resistance-training programmes are safe and effective (Fiatarone et al., 1990; Frontera et al., 1988). The 1998 American College of Sports Medicine (ACSM) stand (Mazzeo et al., 1998) concluded that the capacity to adapt to resistance-training exercise is well preserved in older men and women but did not indicate specific training routines. The 2002 ACSM stand (Kraemer et al., 2002) recommended resistance-exercise progression models for healthy older adults. It suggested the use of both single-joint (e.g., biceps curl) and multijoint (e.g., lifting a weight from the floor and up over the head) movements, slow to moderate movement and 1 to 3 sets per exercise at 60% to 80% 1RM for 8 to 12 repetitions. Furthermore, it suggested that resistance-training programmes should include light to moderate (40%-60% 1RM) high-velocity movements for 6 to 10 repetitions (or 10-15 repetitions for endurance). The stand also recommended gradual overload, varied and specific exercises and adequate recovery times during and between exercise sessions.

A recent meta-analysis of resistance-training studies in older men and women in which training intensities ranged from 40% to 90% 1RM showed an approximately 25% increase in upper-body strength and an approximately 30% increase in lower-body strength (Peterson et al., 2010). Importantly, the study suggested that when the training intensities were grouped as less than 60% 1RM, 60% to 69% 1RM, 70% to 79% 1RM and greater than 80% 1RM, the higher-intensity resistance-exercise programmes were superior for improving strength. In this regard, most studies suggest that moderate- to heavy-intensity resistance exercises (>60% 1RM) are necessary to optimise improvements in strength and that exercising 2 days/wk is as beneficial as 3 days/wk given that the intensity of exercise is similar (de Vos et al., 2005; Fatouros et al., 2005; Seynnes et al., 2004). Indeed, it has been shown that even 1 resistance-exercise session/wk can improve muscle strength (Taaffe et al., 1999). Although high-intensity resistance training is well tolerated even by frail older adults (Sullivan et al., 2007), older adults beginning with this type of programme would benefit from a progressive resistance overload approach in order to minimise the risks of injuries (Harris et al., 2004).

As pointed out earlier, the age-related decrease in power could double the actual decrease in muscle strength. Importantly, ADL often require power. According to Granacher and colleagues (2011), if the ability to produce force rapidly is reduced in a fall-risk situation (e.g., an unexpected stop while standing in a moving bus), then the capacity to regain balance will be compromised and the likelihood of a fall increases. In this context, high-velocity resistance training becomes more relevant. Miszko and colleagues (2003) examined the effects of a 16 wk strength-training or power-training intervention (3 times/wk) on maximal strength and peak power of the leg extensors in community-dwelling older adults (mean age 73 yr). The training intensity in the strength training group increased from 50% to 70% of 1RM by week 8 and was further increased and maintained at 80% of 1RM for the remainder of the study. The power-training group exercised at the same intensity as the strength-training group for the first 8 wk and then the training programme was changed to 3 sets of 6 to 8 repetitions at 40% of 1RM at the highest possible speed. The results showed that although both programmes were equally effective in improving maximal strength, power training was more effective than strength training in improving whole-body physical function (measured using a scale of physical functional

performance that evaluated 16 activities that involved the lower body, upper body, balance, coordination and endurance). Similarly, Fielding and colleagues (2002) compared the effects of 16 wk low-velocity and high-velocity resistance-training programmes. They showed that the strength of the leg extensors increased in both training groups by approximately 35% and that leg-press peak muscle power increased significantly more in the high-velocity group (97%) compared with the low-velocity group (45%).

It has been proposed that eccentric resistance-training programmes are well suited for older adults because they can handle high loads at low energetic costs (Granacher et al., 2011). The available data show that older adults can obtain substantial strength gains at a relatively low cardiovascular cost (Paterson, Jones & Rice, 2007). However, limitations of this type of training are that it requires special training equipment (e.g., an isokinetic device) and supervision by qualified personnel (Granacher et al., 2011) and increases the likelihood of injury to muscle, tendon and joints (Paterson, Jones & Rice, 2007). Nevertheless, proper supervision and careful progression should minimise these concerns. More controlled studies are required before guidelines for this type of programme can be established (Paterson, Jones & Rice, 2007).

Despite the demonstrated improvements in strength and power with resistance-training programmes in older adults and the improvement on tests of physical performance related to lifting, some question whether these gains are transferable to a range of functional outcomes and, specifically, to the maintenance of functional independence. Indeed Latham and colleagues (2004) concluded from their review that the effect on outcomes of disability is not clear. One approach to using resistance exercise to improve functional abilities has been to wear a weighted vest (e.g., an additional 10% of body weight) while performing callisthenic exercises that mimic various ADL (e.g., rising from a chair or climbing stairs).

Although studies of strength training have generally examined changes in strength and power, some have also looked at changes in cardiorespiratory fitness $\dot{V}O_2$max. Changes in $\dot{V}O_2$max in men and women in their 60s and 70s in response to programmes of 9 to 24 wk in duration generally range from 0 to less than 10% (see Paterson, Jones & Rice, 2007). Other studies have compared combined aerobic and strength training with aerobic training alone. Increases in $\dot{V}O_2$max have generally been similar for the two programmes; some differences have been found in other physiological adaptations. Recent evidence has shown that a resistance-training programme combined with aerobic training has a greater effect on functional outcomes (Davidson et al., 2009). Thus, resistance training complements the benefits of aerobic exercise and is a recommended adjunct to the physical activity programme of older adults.

7 Exercise-Training Interventions and Cognitive Function

Although cognitive function declines with age, some evidence shows that physically active older adults are less likely than their sedentary counterparts to develop Alzheimer's disease and other forms of dementia (see also chapter 10). Larson and colleagues (2006) studied 1,740 men and women over the age of 65 yr who did not have cognitive impairment. After an average follow-up period of 6.2 yr, 158 individuals developed Alzheimer's dementia. The incidence rate of Alzheimer's disease was significantly higher for those who exercised fewer than 3 times/wk (19.7/1,000 person years) compared with those who exercised more than 3 times/ wk (13.0/1,000 person years) and performed different types of physical activities (i.e., walking, hiking, bicycling, aerobics, swimming, water aerobics or weight training) for at least 15 min/ session. This suggests that exercise interventions may be useful in preventing or slowing age-related decline in cognitive function. As expressed in the ACSM stand of 1998 (Mazzeo et al., 1998), the underlying rationale that justifies this type of intervention is that the brain of older

adults operates under more hypoxic conditions due to age-related reductions in cardiovascular performance and that exercise could reverse this situation. However, even though some studies have shown positive effects of exercise training on cognitive function in the elderly, data on this topic are still equivocal.

Erickson and Kramer (2009) reported that 6 mo of aerobic training (walking) in a group of older adults resulted in improvements in aerobic fitness as well as enhanced executive function (as shown by task switching, stopping and selective attention tasks) compared with the control group that performed stretching and toning activities. Despite these positive effects, the intervention did not change other cognitive tasks that involved nonexecutive processes such as processing speed. The authors concluded that 6 mo of moderate aerobic exercise could reverse some of the age-related decline in cognitive function and that the brains of older adults still retain the plasticity required to improve performance of executive processes. Similarly, Hawkins, Kramer and Capaldi (1992) studied older adults who were randomised into an aerobic exercise group or a waitlist control. In this study, participants were tested with a series of single and dual auditory- and visual-perception tasks before and after the 10 wk aerobic exercise programme. Only the individuals in the aerobic-training group showed significant improvement in dual-task performance. Both groups displayed similar improvements in single-task performance.

Muscari and colleagues (2010) reported that healthy older adults undertaking endurance-exercise training for 1 yr showed a reduction in age-related cognitive decline as assessed by the Mini Mental State Examination. The data showed that the control group had a significant decrease in Mini Mental State Examination score compared with the exercise-training group. Additionally, the odds ratio of having a stable cognitive status after 1 yr was greater in the older adults who performed aerobic exercise than in the control group. The authors speculated that some of the mechanisms that mediate the beneficial effects of exercise on cognitive function might include increases in cerebral blood flow and enhanced production of neurotransmitters and neurotrophic and angiotrophic substances such as brain-derived neurotrophic factor, insulin-like growth factor-1 and vascular endothelial growth factor.

A recent meta-analysis (Angevaren et al., 2008) highlighted the positive effects of exercise training on cognitive function. However, it also pointed out that not all of its types of cognitive function showed clear evidence of a positive adaptation in response to exercise interventions. The meta-analysis showed that 8 out of 11 studies reported an increase in aerobic fitness of approximately 14% in the aerobic-exercise intervention group and that this gain coincided with improvements in cognitive function (Angevaren et al., 2008). The largest improvements in cognitive function were related to the areas of motor function (effect size 1.17), auditory attention (effect size 0.52) and delayed memory functions (effect size 0.50; this result is based on a single study). Importantly, this meta-analysis also showed that the effects for cognitive speed (speed at which information is processed) and visual attention were modest (effect size 0.26 for both). Thus, although aerobic exercise had significant effects on some subcategories of cognition, some comparisons yielded no significant results.

In a recent systematic review (Snowden et al., 2011) of the literature regarding the effects of physical activity and exercise-intervention trials on cognitive function in older adults, an expert panel concluded that although some evidence of exercise-induced benefit was not sufficient to assert that physical activity or exercise improves cognition in older adults. Nevertheless, it appears from the overview of the present literature on exercise and cognitive function that aerobic fitness has the capacity to prevent cognitive decline. This suggests the need for physical activities that improve fitness, such as moderately vigorous exercise-training programmes.

Implications for Practice

- It is not too late to start. Improvements in cardiorespiratory fitness ($\dot{V}O_2$max) have been observed in both men and women aged 65 to 79 yr as well as in groups of octogenarians (aged >80 yr).
- Exercise intensity is an important element in the dose response to exercise training. Training studies have generally used exercise intensities in the range of 50% to 70% of the individual's $\dot{V}O_2$max. The more vigorous programmes show greater increases in cardiorespiratory fitness (20% increase in $\dot{V}O_2$max). This level of activity has also been described as a percentage of age-adjusted heart rate reserve (e.g., 75%)
- Short-term (~12 wk) exercise-training programmes are effective in increasing $\dot{V}O_2$max. Therefore, although being physically active is a lifelong pursuit, it is possible to quickly improve fitness and perhaps maintain the gains over the long term.
- The physiological adaptations to exercise differ in men and women. In men the emphasis is on central adaptations (i.e., heart), and in women the emphasis is on peripheral adaptations (i.e., specific muscles used). Thus, it is particularly advisable for women to tailor the exercise programme to activities of daily living (essential mobility).
- Older men and women adapt to resistance training with gains in muscle strength and power. The more vigorous programmes in which resistance exercises exceed 60% of 1RM are the most effective.
- Exercise training may be effective in preserving some aspects of cognitive function. It appears that moderate- to vigorous-intensity exercise may be most effective because the changes in cognitive function may be related to the improved fitness or physiological adaptations produced by higher-intensity exercise.

In summary, some of the data reported in the literature tentatively suggest a cause–effect relationship between better fitness and improved cognition. However, more intervention studies seem necessary to further clarify the relationship between fitness status and training protocols (i.e., type of training, intensity and duration) and aspects of cognitive function. "Implications for Practice" summarises key concepts for exercise recommendations for older adults gleaned from the cardiorespiratory- and resistance-training intervention studies.

8 Exercise Programmes for Older Adults

How should one start a programme? Is it safe to exercise? Should one seek medical clearance? In general, the answer to these questions is not clear. Widespread use of the Physical Activity Readiness Questionnaire (PAR-Q; see www. CSEP.ca/home/publications) is one approach for screening out those who should seek medical advice before starting an exercise programme. However, the PAR-Q notes that it is designed for those up to age 69 yr and that older adults who are not used to being active should check with their doctor. Given the risks of inactivity, another view is that those who plan to remain inactive should be the ones to consult their physician! A newer version of the PAR-Q that is in press is somewhat more detailed and proceeds through a number of steps that may screen a large number of cases that previously were screened out. Another approach for healthy community-dwelling older adults is to start slowly (e.g., start with 10 min of continuous walking and increase to 30 min and then over a few weeks increase to brisk walking or a moderate intensity before attempting vigorous exercise or greater volume). That said, although a number of authors suggest slow progression in both aerobic- and resistance-

EVIDENCE TO PRACTICE

Epidemiological data and experimental studies of exercise interventions provide the evidence base to inform practice

- in the realms of health and mental health promotion of physical activity,
- in health professions in recommending exercise,
- in the fitness industry in prescribing and programming exercise for older adults, and
- for older adults to adopt lifestyles that include effective physical activity.

What is the appropriate aerobic exercise intensity for older adults?

- For those of average cardiorespiratory fitness for their age, moderate-intensity exercise is achieved through brisk walking (also referred to as fast walking or walking for exercise). Moderate-intensity exercise manifests as an increase in heart rate (to the range of 70%-75% of age-adjusted maximum heart rate reserve), a perceptible increase in breathing rate (such that it would be difficult to sing) or a self-rating that the activity is at a difficulty level of 6 or 7 on a 10-point scale.
- Older adults of below-average to average fitness can accomplish these relative intensities by walking 5 km/h (3 miles/h; moderate intensity) or 6 km/h (4 miles/h; vigorous intensity).

What is the needed amount of these activities?

- It is necessary for continuous periods of exercise of at least 10 min and increasing to at least 30 min/session to accomplish 150 min/wk (more is better).
- Initially it may seem difficult to maintain continuous activity for these time periods. However, as adaptation occurs, the tolerable duration of each exercise session will increase within a few weeks.

training programmes for older adults (in part this is out of caution), little evidence supports a slow progression. In fact, the many shorter training studies cited in this chapter progressed exercise to the desired intensity within the first couple weeks and achieved substantial gains with continued progression. It appears that older adults adapt physiologically over a time frame similar to that observed in young adults.

Many programmes for older adults emphasise stretching or flexibility exercises. However, it is now clear that these exercises produce no known health benefits and little benefit in terms of functional abilities and have smaller effects on functional outcomes than do aerobic or strength programmes. Thus, the efficacy of flexibility exercise has been questioned such that activities that emphasise stretching callisthenics, although not contraindicated for older adults, are not of known benefit. Time pursuing such activity would be better spent pursuing endurance and strength activities.

Additionally, a number of programmes for older adults incorporate exercises that emphasise balance. Indeed, balance is essential for safely performing mobility activities, and good balance will prevent falls. Balance-type activities (e.g., walking on uneven terrain, moving through a course that pivots and turns, carrying objects) can be incorporated into aerobic programmes. For those with mobility limitations it may be advisable to include specific balance exercises.

It is also advisable to include a warm-up and a cool-down in exercise programmes for older adults. The 5 to 10 min warm-up should gradually progress from light exercise to moderate intensity of the activity or muscle groups to be used for the remainder of the session. The 5 to 10 min cool-down should do the opposite. Thus, a typical exercise session for older adults should include the following:

- A 5 min warm-up of the muscle groups to be used during the exercise session that gradually increases in intensity.

- 30 min of aerobic (i.e., rhythmic, dynamic) activities that could take various forms: continuous brisk walking, aerobics routines or interval training that includes periods of vigorous activity alternated with periods of light- to moderate-intensity activity (e.g., 3 min of jogging and 3 min of walking, repeated 5 times). This cardiorespiratory exercise can be prescribed and monitored as detailed in table 7.2. Such intensity guidelines allow for continued exercise progression.

- A 5 min cool-down during which aerobic (i.e., rhythmic, dynamic) activity is continued at a gradually reduced intensity. If stretching exercises are desired, the

Table 7.2   Exercise Prescription for Older Adults

Description[1]	%$\dot{V}O_2$max[2]	%HRmax[3]	Approximate training heart rate (beats/min)
Moderate	50	69	110
Moderate to vigorous	60	75	119
Vigorous	70	82	130

[1]For a 70-yr-old.

[2]%$\dot{V}O_2$max = the maximal oxygen uptake or the maximum volume of oxygen that can be utilized in one minute during maximal or exhaustive exercise. It is measured as milliliters of oxygen used in one minute per kilogram of body weight.

[3]%HRmax = percentage of age-adjusted maximal heart rate. %HRmax = $(0.64 \times$ %$\dot{V}O_2$max$) + 37$ (Swain et al., 1994).

Age-adjusted maximum heart rate = $208 - (0.7 \times$ age$)$ (Tanaka, Monahan & Seals, 2001).

Some practitioners recommend using percentage heart rate reserve (HRR), which is very close to %$\dot{V}O_2$max (i.e., 60% HRR is ~60% $\dot{V}O_2$max). HRR = (maximum HR – resting HR) + resting HR.

Canadian Physical Activity Guidelines

best time to perform these is after the cool-down.

Two additional exercise sessions per week should include resistance exercises that incorporate weights, resistance bands, a weight vest or callisthenics that lift body weight or additional weights. The goal of these sessions should be to perform exercises that are of greater intensity than encountered in usual daily activities and that lead to fatigue in only 10 or so repetitions. These sessions should also include some resistance exercises with fast contractions to promote power development. These resistance-training programmes are referred to as progressive resistance training; therefore, the programme must include progression.

For individuals in whom $\dot{V}O_2max$ has not been measured, exercise intensity may be prescribed by recommending intensity as a percentage of age-adjusted maximal heart rate. This can be converted to an age-adjusted steady-state submaximal exercise heart rate.

9 Summary

Information from epidemiological studies of the effect of physical activity on outcomes of morbidity and functional independence and from experimental interventions of exercise-training programmes in older adults has contributed to evidence-based guidelines for physical activity in older adults. The guidelines recommend at least 150 min/wk of moderate-intensity cardiorespiratory exercise and 2 sessions/wk of muscle-strengthening exercises. A need exists for preventive medicine given the concern that health care costs will become prohibitive with the aging of society. Exercise is powerful preventive medicine. Increased physical activity and fitness of community-dwelling older adults will compress the period of morbidity, thus preventing long-term chronic disease and functional disability and enabling older adults to enjoy high-quality, independent living. Informed health practitioners are needed to promote physical activity to patients and clients and to provide the fitness industry with high-quality programmes and the opportunity to influence and work with older adults.

10 References

Angevaren, M., Aufdemkampe, G., Verhaar, H. J., Aleman, A., & Vanhees, L. (2008). Physical activity and enhanced fitness to improve cognitive function in older people without known cognitive impairment. *Cochrane Database Syst Rev*, 3, CD005381. doi: 10.1002/14651858.CD005381.pub3.

Arbab-Zadeh, A., Dijk, E., Prasad, A., Fu, Q., Torres, P., & Zhang, R. (2004). Effect of aging and physical activity on left ventricular compliance. *Circulation*, 110(13), 1799-1805.

Bassey, E.J. (1978). Age, inactivity and some physiological responses to exercise. *Gerontology*, 24(1), 66-77.

Bassey, E.J., Fiatarone, M.A., O'Neill, E.F., Kelly, M., Evans, W.J., & Lipsitz, L.A. (1992). Leg extensor power and functional performance in very old men and women. *Clinical Science (Lond)*, 82(3), 321-327.

Beere, P.A., Russell, S.D., Morey, M.C., Kitzman, D.W., & Higginbotham, M.B. (1999). Aerobic exercise training can reverse age-related peripheral circulatory changes in healthy older men. *Circulation*, 100(10), 1085-1094.

Bijnen, F.C., Feskens, E.J., Caspersen, C.J., Nagelkerke, N., Mosterd, W.L., & Kromhout, D. (1999). Baseline and previous physical activity in relation to mortality in elderly men: The Zutphen Elderly Study. *American Journal of Epidemiology*, 150(12), 1289-1296.

Blair, S.N., Kohl, H.W. III, Barlow, C.E., Paffenbarger, R.S. Jr., Gibbons, L.W., & Macera, C.A. (1995). Changes in physical fitness and all-cause mortality. A prospective study of healthy and unhealthy men. *Journal of the American Medical Association*, 273(14), 1093-1098.

Blumenthal, J.A., Emery, C.F., Madden, D.J., George, L.K., Coleman, R.E., & Riddle, M.W. (1989). Cardiovascular and behavioral effects of aerobic exercise training in healthy older men and women. *Journal of Gerontology*, 44(5), M147-M157.

Cunningham, D.A., Rechnitzer, P.A., Howard, J.H., & Donner, A.P. (1987). Exercise training of men at retirement: A clinical trial. *Journal of Gerontology*, 42(1), 17-23.

Davidson, L.E., Hudson, R., Kilpatrick, K., Kuk, J.L., McMillan, K., & Janiszewski, P.M. (2009). Effects of exercise modality on insulin resistance and functional limitation in older adults: A randomized controlled trial. *Archives of Internal Medicine*, 169(2), 122-131.

de Vos, N.J., Singh, N.A., Ross, D.A., Stavrinos, T.M., Orr, R., & Fiatarone Singh, M.A. (2005). Optimal load for increasing muscle power during explosive resistance training in older adults. *Journal of Gerontology, A Biological Science Medical Science*, 60(5), 638-647.

Ehsani, A.A., Ogawa, T., Miller, T.R., Spina, R.J., & Jilka, S.M. (1991). Exercise training improves left ventricular systolic function in older men. *Circulation*, 83(1), 96-103.

Ehsani, A.A., Spina, R.J., Peterson, L.R., Rinder, M.R., Glover, K.L., & Villareal, D.T. (2003). Attenuation of cardiovascular adaptations to exercise in frail octogenarians. *Journal of Applied Physiology*, 95(5), 1781-1788.

Erickson, K.I., & Kramer, A.F. (2009). Aerobic exercise effects on cognitive and neural plasticity in older adults. *British Journal of Sports Medicine*, 43(1), 22-24.

Evans, E.M., Racette, S.B., Peterson, L.R., Villareal, D.T., Greiwe, J.S., & Holloszy, J.O. (2005). Aerobic power and insulin action improve in response to endurance exercise training in healthy 77-87 yr olds. *Journal of Applied Physiology* 98(1), 40-45.

Fatouros, I.G., Kambas, A., Katrabasas, I., Nikolaidis, K., Chatzinikolaou, A., & Leontsini, D. (2005). Strength training and detraining effects on muscular strength, anaerobic power, and mobility of inactive older men are intensity dependent. *British Journal of Sports Medicine* 39(10), 776-780.

Ferrucci, L., Izmirlian, G., Leveille, S., Phillips, C.L., Corti, M.C., & Brock, D.B. (1999). Smoking, physical activity, and active life expectancy. *American Journal of Epidemiology*, 149(7), 645-653.

Fiatarone, M.A., Marks, E.C., Ryan, N.D., Meredith, C.N., Lipsitz, L.A., & Evans, W.J. (1990). High-intensity strength training in nonagenarians. Effects on skeletal muscle. *Journal of the American Medical Association*, 263(22), 3029-3034.

Fielding, R.A., LeBrasseur, N.K., Cuoco, A., Bean, J., Mizer, K., & Fiatarone Singh, M.A. (2002). High-velocity resistance training increases skeletal muscle peak power in older women. *Journal of the American Geriatric Society*, 50(4), 655-662.

Fries, J.F. (1980). Aging, natural death, and the compression of morbidity. *New England Journal of Medicine*, 303(3), 130-135.

Frontera, W.R., Meredith, C.N., O'Reilly, K.P., Knuttgen, H.G., & Evans, W.J. (1988). Strength conditioning in older men: Skeletal muscle hypertrophy and improved function. *Journal of Applied Physiology*, 64(3), 1038-1044.

Gass, G., Gass, E., Wicks, J., Browning, J., Bennett, G., & Morris, N. (2004). Rate and amplitude of adaptation to two intensities of exercise in men aged 65-75 yr. *Medicine and Science in Sports and Exercise*, 36(10), 1811-1818.

Granacher, U., Muehlbauer, T., Zahner, L., Gollhofer, A., & Kressig, R.W. (2011). Comparison of traditional and recent approaches in the promotion of balance and strength in older adults. *Sports Medicine* 41(5), 377-400.

Hagberg, J.M., Graves, J.E., Limacher, M., Woods, D.R., Leggett, S.H., & Cononie, C. (1989). Cardiovascular responses of 70- to 79-yr-old men and women to exercise training. *Journal of Applied Physiology*, 66(6), 2589-2594.

Hakim, A.A., Petrovitch, H., Burchfiel, C.M., Ross, G.W., Rodriguez, B.L., & White, L.R. (1998). Effects of walking on mortality among nonsmoking retired men. *New England Journal of Medicine*, 338(2), 94-99.

Harris, C., DeBeliso, M.A., Spitzer-Gibson, T.A., & Adams, K.J. (2004). The effect of resistance-training intensity on strength-gain response in the older adult. *Journal of Strength and Conditioning Research*, 18(4), 833-838.

Hawkins, H.L., Kramer, A.F., & Capaldi, D. (1992). Aging, exercise, and attention. *Psychology and Aging*, 7(4), 643-653.

Kohrt, W.M., Malley, M.T., Coggan, A.R., Spina, R.J., Ogawa, T., & Ehsani, A.A. (1991). Effects of gender, age, and fitness level on response of VO_2max to training in 60-71 yr olds. *Journal of Applied Physiology*, 71(5), 2004-2011.

Kraemer, W.J., Adams, K., Cafarelli, E., Dudley, G.A., Dooly, C., & Feigenbaum, M.S. (2002). American College of Sports Medicine position stand. Progression models in resistance training for healthy adults. *Medicine and Science in Sports and Exercise*, 34(2), 364-380.

Larson, E.B., Wang, L., Bowen, J.D., McCormick, W.C., Teri, L., & Crane, P. (2006). Exercise is associated with reduced risk for incident dementia among persons 65 years of age and older. *Annals of Internal Medicine*, 144(2), 73-81.

Latham, N.K., Bennett, D.A., Stretton, C.M., & Anderson, C.S. (2004). Systematic review of progressive resistance strength training in older adults. *Journal of Gerontology: A Biological Science Medical Science*, 59(1), 48-61.

Lee, I.M., Hsieh, C.C., & Paffenbarger, R.S. Jr. (1995). Exercise intensity and longevity in men. The Harvard Alumni Health Study. *Journal of the American Medical Association* 273(15), 1179-1184.

Macaluso, A., & De Vito, G. (2004). Muscle strength, power and adaptations to resistance training in older people. *European Journal of Applied Physiology* 91(4), 450-472.

Makrides, L., Heigenhauser, G.J., & Jones, N.L. (1990). High-intensity endurance training in 20- to 30- and 60- to 70-yr-old healthy men. *Journal of Applied Physiology,* 69(5), 1792-1798.

Mazzeo, R.S., Cavanagh, P., Evans, W.J., Fiatarone Singh, M.A., Hagberg, J.M., & McAuley, E. (1998). American College of Sports Medicine Position Stand. Exercise and physical activity for older adults. *Medicine and Science in Sports and Exercise*, 30(6), 992-1008.

Meredith, C.N., Frontera, W.R., Fisher, E.C., Hughes, V.A., Herland, J.C., & Edwards, J. (1989). Peripheral effects of endurance training in young and old subjects. *Journal of Applied Physiology*, 66(6), 2844-2849.

Miszko, T.A., Cress, M.E., Slade, J.M., Covey, C.J., Agrawal, S.K., & Doerr, C.E. (2003). Effect of strength and power training on physical function in community-dwelling older adults. *Journal of Gerontology, A Biological Science Medical Science* 58(2), 171-175.

Morris, J.N., Chave, S.P., Adam, C., Sirey, C., Epstein, L., & Sheehan, D.J. (1973). Vigorous exercise in leisure-time and the incidence of coronary heart disease. *Lancet*, 1(7799), 333-339.

Muldoon, M.F., Barger, S.D., Flory, J.D., & Manuck, S.B. (1998). What are quality of life measurements measuring? *British Medical Journal*, 316(7130), 542-545.

Murias, J.M., Kowalchuk, J.M., & Paterson, D.H. (2010a). Mechanisms for increases in VO_2max with endurance training in older and young women. *Medicine and Science in Sports and Exercise* 42(10), 1891-1898.

Murias, J.M., Kowalchuk, J.M., & Paterson, D.H. (2010b). Time course and mechanisms of adaptations in cardiorespiratory fitness with endurance training in older and young men. *Journal of Applied Physiology* 108(3), 621-627.

Muscari, A., Giannoni, C., Pierpaoli, L., Berzigotti, A., Maietta, P., & Foschi, E. (2010). Chronic endurance exercise training prevents aging-related cognitive decline in healthy older adults: A randomized controlled trial. *International Journal of Geriatric Psychiatry*, 25(10), 1055-1064.

Paffenbarger, R.S. Jr., Kampert, J.B., Lee, I.M., Hyde, R.T., Leung, R.W., & Wing, A.L. (1994). Changes in physical activity and other lifeway patterns influencing longevity. *Medicine and Science in Sports and Exercise* 26(7), 857-865.

Paffenbarger, R.S. Jr., Wing, A.L., & Hyde, R.T. (1978). Physical activity as an index of heart attack risk in college alumni. *American Journal of Epidemiology*, 108(3), 161-175.

Pahor, M., Blair, S.N., Espeland, M., Fielding, R., Gill, T.M., & Guralnik, J.M. (2006). Effects of a physical activity intervention on measures of physical performance: Results of the lifestyle interventions and independence for Elders Pilot (LIFE-P) study. *Journal of Gerontology, A Biological Science Medical Science* 61(11), 1157-1165.

Pasco, J.A., Williams, L.J., Jacka, F.N., Henry, M.J., Coulson, C.E., & Brennan, S.L. (2011). Habitual physical activity and the risk for depressive and anxiety disorders among older men and women. *International Psychogeriatrics* 23(2), 292-298.

Paterson, D.H., Govindasamy, D., Vidmar, M., Cunningham, D.A., & Koval, J.J. (2004). Longitudinal study of determinants of dependence in an elderly population. *Journal of the American Geriatric Society*, 52(10), 1632-1638.

Paterson, D.H., Jones, G.R., & Rice, C.L. (2007). Ageing and physical activity: Evidence to develop exercise recommendations for older adults. *Canadian Journal of Public Health*, 98(Suppl. 2), S69-S108.

Paterson, D.H., & Warburton, D.E. (2010). Physical activity and functional limitations in older adults: A systematic review related to Canada's Physical Activity Guidelines. *International Journal of Behavioral Nutrition and Physical Activity* 7, 38.

Peterson, M.D., Rhea, M.R., Sen, A., & Gordon, P.M. (2010). Resistance exercise for muscular strength in older adults: A meta-analysis. *Ageing Research Reviews*, 9(3), 226-237.

Pogliaghi, S., Terziotti, P., Cevese, A., Balestreri, F., & Schena, F. (2006). Adaptations to endurance training in the healthy elderly: Arm cranking versus leg cycling. *European Journal of Applied Physiology* 97(6), 723-731.

Seals, D.R., Hagberg, J.M., Hurley, B.F., Ehsani, A.A., & Holloszy, J.O. (1984). Endurance training in older men and women. I. Cardiovascular responses to exercise. *Journal of Applied Physiology* 57(4), 1024-1029.

Seynnes, O., Fiatarone Singh, M.A., Hue, O., Pras, P., Legros, P., & Bernard, P.L. (2004). Physiological and functional responses to low-moderate versus high-intensity progressive resistance training in frail elders. *Journal of Gerontology, A Biological Science Medical Science* 59(5), 503-509.

Snowden, M., Steinman, L., Mochan, K., Grodstein, F., Prohaska, T.R., & Thurman, D.J. (2011). Effect of exercise on cognitive performance in community-dwelling older adults: Review of intervention trials and recommendations for public health practice and research. *Journal of the American Geriatric Society*, 59(4), 704-716.

Spina, R.J., Meyer, T.E., Peterson, L.R., Villareal, D.T., Rinder, M.R., & Ehsani, A.A. (2004). Absence of left ventricular and arterial adaptations to exercise in octogenarians. *Journal of Applied Physiology*, 97(5), 1654-1659.

Spina, R.J., Miller, T.R., Bogenhagen, W.H., Schechtman, K.B., & Ehsani, A.A. (1996). Gender-related differences in left ventricular filling dynamics in older subjects after endurance exercise training. *Journal of Gerontology, A Biological Science Medical Science* , 51(3), B232-B237.

Spina, R.J., Ogawa, T., Kohrt, W.M., Martin, W.H. III, Holloszy, J.O., & Ehsani, A.A. (1993). Differences in cardiovascular adaptations to endurance exercise training between older men and women. *Journal of Applied Physiology*, 75(2), 849-855.

Sullivan, D.H., Roberson, P.K., Smith, E.S., Price, J.A., & Bopp, M.M. (2007). Effects of muscle strength training and megestrol acetate on strength, muscle mass, and function in frail older people. *Journal of the American Geriatric Society*, 55(1), 20-28.

Suominen, H., Heikkinen, E., & Parkatti, T. (1977). Effect of eight weeks' physical training on muscle and connective tissue of the M. vastus lateralis in 69-year-old men and women. *Journal of Gerontology*, 32(1), 33-37.

Swain, D.P., Abernathy, K.S., Smith, C.S., Lee, S.J., & Bunn, S.A. (1994). Target heart rates for the development of cardiorespiratory fitness. *Medicine and Science in Sports and Exercise* 26(1), 112-116.

Taaffe, D.R., Duret, C., Wheeler, S., & Marcus, R. (1999). Once-weekly resistance exercise improves muscle strength and neuromuscular performance in older adults. *Journal of the American Geriatric Society*, 47(10), 1208-1214.

Tanaka, H., Monahan, K.D., & Seals, D.R. (2001). Age-predicted maximal heart rate revisited. *Journal of the American College of Cardiology* 37(1), 153-156.

Wen, C.P., Wai, J.P., Tsai, M.K., Yang, Y.C., Cheng, T.Y., & Lee, M.C. (2011). Minimum amount of physical activity for reduced mortality and extended life expectancy: A prospective cohort study. *Lancet*, 378(9798), 1244-1253.

Impact of Physical Activity on Mental Health in Long-Term Conditions

Sarah Edmunds, PhD
University of Westminster, London, United Kingdom

Angela Clow, PhD
University of Westminster, London, United Kingdom

Chapter Outline

1. Long-Term Conditions and Mental Health Issues
2. Long-Term Conditions and Quality of Life
3. Long-Term Conditions and Physical Activity
4. Chronic Obstructive Pulmonary Disease
5. Diabetes
6. Cancer
7. Summary
8. References

Editors' Introduction

Approximately 30% of the European population has a long-term physical health condition. People with a long-term condition that is comorbid with a mental health problem have worse health outcomes than do people with either of these alone. This chapter explains the important role of physical activity in maintaining physical and mental health in people with long-term conditions. It focusses particularly on chronic obstructive pulmonary disease, diabetes and cancer and reviews evidence of the relationship between physical activity and mental health in people with these conditions as well as the efficacy of exercise interventions for reducing mental health problems in these populations ong-term conditions (LTCs) have been defined as "those conditions that cannot, at present, be cured, but can be controlled by medication and other therapies. The life of a person with an LTC is forever altered—there is no return to normal" (Department of Health, 2008, p. 10). LTCs include diabetes, arthritis, chronic obstructive pulmonary disease (COPD) and a number of cardiovascular diseases. In addition, conditions such as human immunodeficiency virus (HIV), acquired immunodeficiency syndrome (AIDS) and certain cancers that were not traditionally considered LTCs are increasingly being regarded as such (Naylor et al., 2012). Many mental health problems can themselves be considered LTCs. However, in this chapter the term *long-term condition* refers specifically to physical health conditions.

The World Health Organisation's (2011) report on the global burden of noncommunicable diseases (i.e., all previously mentioned LTCs except HIV and AIDS) found that noncommunicable diseases are by far the leading cause of mortality in the world and represent 63% of all deaths. The majority of these deaths are due to cardiovascular disease, diabetes, cancer and chronic respiratory disease. The highest occurrence of deaths from these diseases is in low- and middle-income countries, and the prevalence in these countries is predicted to increase substantially in the future. In Europe 29% of people aged 15 yr or older report a longstanding health problem (TNS Opinion, 2007), and the Office for National Statistics (2005) found that in England approximately 30% of the population (15.4 million people) has a LTC. As populations age, the burden of LTCs is projected to increase even further.

1 Long-Term Conditions and Mental Health Issues

People with LTCs are two to three times more likely than the general population to experience mental health problems. Depression and anxiety are the most frequently reported mental health problems in people with LTCs, but dementia, cognitive decline and some other conditions have also been reported (Naylor et al., 2012). Depression is two to three times more common in people with an LTC than in those with good physical health and occurs in approximately 20% of people with an LTC (National Collaborating Centre for Mental Health, 2010). Conservative estimates suggest that at least 30% of all people with an LTC also have a comorbid mental health problem of some kind (Cimpean & Drake, 2011). Research has shown that having a mental health problem along with an LTC has a stronger negative impact on quality of life and functional status than does either the number of LTCs or the severity of those conditions. For example, quality of life is lower in people with one LTC and depression than in people with two or more LTCs and no depression (Moussavi et al., 2007). Figure 8.1 shows the overlap between LTCs and mental health disorders.

In addition to experiencing psychological distress, patients with an LTC and comorbid mental health problem experience poorer clinical outcomes compared with people with an LTC and no mental health problem (Moussavi et al., 2007). This is partly because self-management is necessary for effectively controlling LTCs, and poor mental health can result in poorer self-management. For example, it may lead to lack of motivation and energy to adhere to treatment plans or attend medical appointments (DiMatteo, Lepper & Croghan, 2000). From a financial perspective, comorbid mental health problems are typically associated with a 45% to 75% increase in care costs for a person with an LTC. These data are based on a wide range of LTCs and are observed after adjustment for severity of physical disease (Unützer et al., 2009; Welch et al., 2009).

2 Long-Term Conditions and Quality of Life

Quality of life is an individual's perception of their ability to function well on physical, mental and social levels. Quality of life can be measured in a reliable and valid manner using self-reported questionnaires, which can be categorised into three main groups: generic, disease specific and domain specific. Generic questionnaires measure quality of life in general terms, independent of the presence of any disease. Disease-specific questionnaires measure the consequences of a specific disease on quality of life. Domain-specific questionnaires focus on certain domains of quality of life (e.g., physical inabilities).

Where it is possible to manage but not cure a disease, such as in LTCs, measures of quality of life are frequently used to help determine

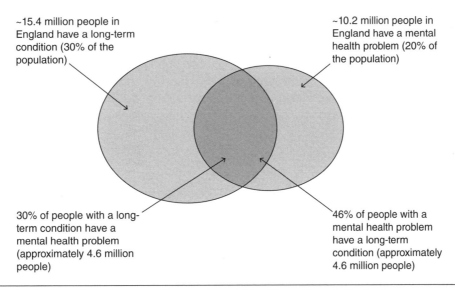

~15.4 million people in England have a long-term condition (30% of the population)

~10.2 million people in England have a mental health problem (20% of the population)

30% of people with a long-term condition have a mental health problem (approximately 4.6 million people)

46% of people with a mental health problem have a long-term condition (approximately 4.6 million people)

Figure 8.1 Overlap between long-term conditions and mental health problems in England.

Adapted, by permission, from C. Naylor et al., 2012, *Long-term conditions and mental health: The cost of co-morbidities* (London: The King's Fund and Centre for Mental Health).

KEY CONCEPTS

- Approximately 30% of people with a long-term condition have a comorbid mental health condition.

- Physical activity is an important part of the management of physical and psychological well-being in people with long-term conditions.

- Pulmonary rehabilitation leads to reduced depression and anxiety and increased quality of life in people with chronic obstructive pulmonary disease. Further research is required to understand the optimal exercise dose; the interaction of exercise training, education and psychosocial support during pulmonary rehabilitation; and how to sustain changes in physical activity behaviour after pulmonary rehabilitation.

- Physical inactivity is associated with greater depression in people with type 2 diabetes. Further research is required to understand the causality of this relationship, although available data suggest that physical activity interventions reduce depression.

- Data that explore the relationship between physical activity and mental health in people with type 1 diabetes are limited.

- Physical activity has been shown to increase quality of life and reduce anxiety and depression in cancer survivors. Data suggest that supervised and group exercise are more beneficial than unsupervised and home-based exercise in this population.

the impact of treatment and disease. They help health professionals make informed judgements about whether treatment is appropriate and, where a choice of treatments exists, which might be the best option. Researchers frequently use these measures to assess the impact of a new intervention.

3   Long-Term Conditions and Physical Activity

Doctors have traditionally advised people with a range of LTCs to rest and not tire themselves out, and this advice persists in the lay psyche. For example, a recent Swedish survey found that the physical activity levels of people with diabetes, rheumatoid arthritis or COPD are lower than those of healthy controls; 73% of people with diabetes, 74% with rheumatoid arthritis and 84% with COPD reported low physical activity levels compared with 60% of controls (Arne et al., 2009). However, modern treatment of LTCs often includes promoting physical activity as part of a healthy lifestyle, and accumulating evidence shows the importance of physical activity in the management of both physical and psychological well-being for people with one or more LTCs. Regular contact between health professionals and people with LTCs provides opportunities for promoting physical activity in this group.

Each LTC presents its own challenges and benefits with regard to physical activity. The remainder of this chapter focusses in particular on the impact of physical activity on mental health and well-being in people with COPD, diabetes and cancer.

4   Chronic Obstructive Pulmonary Disease

COPD is characterised by airflow obstruction that is not fully reversible and usually progressive in the long term. It is predominantly caused by smoking. Symptoms include breathlessness (dyspnoea) on exertion, chronic cough, regular production of sputum and frequent winter bronchitis or wheeze. Exacerbation of symptoms often

occurs in which the patient's symptoms rapidly worsen beyond normal day-to-day variations. Diagnosis relies on a combination of history, physical examination and confirmation of airflow obstruction using spirometry; no single test for COPD exists (National Institute for Health and Clinical Excellence, 2010). Severity of COPD is often classified using the Global Initiative for Chronic Obstructive Lung Disease (GOLD) criteria (I [mild], II [moderate], III [severe] and IV [very severe]) and index of body mass, airway obstruction, dyspnoea and exercise capacity (BODE).

The World Health Organisation has predicted that by 2020 COPD will be the third leading cause of death and fifth leading cause of disability in the world (Murray & Lopez, 1996, 1997). Mortality rates for men in the United Kingdom are at a plateau and mortality rates for women are steadily increasing (Soriano et al., 2000) most likely as a result of the uptake of smoking among women post-World War II. According to the chief medical officer in England, COPD accounts for more than £800 million in direct health care costs (Department of Health, 2005); more than one half of these costs relate to the provision of hospital care. COPD is among the most costly inpatient conditions that the National Health Service treats.

4.1   COPD and Mental Health

People with COPD are at increased risk of depression compared with those without COPD, and those with the most severe COPD have the highest risk of developing depression (Schneider et al., 2010). Research has shown that prevalence of anxiety ranges from 10% to 100% and that the prevalence of panic attacks and panic disorder ranges from 8% to 67% (Hynninen et al., 2005). Qualitative research has found that anxiety, fear and panic are prevalent due to the unpleasant experience of symptom exacerbations and that guilt, denial and regret are common because of patients' feelings about smoking being the cause of COPD (Fraser et al., 2006). Furthermore, having COPD and a comorbid mental disorder is associated with worse health status and breathlessness independent of the severity of COPD (Felker et al., 2010). Felker et al. (2010) assert that the psychological factors in COPD need greater attention in order to improve the quality of the patient experience and reduce costs. The pursuit of nonpharmacological treatment options for depression and anxiety is important because few studies have shown pharmacotherapy to alleviate depression in this patient population (Nguyen & Carrieri-Kohlman, 2005).

4.2 COPD and Physical Activity and Exercise

Overall, people with COPD are physically active for less time and at lower intensity than are people in the healthy population. However, estimates of the extent to which physical activity is reduced compared with healthy controls vary widely; across 47 studies, estimates ranged from 28% to 97%. Lower levels of physical activity are associated with higher levels of airway obstruction, lower levels of physical fitness and high levels of systemic inflammation (Bossenbroek et al., 2011). Garcia-Aymerich and colleagues (2006) followed a cohort of 2,386 individuals with COPD over a 20 yr period and found that individuals who self-reported very low levels of physical activity were at greater risk of hospital admission than were those who reported low, moderate or high levels of physical activity [incidence rate ratio = 0.72, 95% confidence interval (CI) = 0.53-0.97] and had a greater risk of all-cause mortality (hazard ratio = 0.76, 95% CI = 0.65-0.90) and respiratory mortality (hazard ratio = 0.70, 95% CI = 0.48-1.02). More recently, Waschki and colleagues (2011) used objective multisensory armband activity monitors (SenseWear Pro armband) to investigate the extent to which physical activity could predict future mortality in a group of 170 individuals with stable COPD (GOLD stages I-IV) over a 4 yr period. Physical activity was found to be a stronger predictor of all-cause mortality than a wide range of other prognostic assessments that are regularly used in COPD. A linear association existed between physical activity and mortality such that the relative risk of death more than doubled for every decrease of 200 to 250 kcal in active daily energy expenditure.

Exercise training is a key component of pulmonary rehabilitation. Exercise training is a well-established, nonpharmacological, multidisciplinary intervention that aims to restore patients with COPD to the highest possible level of independent function. An interdisciplinary team of health care professionals delivers education and psychosocial support alongside the exercise training. Programmes vary in length (4 wk-18 mo) and in type, dose and location (e.g., home, hospital) of exercise training (Ries et al., 2007). Research has demonstrated the efficacy of pulmonary rehabilitation compared with standard community care, and evidence strongly supports the use of pulmonary rehabilitation in the management of patients with COPD (Lacasse et al., 2009).

4.3 COPD, Physical Activity and Quality of Life

Bossenbroek and colleagues (2011) identified six studies published between 1995 and 2009 that assessed the relationship between physical activity and quality of life; four found a positive correlation and two found a negative correlation. The authors suggested that differences in the physical activity assessment methods and quality-of-life questionnaires accounted for the differences between studies and concluded that the relationship between physical activity and quality of life was not clear. More recently, Esteban and colleagues (2010) reported 5 yr follow-up data for 445 patients with COPD. Each patient completed disease-specific (St. George's Respiratory Questionnaire and Chronic Respiratory Questionnaire) and generic Medical Outcomes Trust Short-Form 36-item health survey (SF-36) measures of quality of life and were interviewed about their physical activity at baseline and 5 yr later. None of the participants participated in pulmonary rehabilitation during the 5 yr follow-up period. Physical activity was classified as low (engaging in light physical activity such as walking for 2 h/wk), moderate (engaging in light physical activity such as walking for 2-4 h/wk) or high (engaging in light physical activity such as walking for 4 h/wk). Patients who consistently engaged in low levels of physical activity and those whose physical activity decreased over the 5 yr period experienced significant declines in quality of life. In contrast, quality of life improved in patients who maintained moderate or high levels of physical activity and in those whose level of physical activity increased.

Objective physical activity monitoring allows for more detailed exploration of the relationship between physical activity intensity and quality of life. Jehn and colleagues (2012) used accelerometers to assess the physical activity of 107 individuals (70% male, aged 65 ± 11 yr) with COPD (GOLD stages II-IV). Quality of life was measured using both the St. George's Respiratory Questionnaire and the SF-36. Walking intensity significantly predicted quality-of-life scores and was a stronger predictor than total distance covered per day, total steps per day or daily energy expenditure. Patients with the lowest walking intensities had the worst outcome in terms of quality of life and the highest disease severity in terms of GOLD stage and BODE index.

4.4 Pulmonary Rehabilitation and Mental Health

Pulmonary rehabilitation has been shown to improve the mental health and well-being of people with COPD. Lacasse and colleagues (2009) reviewed 31 randomised controlled studies that compared pulmonary-rehabilitation programmes of at least 4 wk duration with standard community care. Inpatient, outpatient and home-based pulmonary-rehabilitation programmes were included if they consisted of exercise therapy with or without any form of education or psychological support. Statistically significant improvements were found for quality of life immediately after the intervention. In four important domains of quality of life (Chronic Respiratory Questionnaire scores for dyspnoea,

fatigue, emotional function and mastery) the effect was larger than the minimal clinically important difference. Statistically significant improvements also occurred in two of the three domains (impact and activity but not symptoms) of the St. George's Respiratory Questionnaire. Functional and maximal exercise capacity also increased, but the effect was small and slightly below the level of clinical significance. The long-term impact of pulmonary rehabilitation could not be reviewed because evidence was insufficient. Coventry and Hind (2007) reviewed the impact of pulmonary rehabilitation on symptoms of anxiety, depression and quality of life. They identified six randomised controlled trials that compared comprehensive pulmonary rehabilitation with standard care or education. All studies included patients over age 60 yr with stable COPD and moderate to severe symptoms. The six pulmonary-rehabilitation programmes were outpatient based, lasted at least 4 wk and included at least 2 supervised sessions/wk of low-intensity or incremental, high-intensity exercise training. Overall, comprehensive pulmonary rehabilitation was more effective than standard care for reducing anxiety (standardised mean difference (SMD) = –0.33, 95% CI = –0.57 to –0.09), depression (SMD = –0.58, 95% CI = –0.93 to –0.23) and generic and disease-specific quality of life, although these gains were not sustained at the 12 mo follow-up. The evidence suggests that pulmonary rehabilitation is effective, at least in the short term, for people with less favourable psychosocial health, but evidence about its efficacy for people with severe anxiety and depression was limited. More attention to the development of long-term improvements in mental health is warranted.

The majority (90%) of research on pulmonary rehabilitation has been conducted in community programmes. Inpatient programmes also exist; these are considered best suited for older patients and those with more severe COPD symptoms. Bratås and colleagues (2010) evaluated the impact of a 4 wk inpatient pulmonary-rehabilitation programme on 161 patients (79) male, and 82 female aged 65 ±9 yr) with COPD ranging from mild to very severe (6% GOLD I, 34% II, 26% III and 34% IV). Follow-up data were available for 136 participants, pre–post comparisons showed significant increases in St. George's Respiratory Questionnaire symptom and impact scores but no significant change in physical activity score. A significant reduction occurred in depression as measured by the Hospital Anxiety and Depression Scale (HADS), but no significant change in anxiety occurred. The authors suggest that the measure of general anxiety used in the HADS may not be sensitive to the panic and anxiety related to dyspnoea, which occurs frequently in people with COPD. Regression analyses showed that patients with mild to moderate COPD symptoms were more likely to have a clinically significant improvement in health-related quality of life at the end of the 4 week intervention programme compared with patients with severe or very severe symptoms [odds ratio (OR) = 4.2, 95% CI = 1.7-10.3]. Sex, age, comorbidity, anxiety and depression were not significantly associated with clinically significant improvement in health-related quality of life over the intervention period. This suggests that it might be important to refer patients to pulmonary rehabilitation at an early stage of the disease in order to achieve improvements in health-related quality of life.

Studies that compare comprehensive pulmonary rehabilitation with standard care do not allow one to understand the relative impact of each component of the programme (i.e., exercise training, education and psychological support) individually. An early study by Cockcroft and colleagues (1982) compared the impact of a 6 wk graduated exercise programme that included walking, swimming, a rowing machine and cycle tests with the impact of standard care. A total of 34 men with COPD were randomly allocated to experimental (n = 18) and control (n = 16) groups. The intervention had no significant effect on either anxiety or depression. However, the small scale and incomplete reporting of this trial make it difficult to draw firm conclusions about whether exercise training alone is insufficient to improve anxiety and depression

in COPD patients. A further study by Emery and colleagues (1998) compared a programme consisting of exercise, education and stress management (n = 30) with a programme consisting of education and stress management only (n = 24) and a waiting-list control group (n = 25). The exercise programme was intensive and lasted for 10 wk. At the end of the programme the exercise group experienced significant improvements in endurance, anxiety and verbal fluency compared with the other two groups. Changes in depression and quality of life were not significantly different in the exercise group compared with the control group. Given the widespread use of pulmonary-rehabilitation programmes, surprisingly little research has tested the efficacy of each component of pulmonary rehabilitation separately. This limits the extent to which one can make evidence-based judgements about which aspects of pulmonary rehabilitation lead to improved psychological outcomes.

4.4.1 Optimal Dose of Exercise Training During Pulmonary Rehabilitation

Defining and prescribing optimal exercise intensity for people with COPD are challenging due to the nature of the illness. Guidelines for exercise in COPD recommend a minimum intensity of 40% of peak oxygen uptake ($\dot{V}O_2$peak) (American College of Sports Medicine, 2006; Cooper, 2001), and the consensus is that higher-intensity training elicits greater physiological benefits (Nici et al., 2006; Troosters et al., 2005). However, many patients with COPD are unable to maintain high-intensity exercise for a sustained period due to intolerable symptoms. Therefore, interval training (repeated short bouts of high-intensity exercise interspersed with recovery periods) has been suggested as way for patients with COPD to gain the benefits of high-intensity training without experiencing intolerable symptoms. A recent Cochrane review assessed the effects of training intensity (higher versus lower) or type (continuous versus interval) on quality of life, exercise capacity and functional exercise capacity in people with COPD (Zainuldin, Mackey &

Alison, 2011). The review included 3 studies (231 participants) that compared the impact of higher- and lower-intensity exercise (2 studies measured quality of life) and 8 studies (367 participants) that compared continuous training with interval training (3 studies measured quality of life). The studies were classified as low to moderate quality. Training intensity (high or low) did not significantly influence improvement in endurance time or 6 min walk distance, and data were insufficient to draw any conclusions on exercise capacity, symptoms and quality of life. Continuous and interval training appear to be equally effective in improving exercise capacity, symptoms and quality of life. These findings concur with those of a previous systematic review of interval versus continuous training for individuals with COPD (Beauchamp et al., 2010). This review included 2 studies that compared the impact of high-intensity interval training and continuous moderate-intensity training on anxiety and depression and found no significant difference between training protocols. Further research is needed to understand psychological outcomes of training intensity in patients with COPD. For example, allowing patients to exercise at their preferred exercise intensity may be more important than absolute intensity for psychological outcomes, but this has not been tested with COPD patients.

4.4.2 Mental Health and Pulmonary Rehabilitation in Unstable COPD

The previously discussed studies focus mainly on patients with stable COPD symptoms. A more recent Cochrane review examined the impact of pulmonary rehabilitation in people who had recently been hospitalised with an exacerbation of COPD (Puhan et al., 2011) on future hospital admissions, mortality, health-related quality of life and exercise capacity. The review included 9 randomised controlled trials that compared pulmonary rehabilitation of any length with standard care. The findings showed that pulmonary rehabilitation significantly reduced hospital admissions (OR = 0.22, 95% CI = 0.08-0.58) and mortality (OR = 0.28, 95% CI = 0.10-0.84).

Effects on health-related quality of life were well above the minimal clinically important difference when measured by the Chronic Respiratory Questionnaire (dyspnoea, fatigue, emotional function and mastery domains) and the St. George's Respiratory Questionnaire (total score, impacts and activity limitations domains but not symptoms domain). A clinically important and statistically significant increase in exercise capacity was found, and no adverse effects of pulmonary rehabilitation were reported. These results suggest that the impact of pulmonary rehabilitation is similar for stable patients and patients who have had an exacerbation of COPD. However, the large increases in exercise capacity and reduction in hospital admissions suggest that pulmonary rehabilitation may be particularly beneficial for patients after a COPD exacerbation.

4.5 Implications for Practice

The National Institute for Health and Clinical Excellence (2010) guideline on the management of adults with COPD in primary and secondary care recommends that pulmonary rehabilitation should be made available to all appropriate people with COPD, including those who have had a recent hospitalisation for an acute exacerbation. Pulmonary rehabilitation is not suitable for people who cannot walk, have unstable angina or have had a recent myocardial infarction.

Recent research has been interested in the extent to which exercise training affects daily physical activity during and after pulmonary-rehabilitation programmes (i.e., the extent to which changes in physical activity are sustained). A review by Ng and colleagues (2012) found no randomised controlled trials on this topic but found two controlled trials and five single-group studies. Overall, they found a small effect of exercise training on daily physical activity (overall mean effect = 0.12, $p < .01$). Ng and colleagues suggest that increased physical activity is more likely to occur when supervised exercise training is offered at least 3 times/wk and when the intervention period is extended for participants who experience an acute exacerbation of their disease. A greater focus on domestic physical activity and a structured approach to promoting home-based exercise using behaviour-change techniques might be required to increase physical activity during and after a course of rehabilitation (Singh & Morgan, 2012). A similar review by Casaburi (2011) emphasised that increased exercise tolerance does not mean that people will necessarily participate in increased physical activity and recommended that there needs to be a shift in thinking so that the importance of change in physical activity behaviour as a long-term outcome is emphasised in addition to change in functional exercise capacity. Like Ng and colleagues (2012), Casaburi (2011) suggests that future efforts should link interventions for improving exercise tolerance to evidence-based behaviour-modification approaches to promoting physical activity. Troosters and colleagues (2010) also emphasised the importance of promoting lasting increases in physical activity through pulmonary rehabilitation, which they described as the cornerstone to long-lasting benefits.

5   Diabetes

Diabetes is a chronic metabolic disorder. Two main types of diabetes exist. Each has a different underlying cause, but the role of insulin is central to both. Insulin is a hormone that facilitates the uptake of glucose from the blood into cells, where it can be used immediately for energy or stored as glycogen, protein or adipose tissue. Individuals with type 1 diabetes are unable to produce insulin, and individuals with type 2 diabetes produce insufficient insulin or the cells become insensitive to it. Both conditions result in high blood glucose levels (hyperglycaemia) if untreated. Over time hyperglycaemia can lead to retinopathy, neuropathy (disorder of the peripheral nerves that sometimes results in amputation), nephropathy (disease of the kidney), heart problems and other disorders.

Type 2 diabetes, the most common form of diabetes, typically affects people over age 45 yr who are overweight. Physical activity, along with a healthy diet, is an important component of managing type 2 diabetes, although people commonly need medication (taken as tablets or insulin injections) in addition to healthy lifestyle changes to help keep blood glucose levels within the normal range. People with type 1 diabetes are unable to produce endogenous insulin because their pancreatic cells (which produce insulin in healthy individuals) have been destroyed by their body's immune system. The cause of this autoimmune response is still not fully understood. Patients typically develop type 1 diabetes in childhood or adolescence, and treatment includes insulin injections. Managing the condition involves constantly balancing exercise, dietary intake and insulin in order to maintain blood glucose levels that are within a normal range.

According to the International Diabetes Federation (2011), 366 million people (~8.5% of the global population) currently have diabetes, and estimates predict that the number will increase to 552 million by 2030. Therefore, diabetes it is a high priority for public health. The worldwide incidence of type 1 diabetes varies at least 100-fold among countries. The incidence is highest in Finland ($>40/10^5$) and lowest in Venezuela ($0.1/10^5$) and China (0.1–$4.5/10^5$) and has been increasing worldwide at a rate of approximately 3%/yr (Borchers, Uibo & Gershwin, 2010). The costs associated with treating diabetes are large and are also increasing. For example, in the United Kingdom the National Health Service currently spends £9.8 billion/yr on diabetes, and this figure is predicted to increase to £16.8 billion over the next 25 yr. In addition, the cost of treating secondary complications related to diabetes is currently £7.7 billion/yr and is predicted to increase to £13.5 billion by 2036 (Hex et al., 2012).

5.1   Diabetes and Mental Health

Patients with either type 1 or type 2 diabetes are two times more likely to experience clinically relevant depression in their lifetime than are individuals without diabetes (Ali et al., 2006;

Anderson et al., 2001). A recent World Health Organisation study found an interactive effect between depression and diabetes such that having both together causes a negative effect on self-rated overall health that goes beyond the simple addition of the impact of each of the two conditions separately (Moussavi et al., 2007). Comorbid depression has also been associated with reduced quality of life (Schram, Baan & Pouwer, 2009), treatment nonadherence (Gonzalez et al., 2008), clinically significant microvascular and macrovascular complications (Lin et al., 2010) and increased mortality (Katon et al., 2005). People with depression may have lower motivation for self-managing their diabetes, thus leading to poorer health outcomes.

Data from the U.S. 2006 Behavioral Risk Factor Survey showed that the overall age-adjusted prevalence of lifetime diagnosis of anxiety was 19.5% and 10.9% in people with and without diabetes, respectively (Li et al., 2008). After adjusting for educational level, marital status, employment status, current smoking, leisure-time physical activity and body mass index, the prevalence of lifetime diagnosis of anxiety was 20% higher in people with diabetes than in people without diabetes (prevalence ratio = 1.20, 95% CI = 1.12-1.30). A study of 2,049 patients with diabetes in Ireland (Collins, Corcoran & Perry, 2009) found that 32% of the patients exceeded the HADS threshold cutoff score for mild to severe anxiety and 22.4% exceeded the HADS cutoff score for mild to severe depression; this was more than double the estimate for the general population.

5.2 Type 2 Diabetes, Physical Activity and Mental Health

Physical activity is an important self-management behaviour in people with type 2 diabetes. It is associated with improvements in blood glucose control, reduces risk for diabetes-related complications and reduces risk factors for cardiovascular disease and the mortality risk associated with them (American Association of Diabetes Educators, 2012). The 2007 Behavioural Risk

Factor Survey found that adults with type 2 diabetes who reported taking part in regular physical activity had a 32% greater likelihood of reporting optimal self-rated health compared with adults who reported being inactive. Of the active participants who had optimal self-rated health, 90% reported engaging in moderate or vigorous physical activity or a combination of both at least 5 days/wk (Tsai et al., 2010).

Research has found that depression is significantly and independently associated with physical inactivity in patients with diabetes (Geulayov et al., 2010). Given that both physical inactivity and depression are associated with a greater risk of diabetes complications in adults with type 2 diabetes, researchers have begun to investigate the causality of the relationship between physical activity and depression in this group. A review of the literature on physical activity and depression in adults with type 2 diabetes included 12 studies published between 1996 and 2007 (Lysy, Da Costa & Dasgupta, 2008). Of these, 10 were cross-sectional and 2 were randomised intervention trials. Overall, inactive adults with type 2 diabetes were 1.72 to 1.75 times more likely to be depressed than those who were more active, and the depressed were 1.22 to 1.9 times more likely to be physically inactive than the nondepressed. However, the studies were limited by the use of subjective rather than objective measures of physical activity, and causality cannot be inferred from cross-sectional data. The two intervention studies used depression-management programmes and assessed their impact on physical activity and other health-related outcomes. Both trials improved mood but only one demonstrated increased physical activity. A longitudinal study of 2,759 patients (Katon et al., 2010) found that over a 5 yr period those with either no depression or improved depression at the 5 yr follow-up showed greater improvement or maintenance of physical activity than those whose depression worsened or persisted over the follow-up period. Physical activity levels declined over time in those whose depression improved compared with those who were never depressed, suggesting that levels of physical activity continue to decline once depression develops even if improvements in mood symptoms are achieved.

Piette and colleagues (2011) randomised 291 patients with type 2 diabetes and elevated depressive symptoms to either a 12 wk telephone-based cognitive behavioural therapy counselling programme that focussed on reducing depressive symptoms and increasing walking using pedometers or a control group that received usual care. Fifty-eight percent of patients in the intervention group reported reduced depressive symptoms compared with 39% of patients in the control group. The intervention group also achieved an increased number of steps per day, measured by pedometer, and a reduction in systolic blood pressure. No change occurred in average blood glucose levels over the previous 3 months (measured using haemoglobin A_{1c} at the 12 month follow-up). De Groot and colleagues (2012) also implemented a combined 12 wk cognitive behavioural therapy and exercise programme for 50 depressed adults with type 2 diabetes. The study was a single-group design, so the findings are limited by the absence of a control group. Depression in participants was significantly reduced immediately after the programme, and this was sustained 3 months later. Diabetes-specific and general quality of life increased significantly after the programme. A small but significant reduction in haemoglobin A_{1c} occurred immediately after the programme, but this was not maintained 3 mo later. The available evidence suggests that exercise can be used as an intervention to reduce depression in people with type 2 diabetes; however, the number of published studies is relatively small.

Nicolucci and colleagues (2011) found that participation in supervised aerobic- and resistance-exercise training combined with structured exercise counselling was associated with significant improvements in physical and mental health-related quality-of-life measures (SF-36), whereas all scores worsened in individuals who participated in exercise counselling alone. They concluded that the type of exercise intervention implemented has a major impact on quality of life. The data from this trial were further analysed to investigate the relationship between volume of exercise and quality of life (Nicolucci et al., 2012). There was a trend for increased quality of life with increased exercise volume. Significant improvement in the SF-36 physical component summary measure occurred only in people who exercised above 17.5 metabolic equivalents (METs)·h^{-1}·wk and a positive relationship was found between volume of exercise and the SF-36 mental component summary measure. A positive relationship between quality of life and volume of physical activity also was observed in the control group despite an overall deterioration of all scores.

The Diabetes Aerobic and Resistance Exercise Study (DARE) is a randomised controlled trial that determined the effects of aerobic exercise, resistance exercise and a combination of both on patients aged 39 to 70 yr with type 2 diabetes. The intervention consisted of exercise 3 times/ wk for 6 mo; the intensity and duration of each session gradually increased. Both aerobic- and resistance-exercise training improved glycaemic control, and a combination of both was superior to either type of exercise training alone (Sigal et al., 2007). In the same study, well-being outcomes were assessed using the SF-36 and Well-Being Questionnaire 12-item version (WBQ-12). A clinically, but not statistically, significant increase in SF-36 physical component score occurred in the resistance-exercise group compared with the aerobic- or combined-exercise groups. Contrary to the hypothesis, mental health component scores improved more in the no-exercise control group than in the combined aerobic- and resistance-exercise group or the resistance-exercise-only group. The authors suggest that this is due to regression to the mean because the control group had lower mental health component scores at baseline than the other groups. No significant changes in WBQ-12 scores occurred in any group (Reid et al., 2010).

In contrast to the previous studies that looked at trait measures of well-being and quality of life, a recent study by Kopp and colleagues (2012) investigated the acute effect of a 20 min brisk walk on affect during and after the exercise compared with a sedentary control condition for patients with type 2 diabetes. Participants in the exercise condition reported increased energy, more pleasure, reduced tension and higher activation. Increases in self-perceived activation after a single bout of exercise lasted for up to 3 h.

5.3 Type 1 Diabetes, Physical Activity and Mental Health

Physical activity is recommended as part of the treatment regimen for people with type 1 diabetes. However, compared with type 2 diabetes, the relationships between physical activity and glycaemic control and between physical activity and mental health are much less clear.

Chimen and colleagues (2012) reviewed the evidence of the health benefits of physical activity in type 1 diabetes. Their review included 48 intervention studies that aimed to increase physical activity. Increased physical activity led to increased physical fitness, reduced cardiovascular risk factors and reduced insulin requirements but had a limited effect on glycaemic control measured using haemoglobin A_{1c}. Studies typically had small sample sizes and short intervention duration and were not controlled for confounding factors such as diet or adjustment of insulin dosage.

Physical activity has been associated with significantly greater satisfaction with life and well-being in adults with type 1 diabetes (Zoppini, Carlini & Muggeo, 2003) but not in children (Edmunds et al., 2007). A large cross-sectional study of 2,036 adolescents (mean age 14.5 yr) from 21 paediatric diabetes centres across 19 countries (Aman et al., 2009) found statistically significant relationships between physical activity and well-being ($r = .05$), physical symptoms ($r = .05$), psychological symptoms ($r = .06$), perception of health ($r = .15$) and quality of life ($r = .1$). However, although statistically significant, the correlation coefficients were small, suggesting that the clinical significance of these relationships may be limited. In their review of the literature

of physical activity and health outcomes in type 1 diabetes, Chimen and colleagues (2012) concluded that physical activity is beneficial for well-being but that the evidence was weak because it was only from cross-sectional surveys. A randomised controlled 20 wk exercise-intervention study in children with type 1 diabetes published since the review by Chimen and colleagues found no significant effects on quality of life (D'hooge et al., 2011). However, the sample size was small (8 participants/group), which reduces the generalisability of the findings, and, although power calculations were not described, it is likely that the study was underpowered to detect significant differences in quality of life. Further research is required to investigate the relationships between physical activity, mental health and well-being in people with type 1 diabetes.

5.4 Implications for Practice

The American Association of Diabetes Educators (2012) recently published a position statement on diabetes and physical activity. They concluded that given the many health benefits of physical activity, participation in a regular physical activity routine is of primary importance and should be encouraged for individuals with type 1 and type 2 diabetes. Exercise recommendations have shifted away from a narrow focus on structured aerobic exercise and toward promoting moderate-intensity, unstructured lifestyle activity. This broad approach offers options for physical activity that are feasible for even the most deconditioned, sedentary population.

However, individuals with diabetes should undergo a thorough medical examination before initiating an exercise programme (American Association of Diabetes Educators, 2012). Despite the health benefits, exercise also carries potential risks for people with diabetes. For example, exercise can exacerbate severe micro- and macrovascular complications or can lead to significant variability in blood glucose (hyperglycaemia or hypoglycaemia) in those who require exogenous insulin and result in challenges for diabetes management.

6 Cancer

Advances in cancer treatment and earlier detection rates have led to an increase in survival rates and a growing population of people living with or beyond cancer. For example, there are approximately 2 million cancer survivors in the United Kingdom and the number is increasing by 3%/yr (Maddams et al., 2009). Cancer is a disease largely associated with aging, so the aging of the population also contributes to the increasing population of cancer survivors. In the United Kingdom, the most common cancer sites are the breast and prostate, which account for 46% and 31% of all female and male cases, respectively (Campbell, Stevinson & Crank, 2011). The population of people living with or beyond cancer, often called cancer survivors, faces unique challenges, including risk of recurrent cancer, other chronic diseases and persistent adverse effects on physical functioning and quality of life (Schmitz et al., 2010).

6.1 Psychological Comorbidity

Harrington and colleagues (2010) found that prolonged fatigue, cognitive limitations, depression, anxiety, sleep problems and pain were consistently present in heterogeneous cancer survivors for up to 10 yr after primary treatment. Fatigue and symptoms of depression and anxiety were the symptoms most commonly reported across 50 studies regardless of cancer type and treatment. Fatigue is often described as the most distressing symptom—more distressing than pain, nausea or vomiting—related to cancer or cancer treatment. Studies have found both increased incidence of depression and anxiety in cancer survivors compared with healthy populations (Costanzo, Ryff & Singer, 2009) and similar incidence of depression and anxiety (Boyes et al., 2009). Constanzo and colleagues (2009) found that younger cancer survivors experience more adverse psychological responses than do older survivors. Depression and anxiety may also lead to reduced compliance with cancer treatment, increased rates of obesity or reduction in other self-care behaviours and thus negatively affect physical health.

6.2 Cancer, Physical Activity and Mental Health

A relatively new but rapidly growing body of evidence shows that physical activity has physical and psychological benefits for cancer survivors. Courneya (2009) described the reasons why this field is rapidly expanding. First, as cancer survival rates have increased, the impact of lifestyle factors on survivorship has become relevant. Second, quality of life has become a legitimate target for interventions. Third, therapies have improved so that side effects (e.g., nausea, diarrhoea and anaemia) have been controlled and physical activity is now a realistic option for people during and soon after treatment. A series of recently published systematic reviews and meta-analyses has accompanied the increase in physical activity research. The following sections describe the findings from these reviews and qualitative studies, particularly the impact of physical activity on mental health and well-being.

Speck and colleagues (2010) conducted a comprehensive systematic review and meta-analysis of controlled trials of physical activity interventions for cancer survivors during and after treatment. This review included studies with psychosocial outcome variables, although it was not limited to such studies. The review included studies that were published in English, focussed on adults diagnosed with cancer, included an intervention for increasing physical activity outside the physical therapy setting and included a parallel control group. A total of 66 studies met these criteria and were judged to be of high quality. Of these studies, 83% included patients with breast cancer only, 11% included patients with lung cancer only, 10% included patients with prostate cancer only and 9% included patients with colon cancer only. Effect sizes (ES) were reported for psychological and physiological outcome variables. Interventions during treatment resulted in small to moderate positive effects on physical activity level, aerobic fitness, muscular strength, functional quality of life, anxiety and self-esteem. Overall, posttreatment physical activity interventions affected overall quality of life (ES = 0.29, p = .03), breast cancer-specific concerns (ES = 0.62, p = .003), perception of physical condition (ES = 0.57, p = .04), mood disturbance (ES = −0.39, p = .04), confusion (ES = −0.57, p = .05), body image (ES = −0.26, p = .03) and fatigue ES = (−0.54, p = .003). Overall, few adverse events related to physical activity were reported, suggesting that this group can safely undertake physical activity.

More recently, Fong and colleagues (2012) published a review that focussed exclusively on physical activity interventions for cancer survivors who had completed their main cancer treatment. The review included 34 randomised controlled trials that encompassed a range of cancer types, but the majority of studies were conducted on women with breast cancer. Overall physical activity was associated with significantly reduced fatigue, depression, body mass index and body weight. Physical activity was also associated with clinically important increases in quality of life (physical, social and mental health domains), increased aerobic fitness and measures of physical strength. The studies did not consistently report intensity of physical activity, making it difficult to assess its impact. However, significantly larger effects were reported in studies that used aerobic- plus resistance-exercise training compared with studies that used aerobic training alone; this might indicate a potential benefit of higher-intensity training. Similarly, a review that focussed specifically on the effect of exercise interventions on cancer-related fatigue (Brown et al., 2011) found that moderate-intensity resistance exercise (3-6 METs, 60%-80% of 1 RM) reduced cancer-related fatigue more than did lower-intensity resistance exercise or aerobic exercise of any intensity.

The reviews previously discussed focussed only on exercise interventions. A review by Duijts and colleagues (2011) compared the impact of exercise, behavioural and combined (exercise and behavioural) interventions on psychosocial outcomes in breast cancer survivors during and after treatment. The review included 42 randomised controlled behavioural interventions,

17 randomised controlled exercise interventions and 3 randomised controlled combined interventions. For physical exercise interventions, statistically significant and moderate effects were observed for fatigue, depression, body image and health-related quality of life. Reductions in anxiety were reported but these were not statistically significant. Because only one study assessed the effect of physical exercise on stress, a summary effect size could not be calculated. Statistically significant but modest results were found for the effect of behavioural techniques on fatigue and stress, and stronger effects were found for the effect of behavioural techniques on depression and anxiety. No significant effects were observed for body image or health-related quality of life. Exercise frequency and duration of the intervention influenced the effectiveness of exercise interventions on depression, anxiety and body image. Further research that compares the combined effect of exercise and behavioural interventions is required.

The standard treatments for depression in cancer survivors are medication and psychotherapy. These are effective for many people, but depression medication can be contraindicated for people undergoing certain cancer treatments (Kelly et al., 2010), and certain types of cancer (e.g., neck and throat cancers) may impede communication. Craft and colleagues (2012) recently reviewed a number of intervention studies that investigated the efficacy of exercise in treating depression in cancer survivors. The review included 15 randomised controlled trials that compared an aerobic-exercise or aerobic-plus resistance-exercise programme of at least 4 wk duration with usual care for cancer survivors and that reported depressive symptoms as an outcome measure. Overall, exercise was found to have a modest positive effect on depression across cancer types, treatment status at baseline and baseline severity of depressive symptoms (ES = −0.22, p = .04, CI −0.43 to −0.009). Exercise was effective in both the active treatment and posttreatment phases. Although all the studies in this review included depression as an outcome measure, most did not select depressed cancer survivors or subgroups at risk of depression. The effects of exercise on depression may be even larger for survivors who experience significant levels of depression. Further analyses investigated which factors moderated the relationship between exercise and depression. Interventions with exercise sessions that were longer than 30 min had a greater effect on depression than did those with shorter sessions. The largest effects were found for programmes that used supervised exercise and those that were based in exercise facilities rather than in patients' homes. Unsupervised and home-based exercise actually resulted in an increase in depressive symptoms, suggesting that it is important to further investigate how to best deliver exercise interventions (ES of home-based exercise = 0.16; ES of community facility-, gym- or laboratory-based exercise = −0.45; ES of supervised exercise = −0.67, ES of unsupervised exercise = 0.25, ES of mixed exercise = −0.32). This suggests that supervised and group exercise may have therapeutic aspects such as working with an exercise instructor to learn new skills, collaboratively setting and achieving exercise goals and receiving positive feedback and social interaction.

Qualitative studies allow researchers to understand the experiences of cancer survivors in exercise programmes in more depth. They have also been used to gain insight into the experiences of patients with less-common cancers and those with poorer prognoses for whom randomised controlled interventions are not feasible. Adamsen and colleagues (2011) investigated the experiences of 15 people with advanced-stage lung cancer who had participated in an exercise- and relaxation-training programme while undergoing chemotherapy. The participants exercised 2 times/wk for 2 h at the hospital. They had not been active before the cancer diagnosis and said that being offered the exercise programme during the period of shock and anxiety about their diagnosis complemented their need to take action regarding their diseased bodies. This complements previous research that has described a cancer diagnosis as an opportune moment for behaviour change, or a "teachable moment" (Saxton & Daley, 2010). In the study of Adamsen and colleagues (2011), some patients felt that gains in physical strength offered them more strength to fight their cancer. For example, a 47-yr-old male said, "I felt physically weak. The more strength I get from training, the more resistance I will have to use against my illness." The physical training helped patients surpass some of the limitations brought on by the chemotherapy treatment and achieve a sense of well-being. In addition, patients described experiencing more energy as a result of exercising and interpreted soreness, muscle pain and fatigue in a positive, action-orientated light rather than a negative, illness-related context. For example a 65-yr-old female said, "First I had to see how I would react to the training, and I think that it is great. I feel really good afterwards. Also, I was tired and really sore, but I think that was good … really good." Exercising in a group was seen as providing valuable social support. Interestingly, participants said that they rarely engaged in exercise at home, which was part of the exercise programme, despite perceiving that exercise offered valuable benefits.

Spence and colleagues (2011) used interviews to explore experiences in an exercise programme for a group of patients with colorectal cancer who had recently completed treatment. Patients reported reduced fatigue and an increased sense of health, well-being and mental health. The exercise sessions were one-on-one with a trainer, and participants said that the social relationship with the trainer was a key part of their enjoyment of the sessions. They also liked that the sessions were flexible and tailored to their needs and saw the trainer as someone who held them accountable. They felt that the social support was necessary to help them overcome the low confidence they had for exercise before the programme.

6.3 Implications for Practice

The American College of Sports Medicine developed a roundtable consensus statement about exercise for cancer survivors (Schmitz et al., 2010). They provided exercise guidelines and reviewed the evidence on the safety and efficacy of exercise training during and after adjuvant cancer therapy. Overall, the expert panel concluded that exercise is safe during and after cancer treatment. They found that breast cancer survivors with and at risk for lymphedema can safely perform resistance training. However, survivors need to consider some specific risks associated with cancer treatments (e.g., increased risk for fractures and cardiovascular events, neuropathies related to certain types of chemotherapy and treatment-related cardiotoxicity) when exercising. The expert group recommended that exercise prescriptions should be individualised according to a cancer survivor's pretreatment aerobic fitness, medical comorbidities, response to treatment and the immediate or persistent negative effects of treatment that are experienced at any given time.

In 2011 the British Association of Sport and Exercise Sciences produced their own expert statement on exercise and cancer survivorship (Campbell, Stevinson & Crank, 2011). They concluded that evidence shows that exercise can be performed safely during and after cancer treatment provided that individual limitations and specific side effects associated with cancer therapies are considered and monitored. They also concluded that cancer survivors should follow the UK physical activity guidelines and that all survivors, including those undergo-

ing difficult treatments or those with existing disease, should at a minimum avoid being sedentary.

According to the qualitative study by Adamsen and colleagues (2011), the fact that an exercise programme was integrated into their overall treatment protocol and that information was relayed thoroughly between members of the clinical team gave patients the trust and sense of security to break through the barriers of beginning to exercise despite their advancing disease and physical limitations. This suggests that health professionals and oncologists have an important role in recommending exercise during and after treatment.

7   Summary

Mental health problems are two to three times more prevalent in people with LTCs than in the general population; depression and anxiety are the comorbid mental health problems most commonly reported. Having an LTC along with a mental health problem is associated with poorer self-care and worse prognosis than is having an LTC but no mental health problem. Research has shown that increased physical activity can be a route to improved mental health; this is important in its own right but also has benefits for self-care and disease progression. In some LTCs (e.g., diabetes), regular physical activity is an

EVIDENCE TO PRACTICE

- The onset of an LTC may be a teachable moment for changing health behaviour (e.g., increasing physical activity).
- Regular contact between people with LTCs and health professionals provides opportunities to promote the uptake and maintenance of physical activity.
- Physical activity is safe for the majority of people with an LTC, but practitioners working in this area should be aware of specific contraindications and risk factors of physical activity in each condition.

- COPD, diabetes and cancer each present different challenges with regard to physical activity (e.g., breathlessness, blood glucose variability and fatigue, respectively).
- In the absence of disease-specific physical activity guidelines, exercise professionals should tailor the generic guidelines for each patient based on the patient's needs and functional ability.

important part of self-care, and increased physical activity may lead to feelings of empowerment and mastery of the illness. Physical activity has been shown to reduce mental health problems and increase quality of life in COPD, diabetes and cancer. Further research is required to clarify the optimal dose and type of exercise required to gain these benefits. Some evidence indicates that both aerobic and resistance exercise are beneficial and that exercise of higher intensity and frequency may lead to greater positive effects. However, dose–response effects have also shown that performing any activity is better than being sedentary. Physical activity is safe for the majority of people with LTCs, but practitioners and researchers working with these groups should be aware of the specific risks and contraindications for exercise relevant to each LTC. Overall, physical activity has a positive impact on physical and mental health for people with LTCs.

8 References

Adamsen, L., Stage, M., Laursen, J., Rørth, M., & Quist, M. (2011). Exercise and relaxation intervention for patients with advanced lung cancer: A qualitative feasibility study. *Scandinavian Journal of Medicine and Science in Sports*, 22(6), 804-815. no.

Ali, S., Stone, M.A., Peters, J.L., Davies, M.J., & Khunti, K. (2006). The prevalence of co-morbid depression in adults with Type 2 diabetes: A systematic review and meta-analysis. *Diabetic Medicine*, 23(11), 1165-1173.

Aman, J., Skinner, T.C., De Beaufort, C.E., Swift, P.G.F., Aanstoot, H.J., Cameron, F., et al. (2009). Associations between physical activity, sedentary behavior, and glycemic control in a large cohort of adolescents with type 1 diabetes: The Hvidoere Study Group on Childhood Diabetes. *Pediatric Diabetes*, 10(4), 234-239.

American Association of Diabetes Educators. (2012). Diabetes and physical activity. *The Diabetes Educator*, 38(1), 129-132.

American College of Sports Medicine. (2006). Other clinical conditions influencing exercise prescription: Pulmonary diseases. In *ACSM's guidelines for exercise testing and prescription* (7th ed.) (pp. 227-229). Baltimore: Lippincott Williams & Wilkins.

Anderson, R.J., Freedland, K.E., Clouse, R.E., & Lustman, P.J. (2001). The prevalence of comorbid depression in adults with diabetes. *Diabetes Care*, 24(6), 1069-1078.

Arne, M., Janson, C., Janson, S., Boman, G., Lindqvist, U., Berne, C., et al. (2009). Physical activity and quality of life in subjects with chronic disease: Chronic obstructive pulmonary disease compared with rheumatoid arthritis and diabetes mellitus. *Scandinavian Journal of Primary Health Care*, 27(3), 141-147.

Beauchamp, M.K, Nonoyama, M., Goldstein, R.S., Hill, K., Dolmage, T.E., Mathur, S., et al. (2010). Interval versus continuous training in individuals with chronic obstructive pulmonary disease—A systematic review. *Thorax*, 65(2), 157-164.

Borchers, A.T., Uibo, R., & Gershwin, M.E. (2010). The geoepidemiology of type 1 diabetes. *Autoimmunity Reviews*, 9(5), A355-A365.

Bossenbroek, L., de Greef, M.H.G., Wempe, J.B., Krijnen, W.P., & ten Hacken, N.H.T. (2011). Daily physical activity in patients with chronic obstructive pulmonary disease: A systematic review. *Journal of Chronic Obstructive Pulmonary Disease*, 8(4), 306-319.

Boyes, A.W., Girgis, A., Zucca, A.C., & Lecathelinais, C. (2009). Anxiety and depression among long-term survivors of cancer in Australia: Results of a population-based survey. *The Medical Journal of Australia*, 190(7 Suppl.), S94-S98.

Bratås, O., Espnes, G.A., Rannestad, T., & Walstad, R. (2010). Pulmonary rehabilitation reduces depression and enhances health-related quality of life in COPD patients—especially in patients with mild or moderate disease. *Chronic Respiratory Disease*, 7(4), 229-237.

Brown, J.C., Huedo-Medina, T.B., Pescatello, L.S., Pescatello, S.M., Ferrer, R.A., & Johnson, B.T. (2011). Efficacy of exercise interventions in modulating cancer-related fatigue among adult cancer survivors: A meta-analysis. *Cancer Epidemiology Biomarkers and Prevention*, 20(1), 123-133.

Campbell, A., Stevinson, C., & Crank, H. (2011). The BASES expert statement on exercise and cancer survivorship. *The Sport and Exercise Scientist*, 28, 16-17.

Casaburi, R. (2011). Activity promotion: A paradigm shift for chronic obstructive pulmonary disease therapeutics. *Proceedings of the American Thoracic Society*, 8(4), 334-337.

Chimen, M., Kennedy, A., Nirantharakumar, K., Pang, T., Andrews, R., & Narendran, P. (2012).

What are the health benefits of physical activity in type 1 diabetes mellitus? A literature review. *Diabtologia*, 55(3), 542-551.

Cimpean, D., & Drake, R.E. (2011). Treating co-morbid chronic medical conditions and anxiety/depression. *Epidemiology and Psychiatric Sciences*, 20(2), 141-150.

Cockcroft, A., Berry, G., Brown, E.B., & Exall, C. (1982). Psychological changes during a controlled trial of rehabilitation in chronic respiratory disability. *Thorax*, 37(6), 413-416.

Collins, M.M., Corcoran, P., & Perry, I.J. (2009). Anxiety and depression symptoms in patients with diabetes. *Diabetic Medicine*, 26(2), 153-161.

Cooper, C.B. (2001). Exercise in chronic pulmonary disease: Aerobic exercise prescription. *Medicine Science Sports and Exercise*, 33(7 Suppl.), S671-S679.

Costanzo, E.S., Ryff, C.D., & Singer, B.H. (2009). Psychosocial adjustment among cancer survivors: Findings from a national survey of health and well-being. *Health Psychology*, 28(2), 147-156.

Courneya, K.S. (2009). Physical activity in cancer survivors: A field in motion. *Psycho-Oncology*, 18(4), 337-342.

Coventry, P.A., & Hind, D. (2007). Comprehensive pulmonary rehabilitation for anxiety and depression in adults with chronic obstructive pulmonary disease: Systematic review and meta-analysis. *Journal of Psychosomatic Research*, 63(5), 551-565.

Craft, L.L., VanIterson, E.H., Helenowski, I.B., Rademaker, A.W., & Courneya, K.S. (2012). Exercise effects on depressive symptoms in cancer survivors: A systematic review and meta-analysis. *Cancer Epidemiology Biomarkers and Prevention*, 21(1), 3-19.

de Groot, M., Doyle, T., Kushnick, M., Shubrook, J., Merrill, J., Rabideau, E., et al. (2012). Can lifestyle interventions do more than reduce diabetes risk? Treating depression in adults with type 2 diabetes with exercise and cognitive behavioral therapy. *Current Diabetes Reports*, 12(2), 157-166.

Department of Health. (2005). *On the state of the public health: Annual report of the Chief Medical Officer 2004*. London: Department of Health.

Department of Health. (2008). *Raising the profile of long term conditions care: A compendium of information*. London: Department of Health.

D'hooge, R., Hellinckx, T., Van Laethem, C., Stegen, S., De Schepper, J., Van Aken, S., et al. (2011).

Influence of combined aerobic and resistance training on metabolic control, cardiovascular fitness and quality of life in adolescents with type 1 diabetes: A randomized controlled trial. *Clinical Rehabilitation*, 25(4), 349-359.

DiMatteo, M.R., Lepper, H.S., & Croghan, T.W. (2000). Depression is a risk factor for noncompliance with medical treatment: Meta-analysis of the effects of anxiety and depression on patient adherence. *Archives of Internal Medicine*, 160(14), 2101-2107.

Duijts, S.F.A., Faber, M.M., Oldenburg, H.S.A., van Beurden, M., & Aaronson, N.K. (2011). Effectiveness of behavioral techniques and physical exercise on psychosocial functioning and health-related quality of life in breast cancer patients and survivors—A meta-analysis. *Psycho-Oncology*, 20(2), 115-126.

Edmunds, S., Roche, D., Stratton, G., Wallymahmed, K., & Glenn, S.M. (2007). Physical activity and psychological well-being in children with Type 1 diabetes. *Psychology, Health, and Medicine*, 12(3), 353-363.

Emery, C.F., Schein, R.L., Hauck, E.R., & MacIntyre, N.R. (1998). Psychological and cognitive outcomes of a randomized trial of exercise among patients with chronic obstructive pulmonary disease. *Health Psychology*, 17(3), 232-240.

Esteban, C., Quintana, J.M., Aburto, M., Moraza, J., Egurrola, M., Pérez-Izquierdo, J., et al. (2010). Impact of changes in physical activity on health-related quality of life among patients with COPD. *European Respiratory Journal*, 36(2), 292-300.

Felker, B., Bush, K.R., Harel, O., Shofer, J.B., Shores, M.M., & Au, D.H. (2010). Added burden of mental disorders on health status among patients with chronic obstructive pulmonary disease. *Primary Care Companion to the Journal of Clinical Psychiatry*, 12(4), 201-216.

Fong, D.Y.T., Ho, J.W.C., Hui, B.P.H., Lee, A.M, Macfarlane, D.J., Leung, S.S.K., et al. (2012). Physical activity for cancer survivors: Meta-analysis of randomised controlled trials. *British Medical Journal*, 344, e70.

Fraser, D.D., Kee, C.C., & Minick, P. (2006). Living with chronic obstructive pulmonary disease: Insiders' perspectives. *Journal of Advanced Nursing*, 55(5), 550-558.

Garcia-Aymerich, J., Lange, P., Benet, M., Schnohr, P., & Antó, J.M. (2006). Regular physical activity reduces hospital admission and mortality in chronic obstructive pulmonary disease: A population based cohort study. *Thorax*, 61(9), 772-778.

Geulayov, G., Goral, A., Muhsen, K., Lipsitz, J., & Gross, R. (2010). Physical inactivity among adults with diabetes mellitus and depressive symptoms: Results from two independent national health surveys. *General Hospital Psychiatry*, 32(6), 570-576.

Gonzalez, J.S., Peyrot, M., McCarl, L.A., Collins, E.M., Serpa, L., Mimiaga, M.J., et al. (2008). Depression and diabetes treatment nonadherence: A meta-analysis. *Diabetes Care*, 31(12), 2398-2403.

Harrington, C.B., Hansen, J.A., Moskowitz, M., Todd, B.L., & Feuerstein, M. (2010). It's not over when it's over: Long-term symptoms in cancer survivors—A systematic review. *International Journal of Psychiatry in Medicine*, 40(2), 163-181.

Hex, N., Bartlett, C., Wright, D., Taylor, M., & Varley, D. (2012). Estimating the current and future costs of Type 1 and Type 2 diabetes in the UK, including direct health costs and indirect societal and productivity costs. *Diabetic Medicine*, 29(7), 855–862.

Hynninen, K.M.J., Breitve, M.H., Wiborg, A.B., Pallesen, S., & Nordhus, I.H. (2005). Psychological characteristics of patients with chronic obstructive pulmonary disease: A review. *Journal of Psychosomatic Research*, 59(6), 429-443.

International Diabetes Federation. (2011). *Diabetes atlas* (5th ed.). Brussels: International Diabetes Federation.

Jehn, M., Schindler, C., Meyer, A., Tamm, M., Schmidt-Trucksass, A., & Stolz, D. (2012). Daily walking intensity as a predictor of quality of life in patients with COPD. *Medicine and Science in Sports and Exercise*, 44(7), 1212-1218.

Katon, W.J., Russo, J.E., Heckbert, S.R., Lin, E.H.B., Ciechanowski, P., Ludman, E., et al. (2010). The relationship between changes in depression symptoms and changes in health risk behaviors in patients with diabetes. *International Journal of Geriatric Psychiatry*, 25(5), 466-475.

Katon, W.J., Rutter, C., Simon, G., Lin, E.H.B., Ludman, E., Ciechanowski, P., et al. (2005). The association of comorbid depression with mortality in patients with type 2 diabetes. *Diabetes Care*, 28(11), 2668-2672.

Kelly, C.M., Juurlink, D.N., Gomes, T., Duong-Hua, M., Pritchard, K.I., Austin, P.C., et al. (2010). Selective serotonin reuptake inhibitors and breast cancer mortality in women receiving tamoxifen: A population based cohort study. *British Medical Journal*, 340, c69 .

Kopp, M., Steinlechner, M., Ruedl, G., Ledochowski, L., Rumpold, G., & Taylor, A.H. (2012). Acute effects of brisk walking on affect and psychological well-being in individuals with type 2 diabetes. *Diabetes Research and Clinical Practice*, 95(1), 25-29.

Lacasse, Y., Goldstein, R., Lasserson, T.J., & Martin, S. (2009). Pulmonary rehabilitation for chronic obstructive pulmonary disease. *Cochrane Database of Systematic Reviews* 2006, Issue 4. Art. No.: CD003793.

Li, C., Barker, L., Ford, E.S., Zhang, X., Strine, T.W., & Mokdad, A.H. (2008). Diabetes and anxiety in U.S. adults: Findings from the 2006 Behavioral Risk Factor Surveillance System. *Diabetic Medicine*, 25(7), 878-881.

Lin, E.H.B., Rutter, C.M., Katon, W., Heckbert, S.R., Ciechanowski, P., Oliver, M.M., et al. (2010). Depression and advanced complications of diabetes. *Diabetes Care*, 33(2), 264-269.

Lysy, Z., Da Costa, D., & Dasgupta, K. (2008). The association of physical activity and depression in Type 2 diabetes. *Diabetic Medicine*, 25(10), 1133-1141.

Maddams, J., Brewster, D., Gavin, A., Steward, J., Elliott, J., Utley, M., et al. (2009). Cancer prevalence in the United Kingdom: Estimates for 2008. *British Journal of Cancer*, 101(3), 541-547.

Moussavi, S., Chatterji, S., Verdes, E., Tandon, A., Patel, V., & Ustun, B. (2007). Depression, chronic diseases, and decrements in health: Results from the World Health Surveys. *The Lancet*, 370(9590), 851-858.

Murray, C.J.L., & Lopez, A.D. (1996). *The global burden of disease: A comprehensive assessment of mortality and disability from diseases, injuries, and risk factors in 1990 and projected to 2020.* Cambrigde, MA: Harvard School of Public Health on Behalf of the World Health Organization and the World Bank.

Murray, C.J.L., & Lopez, A.D. (1997). Alternative projections of mortality and disability by cause 1990-2020: Global Burden of Disease Study. *The Lancet*, 349(9064), 1498-1504.

National Collaborating Centre for Mental Health. (2010). *Depression in adults with a chronic physical health problem. The NICE guideline on treatment and management.* London: The British Psychological Society and The Royal College of Psychiatrists.

National Institute for Health and Clinical Excellence. (2010). *Chronic obstructive pulmonary disease.*

Management of chronic obstructive pulmonary disease in adults in primary and secondary care (partial update). NICE clinical guideline 101. London: National Collaborating Centre for Acute and Chronic Conditions.

Naylor, C., Parsonage, M., McDaid, D., Knapp, M., Fossey, M., & Galea, A. (2012). Long-term conditions and mental health: The cost of co-morbidities. London: The King's Fund and Centre for Mental Health.

Ng, L., Whye, C., Mackney, J., Jenkins, S., & Hill, K. (2012). Does exercise training change physical activity in people with COPD? A systematic review and meta-analysis. *Chronic Respiratory Disease*, 9(1), 17-26.

Nguyen, H.Q., & Carrieri-Kohlman, V. (2005). Dyspnea self-management in patients with chronic obstructive pulmonary disease: Moderating effects of depressed mood. *Psychosomatics*, 46(5), 402-410.

Nici, L., Donner, C., Wouters, E., Zuwallack, R., Ambrosino, N., Bourbeau, J., et al. (2006). American Thoracic Society/European Respiratory Society statement on pulmonary rehabilitation. *American Journal of Respiratory and Critical Care Medicine*, 173(12), 1390-1413.

Nicolucci, A., Balducci, S., Cardelli, P., Cavallo, S., Fallucca, S., Bazuro, A., et al. (2012). Relationship of exercise volume to improvements of quality of life with supervised exercise training in patients with type 2 diabetes in a randomised controlled trial: The Italian Diabetes and Exercise Study (IDES). *Diabetologia*, 55(3), 579-588.

Nicolucci, A., Balducci, S., Cardelli, P., Zanuso, S., Pugliese, G., & Italian Diabetes Exercise Study Investigators. (2011). Improvement of quality of life with supervised exercise training in subjects with type 2 diabetes mellitus. *Archives of Internal Medicine*, 171(21), 1951-1953.

Office for National Statistics. (2005). *General household survey*. London: Office for National Statistics.

Piette, J.D., Valenstein, M., Himle, J., Duffy, S., Torres, T., Vogel, M., et al. (2011). Clinical complexity and the effectiveness of an intervention for depressed diabetes patients. *Chronic Illness*, 7(4), 267-278.

Puhan, M.A., Gimeno-Santos, E., Scharplatz, M., Troosters, T., Walters, E.H., & Steurer, J. (2011). Pulmonary rehabilitation following exacerbations of chronic obstructive pulmonary disease. *Cochrane Database of Systematic Reviews* 2011, Issue 10. Art. No.: CD005305.

Reid, R., Tulloch, H., Sigal, R., Kenny, G., Fortier, M., McDonnell, L., et al. (2010). Effects of aerobic exercise, resistance exercise or both, on patient-reported health status and well-being in type 2 diabetes mellitus: A randomised trial. *Diabtologia*, 53(4), 632-640.

Ries, A.L., Bauldoff, G.S., Carlin, B.W., Casaburi, R., Emery, C.F., Mahler, D.A., et al. (2007). Pulmonary rehabilitation. *Chest*, 131(5 Suppl.), 4S-42S.

Saxton, J., & Daley, A. (2010). Introduction. In J. Saxton & A. Daley (Eds.), *Exercise and cancer survivorship: impact on health outcomes and quality of life* (pp. 1-16). New York: Springer.

Schmitz, K.H., Courneya, K.S., Matthews, C., Demark-Wahnefried, W., Galvão, D.A., Pinto, B.M., et al. (2010). American College of Sports Medicine roundtable on exercise guidelines for cancer survivors. *Medicine and Science in Sports and Exercise*, 42(7), 1409-1426.

Schneider, C., Jick, S.S., Bothner, U., & Meier, C.R. (2010). COPD and the risk of depression. *Chest*, 137(2), 341-347.

Schram, M.T., Baan, C.A., & Pouwer, F. (2009). Depression and quality of life in patients with diabetes: A systematic review from the European Depression in Diabetes (EDID) research consortium. *Current Diabetes Reviews*, 5(2), 112-119.

Sigal, R.J., Kenny, G.P., Boulé, N.G., Wells, G.A., Prud'homme, D., Fortier, M., et al. (2007). Effects of aerobic training, resistance training, or both on glycemic control in type 2 diabetes. *Annals of Internal Medicine*, 147(6), 357-369.

Singh, S., & Morgan, M. (2012). One step beyond, does rehabilitation influence physical activity? *Chronic Respiratory Disease*, 9, 3-4.

Speck, R., Courneya, K., Mâsse, L., Duval, S., & Schmitz, K. (2010). An update of controlled physical activity trials in cancer survivors: A systematic review and meta-analysis. *Journal of Cancer Survivorship*, 4(2), 87-100.

Spence, R.R., Heesch, K.C., & Brown, W.J. (2011). Colorectal cancer survivors' exercise experiences and preferences: Qualitative findings from an exercise rehabilitation programme immediately after chemotherapy. *European Journal of Cancer Care*, 20(2), 257-266.

Soriano, J.B., Maier, W.C., Egger, P., Visick, G., Thakrar, B., Sykes, J., & Pride, N.B. (2000) Recent trends in physician diagnosed COPD in women and men in the UK. *Thorax*, 55(9), 789-794.

TNS Opinion. (2007). *Health in the European Union*. Brussels: European Commission.

Troosters, T., Casaburi, R., Gosselink, R., & Decramer, M. (2005). Pulmonary rehabilitation in chronic obstructive pulmonary disease. *American Journal of Respiratory and Critical Care Medicine*, 172(1), 19-38.

Troosters, T., Gosselink, R., Janssens, W., & Decramer, M. (2010). Exercise training and pulmonary rehabilitation: New insights and remaining challenges. *European Respiratory Review*, 19(115), 24-29.

Tsai, J., Ford, E., Li, C., Zhao, G., & Balluz, L. (2010). Physical activity and optimal self-rated health of adults with and without diabetes. *BMC Public Health*, 10(1), 1-9.

Unützer, J., Schoenbaum, M., Katon, W.J., Fan, M.-Y., Pincus, H.A., Hogan, D., et al. (2009). Healthcare costs associated with depression in medically ill fee-for-service Medicare participants. *Journal of the American Geriatrics Society*, 57(3), 506-510.

Waschki, B., Kirsten, A., Holz, O., Müller, K.-C., Meyer, T., Watz, H., et al. (2011). Physical activity is the strongest predictor of all-cause mortality in patients with COPD. *Chest*, 140(2), 331-342.

Welch, C.A., Czerwinski, D., Ghimire, B., & Bertsimas, D. (2009). Depression and costs of health care. *Psychosomatics*, 50(4), 392-401.

part

Physical Activity and Mental Health Conditions

Part III examines the role of physical activity in the full range of mental health conditions, including depression and anxiety, dementia, Alzheimer's disease, schizophrenia and addictive behaviour. This part also examines exercise dependence and its relationship with eating disorders and body dysmorphia. Each chapter reviews current knowledge and theory and includes easy-to-follow "Key Concepts" and "Evidence to Practice" sections that are specific to each mental health condition. Physical activity can have a remarkable impact across a range of conditions with different underlying pathologies. Together these chapters provide a powerful testament to the utility of physical activity in attenuating the impact of potentially debilitating mental health conditions. Raising awareness in this area can help others tap into physical activity as a resource for promoting well-being and mental health.

Depression and Anxiety

Amanda Daley, PhD
University of Birmingham, Birmingham, United Kingdom

Chapter Outline

Editors' Introduction

This chapter summarises the evidence for the effectiveness of exercise interventions in the treatment of depression. It provides an accessible overview of the many published reviews and meta-analyses and describes in more detail some recent intervention studies that will be useful for researchers. Its examination of the impact of exercise on women with postnatal and antenatal depression as a special population is especially helpful. This chapter also points to the need for clinicians and health professionals to consider promoting physical activity as a treatment option for depression, includes helpful hints about the dose and type of physical activity that is most beneficial for people with depression and discusses practical considerations for working with this population.

Mental illness is the fourth leading cause of disability worldwide and is predicted to be the second leading cause of disability in developed countries by 2020 (World Health Organisation, 2001). Depression and anxiety are the most common forms of mental disorder, and their prevalence is increasing. Clinical depression presents an important challenge to both primary and secondary health care services (Lester & Howe, 2008) because it is associated with disability, morbidity and mortality (Moussavi et al., 2007) (see "Key Concepts"). In adults, the incidence of depression is estimated to be approximately 3% to 5%/yr (Andrews, Henderson & Hall, 2001; Blazer et al., 1994), and the lifetime prevalence in Western countries is approximately 17% (Lepine et al., 1997). Anxiety disorders are also highly prevalent in adults (Ansseau et al., 2005; Wittchen, 2002). The estimated prevalence of generalised anxiety disorder is 5% to 16% (Wittchen, 2002) and that of panic disorder is between 1.5% and 13% (Craske et al., 2002).

Common treatments for clinical depression are similar to those for anxiety disorders, and it has been shown that about 75% of people who are affected by clinical depression are also affected by anxiety disorder (Myers et al., 1984). The two most common treatments for these disorders are medication (antidepressants) and psychotherapy. In recent years prescription rates for antidepressant medications have dramatically increased, and concern exists about the safety of these medications (Gunnell & Ashby, 2004). Common side effects associated with antidepressants include weight gain, increased blood pressure, hyperglycaemia and sexual dysfunction. Many people do not want to take medication or do not comply with this approach to treatment (Byrne, Regan & Livingston, 2006) and consequently are keen to try alternative, nonpharmacological interventions. Exercise has been proposed as an alternative treatment that potentially could reduce depression and anxiety through biochemical, physiological, psychological and psychosocial mechanisms and pathways.

The new physical activity guidelines "Start Active Stay Active" (see "Physical Activity Guidelines in the United Kingdom" and chapter 2 in this text) published by the chief medical officers of England, Scotland, Wales, and Northern Ireland (2011) state that participation in physical activity can have an important role in promoting mental health and well-being. Over the past three decades there has been considerable research interest in the effects of exercise on depression outcomes. The evidence was so encouraging that in 2007 the National Institute for Health and Clinical Excellence in England (2007) recommended that people with persistent subthreshold depressive symptoms or mild to moderate depression should be advised about the benefits of exercise. Although researchers have studied anxiety disorders less frequently, the evidence reviewed here

Physical Activity Guidelines in the United Kingdom for Adults (19-64 yr)

- Adults should aim to be active daily and should perform at least 150 min/wk of moderate-intensity activity in bouts of 10 min or more. One way to approach this is to perform 30 min at least 5 days/wk.
- Alternatively, comparable benefit can be achieved through 75 min/wk of vigorous-intensity activity or a combination of mod-

erate- and vigorous-intensity activity.
- Adults should also undertake physical activity that improves muscle strength at least 2 days/wk.
- All adults should minimise being sedentary (sitting) for extended periods

Adapted from Chief Medical Officers of England, Scotland, Wales, and Northern Ireland 2011.

indicates that physical activity and exercise also have positive effects on anxiety.

This chapter reviews the evidence about the effectiveness of exercise for reducing depression and anxiety and provides an up-to-date synthesis of what is currently known. This chapter focusses on and emphasises findings from systematic reviews and meta-analyses of randomised controlled trials (RCTs) because these studies provide the best evidence from which to draw conclusions. Furthermore, this chapter is primarily concerned with the effects of exercise on depression because specific clinical guidance exists for this disease. However, it references studies of anxiety disorders where appropriate and relevant. It is important to highlight from the outset that data

KEY CONCEPTS

Psychological Symptoms of Depression

- Continuous low mood or sadness
- Feelings of hopelessness and helplessness
- Low self-esteem
- Tearfulness
- Feelings of guilt
- Feeling irritable and intolerant of others
- Lack of motivation and little interest in things
- Difficulty making decisions
- Lack of enjoyment
- Suicidal thoughts or thoughts of harming oneself
- Feeling anxious or worried
- Reduced interest in sexual intercourse

Psychological Symptoms of Anxiety

- Restlessness
- A sense of dread
- Feeling constantly "on edge"
- Difficulty concentrating
- Irritability
- Impatience
- Being easily distracted

Physical Symptoms of Depression

- Slowed movement or speech
- Change in appetite or weight (usually decreased, but sometimes increased)
- Constipation

- Unexplained aches and pains
- Lack of energy
- Lack of interest in sexual intercourse
- Changes in the menstrual cycle
- Disturbed sleep patterns (e.g., problems going to sleep, waking in the early hours of the morning)

Physical Symptoms of Anxiety

- Dizziness
- Drowsiness and tiredness
- Palpitations
- Muscle aches and tension
- Dry mouth
- Excessive sweating
- Shortness of breath
- Stomach ache
- Nausea
- Diarrhea
- Headache
- Excessive thirst
- Insomnia

Social Symptoms of Depression and Anxiety

- Not doing well at work
- Taking part in fewer social activities and avoiding contact with friends
- Participating in fewer hobbies and interests
- Having difficulties in home and family life

on the effects of exercise on anxiety disorders are far less abundant than are data on the effects of exercise on depression. Chapter 1 reviews physiological mechanisms that have been suggested to underlie the relationships between exercise, depression and anxiety.

1 Evidence Linking Depression and Exercise

Early meta-analyses (McDonald & Hodgson, 1991; North, McCullagh & Tran, 1990) have reported moderate to large effects of exercise on reducing depression. However, because these meta-analyses included non-RCTs and studies in which nondepressed populations were recruited, one must take caution when interpreting their conclusions. Several years later, Craft and Landers (1998) published an updated review and included studies that had recruited individuals experiencing depression as either a primary or secondary disorder. The review included 30 studies (observational and experimental), although several were unpublished dissertations. Analyses showed that exercise resulted in a moderate to large reduction in depression (effect size −0.72). However, the inclusion of observational studies and trials that did not use random allocation of participants to trial groups does restrict the conclusions that one can draw from this particular review. Table 9.1 provides a definition of

effect sizes, and "Methodological Terminology" explains some of the key methodological terminology that is used in this chapter.

Later systematic reviews and meta-analyses have included only RCTs. One of the most influential reviews in this regard, conducted by Lawlor and Hopker (2001), included a total of 14 RCTs and found that exercise exerted a large effect in terms of reducing depression (effect size −1.1) relative to the effect of comparison groups on depression. However, despite this large effect, the authors concluded that the effectiveness of exercise could not be determined because most trials included in their review were of poor quality and had inadequate follow-up outcomes. Several years later, a meta-analysis by Stathopoulou and colleagues (2006) aimed to update and refine the review by Lawlor and Hopker (2001). It included four RCTs that were not available at the time of Lawlor and Hopker's review and excluded studies that did not target clinical levels of depression, were not published in peer-reviewed journals and

Table 9.1 Cohen's Effect Sizes: Difference Between Two Means

Size of effect	d
Small	0.2
Medium	0.5
Large	0.8

Methodological Terminology

An effect size (Cohen's d) measures the magnitude of a treatment effect and is independent of sample size. Effect sizes are commonly used in meta-analysis studies that summarise findings from research studies.

A meta-analysis combines the results of several studies that address a particular research hypothesis. The general aim of a meta-analysis is to estimate the true effect size of studies investigating that hypothesis as opposed to a smaller effect size that is derived in a single study. Meta-

analyses are usually important components of a systematic review.

In meta-analyses, heterogeneity refers to variability or differences between individual studies in the estimates of effects. When excessive variation occurs, it is called statistical heterogeneity. Statistical tests of heterogeneity are used to assess whether the observed variability in study results (effect sizes) is greater than that expected to occur by chance.

did not include a nonactive comparison group. Similar to Lawlor and Hopker, Stathopoulou and colleagues reported a very large treatment (11 trials included) effect (effect size −1.42) in favour of exercise compared with control conditions.

The most recent Cochrane Library systematic review (Mead et al., 2008), which included 23 trials (907 participants) that compared exercise with no treatment or control, reported a large effect size of −0.82. It is important to note that this Cochrane review adopted very broad inclusion criteria in terms of types of participants included (as do other reviews). As a result, it included a number of trials that were conducted with volunteer samples who have been defined as experiencing depression on the basis of applied cut-off scores from self-completed questionnaires and who had not been recruited from clinical settings with a diagnosis of depression.

After the publication of the Cochrane Library review, Krogh and colleagues (2011) argued that reviews should include only studies that have recruited people who had presented to clinical services and been diagnosed with depression by a health professional or participants who had been given a primary diagnosis of depression according to a diagnostic system (e.g., the International Classification of Diseases; World Health Organisation, 2007). This argument is based on the premise that these situations are more likely to mirror clinical situations in which doctors might consider prescribing exercise as a treatment for depression. With this in mind, Krogh and colleagues (2011) recently published a systematic review that included 13 RCTs that fulfilled either of the previously mentioned criteria. They reported a much smaller effect (effect size −0.40) compared with earlier reviews. When the analysis was restricted to the 3 trials that included adequate allocation concealment, blind assessment of outcome and intention to treat analysis, the estimated benefit of exercise was substantially smaller (effect size −0.19 and nonsignificant) than it was when all 13 studies were pooled together. Only 5 of the 13 included studies included long-term follow-up

of the participants to examine the effect of the exercise intervention after its completion. Analyses indicated that exercise had little effect on depression in patients with clinical levels of depression beyond the duration of the exercise programme (effect size −0.01). Further analyses also showed that an inverse relationship existed between the length of the exercise intervention and the magnitude of the relationship between exercise and reduced depression (i.e., the longer the intervention, the smaller the effect).

A number of RCTs postdate systematic reviews and meta-analyses; some of these RCTs are included here for discussion. These particular trials have been selected because they provide a vehicle for raising pertinent issues that are relevant to the debate about the effects of exercise on depression.

An issue that reviews consistently raise is the short follow-up period that is typically included in trials examining exercise and depression. That is, studies often do not follow patients over periods of time that are long enough to determine whether any benefits from exercise have been sustained. However, this would be worth doing only if exercise interventions in studies lasted several months. The importance of longer follow-up in studies should not be underestimated, particularly because current reviews have suggested that the effects of exercise on depression may be short lived. Also, the longer-term effect of exercise on depression relative to the longer-term effect of medication on depression has not been examined. Hoffman and colleagues (2011) addressed this concern by reporting findings of a 1 yr follow-up (i.e., posttreatment at 16 months after randomisation) to a 16 wk intervention study (n = 202 randomised) of home-based exercise, supervised exercise, antidepressant (sertraline) or placebo pill in patients with major depressive disorder. At the end of the intervention period and until the 12 month follow-up, all participants were presented with the option to receive an exercise prescription, a consultation with a psychiatrist for medication or both. Participants could choose to discontinue treatment or to seek treatment elsewhere.

At 4 months, the benefits of exercise and sertraline were similar. At the 1 yr follow-up (*n* = 172), analyses revealed no effect of treatment group on depression score or remission status. However, self-reported exercise (regardless of group allocation at baseline) during the follow-up phase was associated with lower depression scores and greater likelihood of improved depression status. The authors also reported a linear inverse relationship between exercise level (0 to ~180 min/wk) and severity of depressive symptoms; the relationship was weaker after 180 min. The difference in depression score between an individual who reported 180 min/wk of exercise and one who reported 0 min/wk was 3.1 points, which is considered to be clinically meaningful.

Previous reviews have not teased out the potential effects of exercise on specific populations with diverse psychological conditions. For this reason, the trial by Mota-Pereira and colleagues (2011) is of particular interest. These researchers randomised 33 people who had treatment-resistant major depressive disorder for between 9 and 15 mo to usual pharmacotherapy (*n* = 11) or usual pharmacotherapy plus aerobic exercise (*n* = 22) for 12 wk. At the end of the intervention follow-up, the depression scores of the exercise group were significantly lower than those of the usual-care group. Interestingly, no participants in the usual-care group showed response (reduction in symptoms) or remission (feeling well as opposed to just better), yet response and remission rates in the exercise group were 21% (*n* = 4) and 26% (*n* = 5), respectively (these differences are nonsignificant). Data regarding dropout (6%) and compliance (91%) were also very encouraging given the population.

It is often the case that patients with major depressive disorder require second-step treatments to achieve remission. The Trial of Exercise and Depression (TREAD) (Trivedi et al., 2011) conducted in the United States investigated the efficacy of aerobic exercise as an additional treatment for 126 people with major depressive disorder who had not remitted with antidepres-

sant treatment. The authors of the trial argued that patients who show some response (but not remission) to their first treatment need augmentation but that pharmacological augmentation treatments (e.g., lithium, tri-iodothyronine, buspirone) are not universally effective, have side effects, come with an increased risk of interactions and require additional monitoring and that, for these reasons, exercise could be a worthy alternative augmentation treatment. Participants were randomised to either 4 or 16 $kcal \cdot kg^{-1} \cdot wk^{-1}$ of exercise expenditure for 12 wks and selective serotonin reuptake inhibitor treatment continued as usual. An expenditure of 16 $kcal \cdot kg^{-1} \cdot wk^{-1}$ equates to walking at 6.4 km/h (4 miles/h) for 210 min/wk and 4 $kcal \cdot kg^{-1} \cdot wk^{-1}$ equates to walking at 4.8 km/h (3 miles/h) for about 75 min/wk. The study found significant improvements over time when data for both exercise groups were combined. Remission (i.e., feeling well) rates were 28.3% for the group that expended 16 $kcal \cdot kg^{-1} \cdot wk^{-1}$ and 15.5% for the group that expended 4 $kcal \cdot kg^{-1} \cdot wk^{-1}$; this finding approached significance ($p < .06$).

2   Exercise and Postnatal Depression

Postnatal depression (PND) is a serious problem that affects about 10% to 15% of women some time in the first year after giving birth (Gaynes et al., 2005; O'Hara & Swain, 1996) (see "Symptoms of Postnatal Depression"). Although some studies suggest that the incidence of depression after childbirth is no greater than that at other points in a woman's life cycle (Cooper et al., 1988), it can be argued that PND is likely to be more problematic because its effects are experienced at a time when exceptional demands are placed on the woman in caring for her baby and family. PND has health consequences not only for the mother but for the child and the family as a whole as well. Symptoms of PND may include anxiety attacks, tearfulness, loss of interest in life, insecurity, inappropriate obsessional thoughts, irritability, fatigue, insomnia, guilt and fear of harming the baby (Beck, 1992, 2002). The child

Symptoms of Postnatal Depression

- Panic attacks
- Sleeplessness
- Extreme tiredness
- Aches and pains
- Feeling generally unwell
- Memory loss or being unable to concentrate

- Feelings of not being able to cope
- Not being able to stop crying
- Loss of appetite
- Feelings of hopelessness
- Not being able to enjoy anything
- Loss of interest in the baby
- Excessive anxiety about the baby

of a woman with PND may display insecure attachment, behavioural problems and impaired cognitive development (Beck, 1995, 1996, 1999; Hay et al., 2001; Murray, 1992; Sharp, Hay & Pawlby, 1995).

Given the reluctance of some women to take antidepressant medication after giving birth (Whitton, Warner & Appleby, 1996), the limited availability of psychological therapies and the potential for prolonged effects of morbidity, researchers and practitioners need to consider novel interventions for treating PND. Exercise has been proposed as a potential treatment for PND. In their 2007 guidance on the management of antenatal and postnatal mental health, the National Institute for Health and Clinical Excellence in England recommended that exercise should be considered as a treatment for women who develop mild or moderate depression during the postnatal period.

A recent meta-analysis (Daley, Jolly & MacArthur, 2009) of RCTs found that exercise significantly reduced symptoms of PND (effect size −0.81) when compared with no exercise, although significant heterogeneity was found and the analysis included only 5 trials involving 221 participants. Importantly, one of the included trials (Armstrong & Edwards, 2003) involved exercise as a cointervention with social support. When this trial was excluded from the meta-analysis, the effect size was reduced considerably and became nonsignificant (effect size −0.42; marginal) and heterogeneity was no longer present (i.e., the remaining studies

were similar in size of effect). Put another way, including or excluding the trial by Armstrong and Edwards (2003) had substantial bearing on the findings of the meta-analysis because Armstrong and Edwards (2003) found a very large effect size, whereas other trials reported more modest effects (see figure 9.1).

A forest plot is a graphic display that illustrates the relative strength of treatment effects (in this case, exercise) in multiple studies that address the same question. Squares represent the measure of effect for each included study and horizontal lines across the square represent confidence intervals. The area of each square is proportional to the weight of the study in the meta-analysis. The overall measure of effect for all the studies is commonly plotted as a diamond at the bottom of the forest plot. A vertical line representing no effect is plotted at zero. If the confidence intervals for individual studies overlap with this line, their effect sizes do not differ from no effect for the individual study at the given level of confidence. The same applies for the meta-analysed measure of effect. If the points of the diamond overlap the line of no effect (at zero), the overall meta-analysed result cannot be said to differ from no effect at the given level of confidence.

One explanation for why the Armstrong and Edwards (2003) trial found such a large effect could be that the intervention involved social support plus exercise and the other trials involved exercise only. Moreover, it is clear from the current literature that social support is in itself an

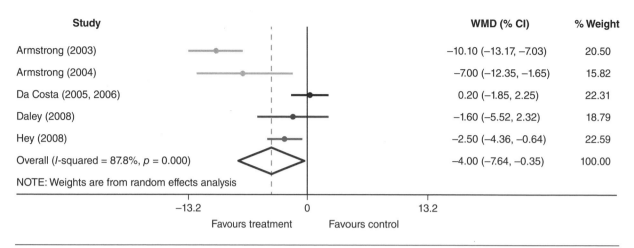

Figure 9.1 Forest plot study summary of the effect of exercise relative to comparators for postnatal depression.
Based on Daley et al. 2009.

effective intervention for depression (Paykel & Cooper, 1992). The systematic review by Daley, Jolly and MacArthur (2009) also highlighted a number of methodological deficiencies in all of the included trials, the most problematic being the inclusion of women who did not have a confirmed diagnosis of PND and the small size of the trials.

In summary, the available evidence suggests that exercise can reduce PND. However, this finding is contingent on the inclusion of one trial that included exercise as a cointervention with social support. Therefore, one should interpret findings from this meta-analysis with some caution. A trial of the effectiveness of exercise as a treatment for PND is ongoing and may resolve some of the uncertainty around this question in due course.

3 Exercise and Antenatal Depression

Although pregnancy is typically portrayed as wonderful, joyful time, about 10% to 20% of women experience antenatal depression (Gaynes et al., 2005). Women who are depressed in pregnancy are more likely to experience obstetric complications and their babies are at greater risk for preterm delivery and low birth weight (Alder et al., 2007). Later in life, these children experience more psychological, behavioural and develop-

mental problems than their peers born to women without depression (World Health Organisation, 2009). Depression during pregnancy is also one of the strongest predictors of PND (Lancaster et al., 2010). The use of antidepressants to treat antenatal depression poses particular problems because these medications can cross the placenta and, because of this, doctors are often reluctant to prescribe them and mothers often do not want to take them (Bonari et al., 2005).

Historically, exercise was discouraged during pregnancy and the prevailing view was that "rest is best." However, this view has been discredited over time as more evidence has emerged to support the role of exercise in improving obstetric outcomes during pregnancy (such as gestational hypertension or diabetes) and reducing the risk of excessive gestational weight gain. Studies have also shown that exercise during pregnancy can promote mental health. A review by Shivakumar and colleagues (2011) identified no studies that had examined exercise in an antenatal population diagnosed with depression but did find six observational studies that had recruited healthy pregnant women and had included assessments of depression, anxiety or related outcomes.

Koniak-Griffin (1994) investigated the effects of a 6 wk aerobic exercise programme on depression and self-esteem levels in 58 pregnant adolescents living in a maternity residential home. The exercise group reported fewer depressive symptoms than the sedentary group. Goodwin, Astbury and McMeeken (2000) compared psychological well-being in exercising (*n* = 25) and nonexercising (*n* = 18) pregnant women. The exercise group had lower anxiety scores over time compared with the nonexercise group. Da Costa and colleagues (2003) examined the association between leisure-time physical activity patterns and psychological well-being during pregnancy. A total of 180 women self-reported through structured interviews the amount of leisure-time physical activity achieved in each trimester. Starting in the third month of pregnancy, data were collected monthly on depressed mood, state anxiety and pregnancy-specific stress. Analyses comparing exercisers and nonexercisers in each trimester showed that exercisers reported significantly less depressed mood, daily hassles, state anxiety and pregnancy-specific stress in the first and second trimesters. Women who exercised in the third trimester reported less state anxiety in that trimester compared with nonexercisers. Two other studies (Poudevigne & O'Connor, 2005; Williams et al., 1988) found no relationship between participation in exercise and mood states in pregnant women.

Because all of the studies identified by Shivakumar and colleagues (2011) were observational, small or very small and contained other methodological concerns, it is not possible to infer cause-and-effect relationships from these studies. Consequently, it is currently unclear whether exercise is an effective treatment for antenatal depression. What is clear, however, is that this question requires further research. Studies that focus on recruiting pregnant women with a diagnosis of antenatal depression would be most useful.

4 Exercise and Anxiety

The effects of exercise on anxiety have been examined by several reviews and meta-analyses (Conn, 2010; Long & Van Stavel, 1995; Petruzzello et al., 1991; Wipfli, Rethorst & Landers, 2008), all of which reported that exercise was associated with a reduction in anxiety. Of particular interest is the review by Petruzzello and colleagues (1991), which divided outcomes of anxiety in studies into three subgroup categories: self-reported state anxiety, self-reported trait anxiety and psychophysiological measures of anxiety. This review included all types of studies. The effect sizes in all categories were associated with a reduction in anxiety (−0.24, −0.34 and −0.56) for self-reported state anxiety, self-reported trait anxiety and psychophysiological measures of anxiety, respectively. The findings from the meta-analysis by Long and Van Stavel (1995) were not dissimilar to those reported by Petruzello and colleagues (1991) and reported an overall effect size of −0.45 for studies using within-gr oup design and −0.36 for those that included a comparison group.

Some reviews have focussed specifically on examining effects in people identified as having high levels of anxiety at the time of study recruitment. In a subgroup analysis, Petruzzello and colleagues (1991) found that the mean effect size was −0.47 in people identified as highly anxious, although a meta-analysis by Stich (1998) reported a much higher effect size (−0.94) from randomised studies in people who demonstrated anxiety scores above the 50th percentile. Within this meta-analysis, the effect size of studies of individuals with formal anxiety disorders was 0.99, which is substantial. In a more recent meta-analysis of only RCTs, Wipfli, Rethorst and Landers (2008) reported an overall effect size of −0.48 (based on 49 studies), which indicates a moderate reduction in anxiety scores in exercisers compared with nonexercisers. The effect size for clinical populations was marginally higher at −0.52, although this was based on data from only 3 studies. The review by Wipfli, Rethorst and Landers (2008) suggests that exercise can be used as an intervention for anxiety, although it must be acknowledged that the vast majority of studies recruited nonclinical populations and not people who were receiving clinical treatment for anxiety disorders. In real terms, those with anxiety disorders are likely to have the most to gain from exercise, and future research should focus on this group.

The majority of previous meta-analyses have included samples with diagnosed anxiety disorders or elevated anxiety and have typically included mental health interventions as the comparator. Conn (2010) conducted a meta-analysis of the anxiolytic effects of physical activity intervention separate from psychological treatments in adults free of clinical anxiety disorders. This review focused on synthesizing anxiety outcomes from physical activity intervention studies among healthy adults on the basis that many people without diagnosed anxiety experience symptoms of anxiety. As such, studies that used interventions to treat anxiety (e.g., relaxation training, stress management) were excluded. Not surprisingly, this meta-analysis reported an overall effect size of −0.22, which is smaller than previously reported by meta-analyses that had included clinically anxious groups. Nevertheless, this finding further confirms that even healthy adults can experience reduced anxiety after participating in an exercise programme.

5   Exercise for Treating Depression and Anxiety

It is important to understand the dose, type and context of exercise that are necessary or ideal for effectively treating depression and anxiety. Information about these prescription parameters is scarce, but it is critical if exercise interventions are to be translated into clinical practice. Asking someone to do something without specifying what they should do or how they should do it would likely make it difficult for the individual to fully comply in a meaningful way. It is also possible that the prescription of exercise for depression and/or anxiety could be different, both in nature and content, than that required for general health benefits.

One trial that is particularly worthy of attention is the Depression Outcomes Study of Exercise (DOSE; Dunn et al., 2005), which attempted to provide evidence about the dose of exercise required to treat depression. In the DOSE study 80 participants were randomised to 1 of 4 exercise groups that varied in total

energy expenditure (7 or 17.5 $kcal \cdot kg^{-1} \cdot wk^{-1}$) and frequency (3 or 5 days/wk) or to a flexibility-exercise placebo control for 12 wk. Exercise at a dose of 17.5 $kcal \cdot kg^{-1} \cdot wk^{-1}$ was effective in reducing depression regardless of frequency, whereas exercise at a dose of 7 $kcal \cdot kg^{-1} \cdot wk^{-1}$ yielded antidepressant effects that were comparable to those of the placebo treatment. The plausible biological reason for why a higher dose of exercise may be more effective than lower doses is that frequent and regular exercise should increase fitness levels such that physical discomfort decreases and exercise becomes a more pleasant and enjoyable experience as the conditioning process progresses. Indeed, findings from both the DOSE and TREAD trials in the United States have indicated that higher doses of exercise are more effective than are lower doses (as defined in the study).

Perraton and colleagues (2010) published a systematic review that attempted to summarise what is currently known about the prescription of exercise for depression. The review is useful because previous reviews of exercise and depression did not synthesise this information in a way that would help guide intervention development. This review included only trials that had reported exercise to be effective in reducing depression in order to analyse the specific dosage parameters and modes of exercise used in these successful trials.

The review found that the most common intensity, frequency and duration of aerobic exercise were 60% to 80% of maximum heart rate, 30 min/session and 3 days/wk over 8 wk. The volume of evidence supporting the use of aerobic exercise programmes to treat depression was greater than that supporting the use of anaerobic exercise programmes. No clear trend showed one mode of aerobic exercise to be the most effective, and a range of activity types appeared to be effective. This is encouraging given that one size does not fit all, and individuals can be encouraged to participate in whatever type of aerobic activity they prefer.

In terms of context of exercise, a number of common trends emerged. A variety of locations were effective in treating depression, although all trials that reported location took place indoors. Both group and individual interventions were effective. However, group exercise may have added benefit by providing social support, which can be pivotal for sustaining compliance and can contribute in its own right to lowering depression. Moreover, exercise might lower depression by several plausible mechanisms, one of which could be interrelations or connections with others (Bailey & McLaren, 2005). Many types of exercise can be performed with other people (depressed or not). Therefore, this exercise could provide social integration and an opportunity to interact with the social world as well as a setting in which to expand social networks and make friends (Stathi, Fox & McKenna, 2002).

Another unresolved question concerns the intensity of exercise at which a reduction in depression might occur. Callaghan and colleagues (2011) compared the effects of preferred intensity with those of prescribed intensity of group-based exercise for 12 sessions over 4 wk in 38 women aged 45 to 65 yr who were receiving treatment for depression from either primary or secondary care services. The preferred-intensity group reported significantly lower depression and higher self-esteem and quality-of-life scores than did the prescribed-exercise group and attended more sessions (66% versus 50%). Similar findings have been found in nondepressed populations (Daley & Maynard, 2003). Several theories, such as self-determination theory (Deci & Ryan, 1985), support the notion that giving people a choice and control over what they do, whether it be exercise or other activities, leads to better adherence and enjoyment of the activity, which in turn leads to enhanced psychological well-being. People experiencing depression are no exception.

Wipfli, Rethorst and Landers (2008) considered the relationship between dose of exercise and anxiety levels as part of their broader meta-analysis of the anxiolytic effect of exercise. The trend in the data from 12 RCTs showed that the effect size increased as exercise approached a dose of 12.5 kcal·kg^{-1}·wk^{-1} (equates to slightly less than the dose recommended for public health) and then began to decrease as exercise dose increased. A combination of aerobic and anaerobic exercise appeared to be better than either type alone, and a frequency of 3 or 4 times/wk appeared more effective than more or less than this amount.

6 Exercise Versus Conventional Treatment for Depression and Anxiety

Comparing the effectiveness of treatments alongside each other can be useful because it allows one to judge the relative merits of the treatments when deciding which might be best and under what circumstances. This can be achieved by comparing effect sizes resulting from treatment(s) or by comparing response and remission rates. This section discusses both of these approaches.

Several studies have evaluated the effectiveness of exercise against the effectiveness of alternative treatments for depression, most notably psychotherapy and antidepressants. In one meta-analysis (Craft & Landers, 1998), exercise was not significantly different from psychotherapy or other types of behavioural and pharmacological interventions. In another meta-analysis (Mead, 2009) the effect of exercise was not significantly different from that of cognitive therapy (152 participants from 6 trials) or antidepressants (201 participants from 2 trials). As discussed earlier, meta-analyses regarding the effect of exercise on depression have reported effect sizes in the region of −0.4 to −1.1, depending on the methodological quality of studies included. An effect size of 0.4 is very much in line with those found for standard treatment of depression and is greater than the effect sizes reported by recent meta-analyses of data from the U.S. Food and Drug Administration of placebo-controlled trials of antidepressants (Kirsch et al., 2008; Turner et al., 2008).

Studies have not always reported their findings in relation to response and remission rates, but this is arguably the best method for assessing whether treatments for depression have been effective for patients in real terms. Dunn and colleagues (2005) reported response and remission rates that were comparable with those of other depression treatments in participants randomised to receive an exercise intervention at the dose recommended for public health.

In a review by Wipfli, Rethorst and Landers (2008), 27 out of 49 studies compared exercise with some other form of treatment for anxiety (e.g., cognitive behavioural therapy, relaxation or meditation and music therapy). Exercise was found to be equal or superior to all other types of treatment for anxiety (effect size 0.19 for all treatments versus −0.48 for exercise). When consideration is given to the effect sizes of individual treatment approaches for anxiety disorders, exercise was as effective as psychotherapy and nearly as effective as medication. This is very encouraging given that psychotherapy and medications are the two most common treatments for anxiety disorders.

On a practical level, exercise is relatively free of side effects and is low cost compared with medication and psychological interventions. Exercise does not have associated negative social stigmas and can be performed when convenient for the individual. In contrast, many psychological treatments include therapy sessions with a counsellor or psychologist. Antidepressants have a latency period of several weeks before they take effect, whereas exercise has potential to provide immediate psychological benefits. Antidepressant medication and psychological treatments cannot offer any direct benefits in terms of improving physical health and well-being. This is an important benefit because depressed patients often demonstrate increased levels of physical illness (Martinsen & Medhus, 1989; Peveler, Carson & Rodin, 2002). Consequently, the rationale for exercise as an intervention may extend beyond the benefits for depression (or anxiety disorders) alone. Also, some symptoms of depression and anxiety (e.g., fatigue, reduced cognitive function) remain resistant despite antidepressant treatment; evidence (Eriksen & Bruusgaard, 2004; Etnier et al., 1997) has shown

that exercise can significantly reduce these types of symptoms as well.

Although systematic reviews and meta-analyses provide evidence of the effectiveness of treatments, they do not provide any information regarding individuals' experiences, perceptions or attitudes about an intervention or treatment. In other words, reviews do not describe what it is like for patients. The next section provides a taste of some of the comments patients have reported as a result of participating in an exercise programme to treat depression.

Searle and colleagues (2011) interviewed 33 patients participating in TREAD, which is an ongoing RCT in England examining the effects of usual care plus physical activity or usual care only. Participants were generally aware that exercise could be an effective treatment for depression, and several described a number of benefits that could be gained from participating. Some examples of things patients said include the following:

"I always feel energised and elevated after I have done something that's caused me hard work, my heart to beat faster. And usually when I've achieved something, you get a sense of euphoria."

"I know that if you increase the amount of movement and your activity then your serotonin level is going to kick in and it's going to make you feel better."

Most participants perceived physical activity to be an acceptable treatment for depression. This is not surprising given that they all had consented to take part in the trial of exercise and depression. A few participants commented that they felt that the effectiveness of physical activity in treating depression would depend on its severity. Most participants stated a preference for physical activity over other treatments, particularly antidepressants.

"I am increasing my confidence, physical activity and some of these more complimentary things need to take over from perhaps some traditional medication, you know…. And I don't want to be considering taking long-term medication, you know."

The preference for physical activity stemmed from the desire to have some autonomy in the longer-term management of their depression, which they thought could be gained from exercise. This suggests that participants appreciated the opportunity to help themselves and, as such, they appeared to be motivated to remain active rather than passive in the treatment process.

Although the benefits of physical activity (e.g., weight loss, social interaction, better sleep) were emphasised during the interviews, some participants (particularly women and those who were low active) discussed negative consequences or aspects of attempting to be physically active; these typically related to their ability. One patient said this:

"I didn't enjoy indoor rock climbing at all. I have absolutely no upper body strength so it was—I didn't like it, it made feel like I was inadequate."

Of interest here is that some participants who were taking antidepressants at the time of the interviews reported that the medication was useful in helping them initiate and maintain their participation in exercise. This issue is critical because a great deal of energy and motivation are required from patients in order for exercise to be an effective treatment for depression. This suggests that it might be better to delay advising patients who are prescribed antidepressants about exercise until their medication has had the opportunity to take effect. One patient explained the interaction between medication and exercise as follows:

"I think I've reached the stage with fluoxetine where it's kick-started the process [of engaging in activity]. I hope I have, I feel as though I have."

The perceived cause of depression seemed to influence the extent to which participants thought physical activity might be helpful. This intimated that physical activity was less helpful if the depression was a function of situational factors rather than biochemical factors. Of note, participants who felt that the cause of depression was a biochemical imbalance (rather than situational) tended to report that physical activity had to be aerobic based in order to be beneficial. In contrast, participants who believed that their depression was related to situational or adverse life events tended to report the benefits of less-intense aerobic activities (e.g., walking).

Several other researchers, albeit some time ago, investigated patients' views about exercise as treatment for mental health disorders. Pelham and Campagna (1991) reported that psychiatric outpatients who participated in a 12 wk exercise-therapy programme expressed positive views about exercise. Similarly, Martinsen and Medhus (1989) asked patients to evaluate the usefulness of an exercise programme compared with other more traditional forms of treatment (i.e., contact with nurses, psychotherapy and medication). Participants who were given the opportunity to participate in the exercise programme rated it the therapeutic element that helped them the most. Those in the control group who did not experience the programme rated individual psychotherapy as most beneficial. These studies challenge commonly held beliefs that patients will not like exercise and will prefer traditional treatments. These studies also emphasise the importance of qualitative research paradigms in understanding what is important to patients when planning treatment for depression and anxiety.

7 Promoting Exercise in the Treatment of Depression and Anxiety

Although the available evidence suggests exercise has a positive effect on depression and anxiety, and although people with these conditions appear to view exercise as treatment favourably, one must remain pragmatic about the complexities surrounding promoting exercise in people experiencing mental illness.

The experience of clinicians and other health professionals who treat major depression is that it is often difficult to motivate seriously depressed people (Seime & Vickers, 2006). Linked to this, a potential incompatibility may exist between exercise and depression or anxiety. People who are feeling depressed or anxious typically experience symptoms such as loss of interest, fatigue, psychomotor agitation, hopelessness, lack of energy, sense of worthlessness, social withdrawal and sleep disturbance; yet a considerable amount of energy, commitment, engagement with surroundings and motivation is required for exercise to be effective in treating these conditions. This might make it very difficult for people who are depressed or anxious to actively engage (spontaneously or prescribed) in exercise as a treatment, and they simply may not have the attributes needed to make the commitment to adhere.

Patients need to adhere to exercise in order to experience therapeutic benefit, and dropout from treatment is a critical factor in determining treatment success. Continued involvement in exercise after remission may also be an important prophylaxis in preventing relapse. Although dropout from exercise programs (rate of ~20%; Stathopoulou et al., 2006) has been identified as a concern in depressed populations (Blumenthal

et al., 1999; Sing, Clements & Fiatarone, 1997), encouragingly this rate is similar to, and in some cases better than, rate of dropout from taking antidepressant medication to treat depression (MacGillivray et al., 2003). As with any type of treatment for depression, patients need to be monitored regularly to ensure adherence.

Regularly achieving the recommended dose of physical activity to obtain health benefits is likely to be challenging, at least initially, for people who are depressed or anxious. Therefore, it may be better to encourage patients to concentrate on achieving short (e.g., 10 min) bouts of exercise and work toward increasing the dose over time. The opportunity to experience success at exercise, regardless of dose or type, is one of the keys factors in determining progress and, ultimately, success. Nevertheless, some consideration should also be given to the studies by Dunn and colleagues (2005), Legrand and Heuze (2007) and Wipfli, Rethorst and Landers (2008), which suggest that the effects of exercise on depression and anxiety may be dose dependent.

As highlighted previously, people with depressive symptoms may find it difficult to overcome

EVIDENCE TO PRACTICE

Practical considerations when working with depressed individuals include the following:

- It can be difficult to motivate people who are depressed.
- People who are depressed often experience fatigue, loss of energy, loss of interest in life, hopelessness and social withdrawal, thus making it difficult for them to initiate and engage in an exercise programme.
- People who choose exercise as a treatment for depression or anxiety disorders need to be monitored regularly by their health care team (as is the case for any treatment).
- It is appropriate to encourage people with depression or anxiety to concen-

trate on achieving small bouts of exercise initially and gradually increase the dose achieved over time.

- People with depression or anxiety may face many barriers to exercise (e.g., accessing exercise facilities) and likely need specific support to overcome these.
- People with depression or anxiety are likely to require ongoing support in order to maintain their level of exercise participation.
- Some people with depression or anxiety may enjoy exercise sessions with other people who are depressed or anxious and may gain additional mental health benefits from such sessions.

barriers to exercise and consequently are less likely to adhere. Interestingly, Vickers and colleagues (2003) found that depressed patients participating in an exercise intervention emphasised that assistance with connecting to the fitness centre was very important. Many felt intimidated by the thought of the fitness centre and having to make the initial appointment and answering questions; support in doing this was instrumental to their decision to initiate exercise. In addition, participants wanted ongoing support for exercise, indicating that these patients often require more input than simply pointing them towards services or instructions or information about exercise.

Although the exact time framework for positive psychological responses to occur from participation in exercise is not known, some studies have shown that changes in mood appear to dissipate within 4 h of completing a bout of exercise (Petruzzello & Landers, 1994; Thayer, 1996). To reinforce and re-establish improvements to mood, therefore, those engaging in exercise as a treatment for depression or anxiety may need to do so on a frequent basis—perhaps several times a day (e.g., regular walking)—thus increasing the time and commitment likely to be required.

For women with PND, complications such as child care responsibilities, fatigue and breastfeeding routines may reduce their opportunities and enthusiasm for exercise (Daley, MacArthur & Winter, 2007). Therefore, any programme that promotes exercise in this population needs to take these factors into account and provide alternative strategies and methods by which women can achieve regular exercise participation. Pregnant women with antenatal depression might find certain types of exercise uncomfortable, and activities such as swimming and walking are likely to be preferred over, and safer than, many other modes of exercise.

8 Summary

Several meta-analyses of the effects of exercise on depression and anxiety have been published over the past two decades. Early reviews reported very positive results regarding exercise for treating depression, but these were based predominantly on observational studies and low-quality controlled trials. A serious question remains about the potential for bias in these included studies. Recent reviews that have utilized more stringent study-inclusion criteria have reported exercise to be effective in reducing depression but have reported smaller effect sizes. In addition, authors of recent reviews have warned against taking their findings at face value because the methodological quality of trials is still not adequate to make any conclusive statement about the effectiveness of exercise as a treatment for clinical depression in the longer term. Evidence supporting the short-term effects of exercise on depression is much more convincing, and exercise appears to be at least as effective as other types of treatment in the short term. Therefore, clinicians and health professionals should consider promoting exercise as a treatment option for depression but should be mindful of the methodological concerns raised by reviews and be aware that current evidence points towards exercise being effective only in the shorter term. Findings from trials involving women experiencing PND have been promising but small, raising concerns about the potential for bias. Evidence regarding antenatal depression is very underdeveloped, and no conclusions on this can be made until further research takes place.

Some evidence supports the role of exercise in reducing clinical and subclinical anxiety, but more research is required, as are data on the dose–response relationship for this outcome. Regardless, participation in exercise has minimal side effects, and exercise has the ability to improve many components of health and well-being. For these reasons alone, health professions should regularly promote exercise.

9 References

Alder, J., Fink, N., Bitzer, J., Hosli, I., & Holzgreve, W. (2007). Depression and anxiety during pregnancy: A risk factor for obstetric, fetal and neonatal outcome? A critical review of the literature. *The Journal of Maternal-Fetal and Neonatal Medicine*, 20, 189-209.

Andrews, G., Henderson, S., & Hall, W. (2001). Prevalence, comorbidity, disability and service utilisation: Overview of the Australian National Mental Health Survey. *British Journal of Psychiatry*, 178(2), 145-153.

Ansseau, M., Fischler, B., Dierick, M., Mignon, A., & Leyman, S. (2005). Prevalence and impact of generalized anxiety disorder and major depression in primary care in Belgium and Luxemburg: The GADIS study. *European Psychiatry*, 20, 229-235.

Armstrong, K., & Edwards, H. (2003). The effects of exercise and social support on mothers reporting depressive symptoms: A pilot randomized controlled trial. *International Journal of Mental Health Nursing*, 12, 130-138.

Bailey, M., & McLaren, S. (2005). Physical activity alone or with others as predictors of sense of belonging and mental health in retirees. *Aging and Mental Health*, 9, 82-90.

Beck, C.T. (1992). The lived experience of postpartum depression: A phenomenological study. *Nursing Research*, 42, 166-170.

Beck, C.T. (1995). The effects of postpartum depression on maternal-infant interaction: A meta-analysis. *Nursing Research*, 44, 298-304.

Beck, C.T. (1996). Postpartum depressed mothers' experiences interaction with their children. *Nursing Research*, 45, 98-104.

Beck, C.T. (1999). Maternal depression and child behaviour problems: A meta-analysis. *Journal of Advanced Nursing*, 29, 623-629.

Beck, C.T. (2002). Postpartum depression: A meta-synthesis. *Qualitative Health Research*, 12, 469-488.

Blazer, D.G., Kessler, R.C., McGonagle, K.A., & Swartz, M.S. (1994). The prevalence and distribution of major depression in a national community sample: The National Comorbidity Survey. *American Journal of Psychiatry*, 15(7), 979-986.

Blumenthal, J.A., Babyak, M.A., Moore, K.A., Craighead, W.E., Herman, H., Khatri, P., et al. (1999). Effects of exercise training on older patients with major depression. *Archives of Internal Medicine*, 159, 2349-2356.

Bonari, L., Koren, G., Einarson, T.R., Jasper, J.D., Taddio, A., & Einarson, A. (2005). Use of antidepressants by pregnant women: Evaluation of perception of risk, efficacy of evidence based counseling and determinants of decision making. *Archives of Women's Mental Health*, 8, 214-220.

Byrne, N., Regan, C., & Livingston, G. (2006). Adherence to treatment in mood disorders. *Current Opinion in Psychiatry*, 19, 44-49.

Callaghan, P., Khalil, E., Morres, I., & Carter, T. (2011). Pragmatic randomised controlled trial of preferred intensity exercise in women living with depression. *BMC Public Health*, 12(11), 465.

Chief Medical Officers of England, Scotland, Wales, and Northern Ireland. (2011). *Start active, stay active. A report on physical activity for health from the four home countries' Chief Medical Officers.* Available: www.dh.gov.uk/en/PublicationsandstatisticsPublications/PublicationsPolicyAndGuidance/DH_128209.

Conn, V.S. (2010). Anxiety outcomes after physical activity interventions: Meta analysis findings. *Nursing Research*, 59(3), 224-231.

Cooper, P., Campbell, E., Day, A., Kennerley, H., & Bond, A. (1988). Non-psychotic psychiatric disorder after childbirth: A prospective study of prevalence, incidence, course and nature. *British Journal of Psychiatry*, 152, 799-806.

Craft, L.L., & Landers, D.M. (1998). The effects of exercise on clinical depression and depression resulting from mental illness: A meta-analysis. *Journal of Sport and Exercise Psychology*, 20, 339-357.

Craske, M.G., Roy-Byrne, P., Stein, M.B., Donald-Sherbourne, C., Bystritsky, A., Katon, W., et al. (2002). Treating panic disorder in primary care: A collaborative care intervention. *General Hospital Psychiatry*, 24, 148-155.

Da Costa, D., Rippen, N., Dritsa, M., & Ring, A. (2003). Self-reported leisure-time physical activity during pregnancy and relationship to psychological well-being. *Journal of Psychosomatic Obstetrics and Gynaecology*, 24, 111-119.

Daley, A.J., Jolly, K., & MacArthur, C. (2009). The effectiveness of exercise in the management of postnatal depression: Systematic review and meta-analysis. *Family Practice*, 26, 154-162.

Daley, A.J., MacArthur, C., & Winter, H. (2007). The role of exercise as a treatment of postnatal depression: A review. *Journal of Midwifery and Women's Health*, 52, 56-62.

Daley, A.J., & Maynard, I.W. (2003). Preferred exercise mode and affective responses in physically active adults. *Psychology of Sport and Exercise*, 4, 347-356.

Deci, E.L., & Ryan, R.M. (1985). *Intrinsic motivation and self-determination in human behavior.* New York: Plenum.

Dunn, A.L., Trivedi, H., Kampert, J.B., & Clark, C.G. (2005). Exercise treatment for depression: Efficacy and dose response. *American Journal of Preventive Medicine*, 28, 1-8.

Eriksen, W., & Bruusgaard, D. (2004). Do physical leisure time activities prevent fatigue? A 15-month prospective study of nurses' aides. *British Journal of Sports Medicine*, *38*, 331-336.

Etnier, J., Salazar, W., Landers, D., Petruzzello, S.J., Han, M., & Nowell, P. (1997). The influence of physical fitness and exercise upon cognitive functioning: A meta-analysis. *Journal of Sport and Exercise Psychology*, 19, 249-277.

Gaynes, B.N., Gavin, N., Melzer-Brody, S., Lohr, K.N., Swinson, T., Gartlehner, G., et al. (2005). Perinatal depression: Prevalence, screening accuracy, and screening outcomes. *Evidence Report Technology Assessment*, 119, 1-8.

Goodwin, A., Astbury, J., & McMeeken, J. (2000). Body image and psychological well-being in pregnancy. A comparison of exercisers and non-exercisers. *Australian and New Zealand Journal of Obstetrics and Gynaecology*, 40, 442-447.

Gunnell, D., & Ashby, D. (2004). Antidepressants and suicide: What is the balance of benefit and risk? *British Medical Journal*, 329(7456), 34-38.

Hay, D., Pawlby, S., Sharp, D., Asten, P., Mills, A., & Kumar, R. (2001). Intellectual problems shown by 11-year-old children whose mothers had postnatal depression. *Journal of Child Psychology and Psychiatry*, 42, 871-889.

Hoffman, B.M., Babyak, M.A., Craighead, W.E., Sherwood, A., Doraiswamy, P.M., Coons, M.J., et al. (2011). Exercise and pharmacotherapy in patients with major depression: One-year follow-up of the SMILE study. *Psychosomatic Medicine*, 73(2), 127-133.

Kirsch, I., Deacon, B.J., Huedo-Medina, T.B., Scoboria, A., Moore, T.J., & Johnson, B.T. (2008). Initial severity and antidepressant benefits: A meta-analysis of data submitted to the Food and Drug Administration. *Public Library of Science Medicine*, 5, e45.

Koniak-Griffin, D. (1994). Aerobic exercise, psychological well-being, and physical discomforts during adolescent pregnancy. *Research in Nursing and Health*, 17, 253-263.

Krogh, J., Nordentoft, M., Sterne, J.A., & Lawlor, D.A. (2011). The effect of exercise in clinically depressed adults: Systematic review and meta-analysis of randomized controlled trials. *Journal of Clinical Psychiatry*, 72(4), 529-538.

Lancaster, C.A., Gold, K.J., Flynn, H.A., Yoo, H., Marcus, S.M., & Davis, M.M. (2010). Risk factors for depressive symptoms during pregnancy: A systematic review. *American Journal of Obstetrics and Gynecology*, 202, 5-14.

Lawlor, D.A., & Hopker, S.W. (2001). The effectiveness of exercise as an intervention in the management of depression: Systematic review and meta-regression analysis of randomized controlled trials. *British Medical Journal*, 322, 1-8.

Legrand, F., & Heuze, J.P. (2007). Antidepressant effects associated with different exercise conditions in participants with depression: A pilot study. *Journal of Sport and Exercise Psychology*, 29, 348-364.

Lepine, J.P., Gastpar, M., Mendlewicz, J., & Tylee, A. (1997). Depression in the community: The first pan-European study DEPRES (Depression Research in European Society). *International Clinical Psychopharmacology*, 12(1), 19-21.

Lester, H., & Howe, A. (2008). Depression in primary care: Three key challenges. *Postgraduate Medical Journal*, 84(996), 545-548.

Long, B.C., & Van Stavel, R. (1995). Effects of exercise training on anxiety: A meta analysis. *Journal of Applied Sports Psychology*, 7, 167-189.

MacGillivray, S., Arnoll, B., Hatcher, S., Ogston, S., Ried, I., Sullivan, F., et al. (2003). Efficacy and tolerability of selective serotonin reuptake inhibitors compared with tricyclic antidepressants in depression treated in primary care: Systematic review and meta-analysis. *British Medical Journal*, 326, 1014.

Martinsen, E.W., & Medhus, A. (1989). Adherence to exercise and patients' evaluation of physical exercise in a comprehensive treatment programme for depression. *Nordic Journal of Psychiatry*, 43, 411-415.

McDonald, D.G., & Hodgson, J.A. (1991). *Psychological effects of aerobic fitness training: Research and theory*. New York: Springer Verlag.

Mead, G.E., Morley, W., Campbell, P., Greig, C.A., McMurdo, M., & Lawlor, D.A. (2009). Exercise for depression. *Cochrane Database of Systematic Reviews*, 4, CD004366.

Mota-Pereira, J., Silverio, J., Carvalho, S., Ribeiro, J.C., Fonte, D., & Ramos, J. (2011). Moderate exercise improves depression parameters in treatment-resistant patients with major depressive disorder. *Journal of Psychiatric Research*, 45(8), 1005-1011.

Moussavi, S., Chatterji, S., Verdes, E., Tandon, A., Patel, V., & Uston, B. (2007). Depression, chronic disease, and decrements in health: Results from the World Health Survey. *Lancet*, 370, 851-858.

Murray, L. (1992). The impact of postnatal depression on infant development. *Journal of Child Psychology and Psychiatry*, 33, 543-561.

Myers, J.K., Weissman, M.M., Tischler, G.L., Holzer, C.E., Leaf, P.J., Orvaschel, H., et al. (1984). Six-months prevalence of psychiatric disorders in three communities: 1980 to 1982. *Archives of General Psychiatry*, 41, 959-967.

National Institute for Health and Clinical Excellence. (2007). *Antenatal and postnatal mental health. Clinical Management and Service Guidance. Clinical guideline 45*. London: NHS.

North, T.C., McCullagh, P., & Tran, Z.V. (1990). Effects of exercise on depression. *Exercise and Sports Science Reviews*, 18, 379-415.

O'Hara, M., & Swain, A. (1996). Rates and risk of postpartum depression—A meta analysis. *International Review of Psychiatry*, 8, 37-54.

Paykel, E.S., & Cooper, Z.C. (1992). Life events and social support. In E.S. Paykel (Ed.), *Handbook of affective disorders* (2nd ed.) (pp. 149-170). Edinburgh: Churchill Livingstone.

Pelham, T., & Campagna, P. (1991). Benefits of exercise in psychiatric rehabilitation of persons with schizophrenia. *Canadian Journal of Rehabilitation*, 4, 159-168.

Perraton, L.G., Kumar, S., Machotka, Z. (2010) Exercise parameters in the treatment of clinical depression: a systematic review of randomized controlled trials. *Journal of Evaluation in Clinical Practice*, 16(3) 597-604.

Petruzzello, S.J., & Landers, D.M. (1994). Varying the duration of acute exercise: Implications for changes in affect. *Anxiety, Stress, and Coping*, 6, 301-310.

Petruzzello, S.J., Landers, D.M., Hatfield, B.D., Kubitz, K.A., & Salazar, W. (1991). A meta- analysis on the anxiety reducing effects of acute and chronic exercise. *Sports Medicine*, 11, 143-182.

Peveler, R., Carson, A., & Rodin, G. (2002). ABC of psychological medicine: Depression in medical patients. *British Medical Journal*, 325, 149-152.

Poudevigne, M., & O'Connor, P. (2005). Physical activity and mood during pregnancy. *Medicine and Science in Sport and Exercise*, 37, 1374-1380.

Searle, A., Calnan, M., Lewis, G., Campbell, J., Taylor, A., & Turner, K. (2011). Patients' views of physical activity as treatment for depression: A qualitative study. *British Journal of General Practice*, 61, 149-156.

Seime, R. J. & Vickers, K. S. (2006), The Challenges of Treating Depression with Exercise: From Evidence to Practice. *Clinical Psychology: Science and Practice*, 13(2), 194–197.

Sharp, D., Hay, D., & P awlby, S. (1995). The impact of postnatal depression on boys' intellectual development. *Journal of Child Psychology and Psychiatry*, 36, 1315-1337.

Shivakumar, G., Brandon, A.R., Snell, P.G., Santiago-Munoz, P., Johnson, N.L., Trivedi, M.H., et al. (2011). Antenatal depression: A rationale for studying exercise. *Depression and Anxiety*, 28(3), 234-242.

Sing, N.A., Clements, K.M., & Fiatarone, M.A. (1997). A randomized controlled trial of progressive resistance training in depressed elders. *Journals of Gerontology Series A: Biological Sciences and Medical Sciences*, 52A, M27-M35.

Stathi, A., Fox, K.R., & McKenna, J. (2002). Physical activity and dimensions of subjective well-being in older adults. *Journal of Aging and Physical Activity*, 10, 76-92.

Stathopoulou, G., Powers, M.B., Berry, A.C., Smiths, J., & Otto, M.W. (2006). Exercise interventions for mental health: A quantitative and qualitative review. *Clinical Psychology: Science and Practice*, 13, 179-193.

Stich FA. (1998). A meta-analysis of physical exercise as a treatment for symptoms of anxiety: adults from the general population. *Journal of Psychosomatic Research*, 33:537-547.

Thayer, R.E. (1996). *The origin of every day moods: Managing energy, tension, and stress*. New York: Oxford University Press.

Trivedi M.H., Greer T.L., Church T.S., Carmody T.J., Grannemann B.D., Galper D.I., Dunn A.L., Earnest C.P., Sunderajan P., Henley S.S., Blair S.N. (2011) Exercise as an augmentation treatment for nonremitted major depressive disorder: a randomized, parallel dose comparison. *Journal of Clinical Psychiatry*, 72(5), 677-84.

Turner, E.H., Matthews, A.M., Linardatos, E., Tell, R.A., & Rosenthal, R. (2008). Selective publication of antidepressant trials and its influence on apparent efficacy. *New England Journal of Medicine*, 358, 252-260.

Vickers, KS, Finnie SB, Hathaway JC, Patten CA, Wheeldon TJ, Reese MM. (2003). Pilot study of a physical activity adherence intervention for depressed patients: study design and baseline characteristics. Poster session presented at the Cooper Institute Conference Series-physical activity and mental health: a multidisciplinary approach. Dallas, TX.

Whitton, A., Warner, R., & Appleby, L. (1996). The pathway to care in post-natal depression: Women's attitudes to post-natal depression and its treatment. *British Journal of General Practice*, 46, 427-428.

Williams, A., Reilly, T., Campbell, I., & Sutherst, J. (1988). Investigation of changes in responses to exercise and in mood during pregnancy. *Ergonomics*, 31, 1539-1549.

Wipfli, B.M., Rethorst, C.D., & Landers, D.M. (2008). The anxiolytic effects of exercise: A meta-analysis of randomized trials and dose-response analysis. *Journal of Sport and Exercise Psychology*, 30, 392-410.

Wittchen, H.U. (2002). Generalized anxiety disorder: Prevalence, burden, and cost to society. *Depression and Anxiety*, 16, 162-171.

World Health Organisation. (2001). *The World Health Report. Mental health: New understanding, new hope*. Geneva, Switzerland: World Health Organisation.

World Health Organisation. (2007). *International statistical classification of disease and related health problems*. Available: www.who.int/classifications/icd/en/.

World Health Organisation. (2009). *Mental health aspects of women's reproductive health: A global review of literature*. Geneva, Switzerland: World Health Organisation.

Dementia and Alzheimer's Disease

Juan Tortosa Martinez, PhD
University of Alicante, Alicante, Spain

Chapter Outline

Editors' Introduction

This chapter reviews the causes and consequences of dementia, focusing particularly on Alzheimer's disease. It evaluates the evidence that physical activity plays a role in delaying the onset of cognitive decline and in attenuating the symptoms and underlying pathophysiology of the disease process. It also makes practical suggestions for developing and using physical activity interventions in patients and provides recommendations for a comprehensive exercise plan that includes aerobic, strength, balance and flexibility training.

Improvements in health care have contributed to an extended average life expectancy, resulting in a significantly increased population of persons 65 yr or older. As a consequence, the incidence of neurodegenerative disease in older people is rapidly increasing and is creating serious concern for families, caregivers, professionals and others in public health systems (Haan & Wallace, 2004). In 2001 there were 24.3 million cases of dementia worldwide (Ferri et al., 2005), and by 2009 the number of cases had increased to 35.6 million. Brookmeyer and colleagues (2007) estimated that in 2006 there were 26 million cases of Alzheimer's disease (AD), the most common subtype of dementia, worldwide. They also estimated that the number of cases of AD worldwide will increase fourfold by 2050.

Vascular dementia is the second most common form of dementia. Other subtypes include dementia due to Lewy body disease, Parkinson's disease, head trauma, human immunodeficiency virus, Huntington's disease, Pick's disease or other general medical conditions; substance-induced dementia; and dementia due to multiple etiologies. Dementia is a progressive condition that includes memory impairment and at least one of the following symptoms: aphasia (communication and language disturbance), apraxia (impaired capacity to perform motor activities despite intact motor function), agnosia (impaired ability to recognise or identify objects despite intact sensory function) or a decline in executive functioning (e.g., planning, organising, sequencing or abstracting) (American Psychiatric Association, 2000). The age of onset may vary depending on the type of dementia, but it is normally late in life. The prevalence of dementia is highest in those aged 85 yr or older (American Psychiatric Association, 2000). AD is divided into early onset (before age 65 yr) and late onset (after age 65 yr) (American Psychiatric Association, 2000). Late-onset AD is by far the predominant type, and the incidence doubles every 5 yr after 65 yr of age (Querfurth & LaFerla, 2010).

In order to classify individuals with AD according to functional decline, the Alzheimer's Association developed a seven-stage framework to describe how a person's abilities change over time.

Seven Stages of AD

1. No impairment: The individual neither experiences memory problems nor shows evidence of other symptoms of dementia.

2. Very mild decline: The individual experiences some memory lapses, but symptoms of dementia are yet undetected.

3. Mild decline: Family, friends or coworkers start to notice some symptoms. Medical professionals may be able to detect some memory or concentration difficulties. At this stage the person may experience trouble coming up with the right name, difficulties performing tasks in social or work settings and trouble with planning and organising.

4. Moderate decline: A medical professional should be able to detect several cognitive difficulties such as forgetfulness of recent events, significant trouble performing challenging mental arithmetic, difficulty performing complex tasks and becoming moody or withdrawn, especially in challenging situations.

5. Moderately severe decline: Difficulties with memory and thinking are now evident. The person already requires some help with daily activities. At this stage the person experiences problems remembering their own address or phone number and becomes confused with where they are or what day it is. The individual does not yet require assistance with eating or using the toilet.

6. Severe decline: The individual requires much more help with daily activities. The person may not remember the name of a spouse of a caregiver, requires help for dressing properly and experiences major changes in sleep patterns, personality and behaviour.

KEY CONCEPTS

Dementia

Dementia describes multiple disorders that are characterised by the development of multiple cognitive deficits, including impaired memory and at least one of the following cognitive disturbances: aphasia (language disturbance), apraxia (impaired capacity to perform motor activities despite intact motor function), agnosia (impaired ability to recognise or identify objects despite intact sensory function) or a decline in executive functioning (e.g., planning, organising, sequencing or abstracting). In order to be considered dementia, the cognitive impairment must be severe enough to disrupt social or occupational functioning and must be considered a decline from previous cognitive functioning (American Psychiatric Association, 2000).

Alzheimer's Disease

Alzheimer's disease (AD) is the most common form of dementia (American Psychiatric Association, 2000). AD is a neurodegenerative disease characterised by a progressive deterioration of higher cognitive functioning in the areas of memory, problem solving and thinking. Also characteristic of AD is the inability to carry out everyday tasks or perform instrumental activities (Rimmer & Smith, 2009).

Plaques of β-Amyloid and Tau Tangles

β-Amyloid proteins build up into plaques in the spaces between nerve cells. Twisted tau proteins build up in tangles inside the cells. Both plaques and tangles are believed to be responsible for blocking communication between cells and causing cell death.

Mild Cognitive Impairment

Mild cognitive impairment (MCI) is usually considered to be a transition phase between normal cognitive aging and dementia, although not all patients with MCI develop dementia (De Carli, 2003). It is characterised by a subjective complaint of memory impairment with objective memory impairment (determined by validated tests in the clinic) following adjustment for age and education but in the absence of dementia (Petersen et al., 1999).

Hippocampus and Amygdala

The hippocampus is an area of the brain that is vital for memory storage and processing as well as for spatial learning (Rothman & Mattson, 2010). The amygdala is important for the processing of emotional stimuli (Scherder et al., 2010). Both regions, which are located in the medial temporal lobe area of the brain, are affected in dementia and AD. The hippocampus is especially affected (Rothman & Mattson, 2010; Scherder et al., 2010).

Neurogenesis

Neurogenesis is the process of generating new neurons in the brain. Neurogenesis is particularly important in the hippocampus.

Plasticity

Neural plasticity is the ability of the neurons to change structurally and functionally and to adapt to the demands of the environment. This process underlies functions such as learning, memory and recovery from brain damage.

Apolipoprotein E Allele 4 Gene

Those who carry the apolipoprotein E allele 4 (APOE e4) gene are at higher risk for AD (Podewils et al., 2005).

Brain-Derived Neurotrophic Factor (BDNF)

Brain-derived neurotrophic factor (BDNF), a molecule that is highly concentrated in the hippocampus, plays a key role in synaptic plasticity and neurogenesis there. Lower levels of BDNF are associated with smaller hippocampus volume, more rapid conversion to dementia and poorer cognitive function (Erikson et al., 2011).

Executive Function

Executive function is a cognitive process that involves planning, organising, scheduling, working memory and multitasking (Foster, Rosenblatt & Kuljiš, 2011).

7. Very severe decline: The person loses the ability to interact properly with the environment, carry on a conversation and control movement. The person now requires help with most daily activities, including eating or using the toilet.

1   Risk Factors and Pathophysiology for Dementia and Alzheimer's Disease

Many risk factors for developing dementia and AD exist, but age is the largest (Querfurth & LaFerla, 2010). Other risk factors include genetic factors such as the APOE e4 lipoprotein of the genetic sequence (Podewils et al., 2005); peripheral risk factors such as obesity, hypertension, cholesterol and type 2 diabetes (Hamer & Chida, 2009; Helzner et al., 2009; Kuller & Lopez, 2011; O'Brien et al., 2003); head trauma (Guo et al., 2000; Magnoni & Brody, 2010); stress (McEwen, 2008; Rothman & Mattson, 2010); depression (Green et al., 2003); inflammatory markers (Kuller & Lopez, 2011; Parachikova et al., 2007) and oxidative stress (Kuller & Lopez, 2011; Rothman & Mattson, 2010). These risk factors can accelerate the progression of the underlying disorder. For example, head trauma and consequent inflammation can induce neurotoxic cascades that facilitate disease progression.

Although the initial causes of dementia and AD are unknown, the underlying pathophysiology is identified as the accumulation of β-amyloid and tau proteins. These proteins accumulate in and between neurons in the brain, forming plaques and tangles, and play a central role in the pathology process (Foster et al., 2011; Kuller & Lopez, 2011). A period of MCI usually precedes dementia. In most common subtypes of dementia a range of changes in brain function is observed, including neuronal atrophy and reduced neurogenesis of the hippocampus (see "Key Concepts" for an explanation of these terms). These changes are associated with reduced levels of the beneficial neuromodulator BDNF and a reduction in the plasticity of the prefrontal cortex (Scherder et al., 2010). Deterioration of executive function, a common characteristic of dementia, results in apathy, agitation and lack of motivation (Scherder et al., 2010).

2   Need for Interventions

Given the projected number of future cases and the social and economic impact of dementia, it is imperative to design feasible strategies for preventing, delaying or treating this disease. Despite encouraging developments in recent research, a cure for dementia has not yet been found. Nevertheless, lifestyle changes may have a positive impact on the prevention of dementia and AD. For example, cognitive stimulation (Fratiglioni, Paillard-Borg & Winblad, 2004; Karp et al., 2006; Wilson et al., 2007), physical activity (Abbott et al., 2004; Karp et al., 2006; Larson et al., 2006; Laurin et al., 2001; Podewils et al., 2005; Rovio et al., 2005, 2010; Simons et al., 2006; Taaffe et al., 2008) and social engagement (Fratiglioni, Paillard-Borg & Winblad, 2004; Solfrizzi et al., 2008) have been shown to be effective for preventing dementia.

Physical activity is one possible nonpharmacological approach for preventing or treating dementia and AD. Physical activity is an inexpensive option that has very few side effects and can be feasible at any stage of the disease. This chapter explores the degree to which exercise may prevent or delay the onset of dementia and AD, slow down progression of the disease and reduce the severity of the symptoms that people suffering from the disease experience. A body of evidence suggests that exercise has significant potential for preventing the development of the disease and for attenuating its progression. This chapter first reviews current research and then offers recommendations for designing and implementing exercise programmes for people with AD. The chapter examines examples of good practices and makes suggestions for practitioners about the type, duration, frequency and intensity of exercise to include according to different prescribed therapeutic goals.

3 Physical Activity and the Prevention of Dementia and Alzheimer's Disease

Physical inactivity is a major cause of increased morbidity and mortality rates (Richardson et al., 2005; Sun et al., 2010). People who are physically active have a decreased risk of developing many cardiovascular risk factors and chronic conditions such as diabetes, obesity, high blood pressure or heart disease (Haskell et al., 2007). Furthermore, physical activity may reduce the risk of developing neurodegenerative diseases such as Parkinson's disease (Smith & Zigmond, 2003) or AD (Abbott et al., 2004; Karp et al., 2006; Larson et al., 2006; Laurin et al., 2001; Podewils et al., 2005; Rovio et al., 2005, 2010; Simons et al., 2006; Taaffe et al., 2008). This section explores the evidence in the literature that supports the role of physical activity in preventing dementia and the positive effects it may have on quality of life in those who already suffer from dementia.

Compelling evidence shows that a positive correlation exists between physical activity and reduced risk of developing the symptoms associated with AD and other dementias. This has important implications for healthy populations but is even more relevant for those who are more at risk of suffering from these diseases. Emery (2011) suggests that memory impairment is a major and recognizable route leading to AD (although not all cases lead to the condition). Research suggests that interventions should take place before memory impairment of any type occurs, or at least before the conversion from memory impairment to full-blown AD, in order to help attenuate the onset of AD (although physical activity also has an impact on the full-blown condition, as discussed later). Brookmeyer and colleagues (2007) estimated that delaying the onset of the disease by 2 yr would result in 22.8 million fewer cases worldwide by the year 2050. This decrease would have tremendous health, social and economic impacts. Strategies for developing healthy lifestyles such as physical activity remain the cornerstone of dementia and AD prevention, as opposed to pharmacological

interventions, which have had modest success so far (Middleton & Yaffe, 2009).

Table 10.1 summarises the characteristics and main findings of studies that examined the role of physical activity in preventing MCI, dementia and AD. Studies were selected from a review of the literature about the association between physical activity and dementia. Articles that appeared in Medline, PubMed and PsycINFO databases over the past 10 yr were selected. One must take into account the sample size, the methods used for measuring physical activity and the follow-up period when considering the relevance of the findings of these types of study. A bigger sample size implies that the results are more robust and generalisable. The methods for measuring physical activity and the follow-up period are of key relevance and are discussed later in this chapter.

The results of the studies are given as hazards ratio or odds ratio, which are similar statistical formulas that measure the effect size of an event and the statistical significance of the associations studied. In these formulas the control group is considered 1.00. For example, in the study of Larson and colleagues (2006) people who exercise 3 or more times/wk have an HR of 0.68. This means that the chance of developing dementia is 32% less in people who exercise 3 or more times/wk (1.00-0.68) compared with people who do not exercise. The confidence interval refers to the validity and variability of the results.

Discerning the causal effects that underlie the correlations is problematic for several reasons, including the number of variables that may have an effect on a multisystemic disease such as dementia or AD. Premorbid inactivity and the fact that a completely accurate diagnosis of AD is made only after death (Friedland et al., 2001) could also influence the results of the studies. Thus, data from case-control studies and short-term (3-5 yr) prospective studies may be influenced by the premorbid (preceding the development of the disease) and morbid (characteristics of the disease) effects of the disease (Friedland et al., 2001). This may be the case for studies by Friedland et al. (2001), Laurin et

Table 10.1 Epidemiological Studies of the Impact of Physical Activity on Dementia and Alzheimer's Disease

Source	Age at baseline (yr)	Sample size (n)	Activities examined	Follow-up (yr)	Main findings
Friedland et al. (2001)	Mean: 72.5 for case group, 71.3 for control group	551 (193 with dementia, 358 without dementia)	Passive, intellectual and physical activity	Case-control study (no follow-up)	Low participation in intellectual, passive and physical activities in midlife is a risk factor for developing Alzheimer's disease. Researchers estimated that inactivity in midlife increases the risk of developing Alzheimer's disease by 250%.
Laurin et al. (2001)	≥65	4,615	Frequency of physical activity (≥ 3 times/wk, 1 time/wk or <1 time/wk); intensity of physical activity (more vigorous than, equal to or less vigorous than walking); and composite score (indicating no, low, moderate or high physical activity)	5	Moderate levels of physical activity reduced the risk of any dementia type (OR: 0.69; 95% CI: 0.50-0.95) and Alzheimer's disease (OR: 0.67; 95% CI: 0.46-0.98). High levels of physical activity reduced symptoms of dementia (OR: 0.63; 95% CI: 0.40-0.98) and Alzheimer's disease (OR: 0.50; 95% CI: 0.28-0.90). When adjusted for sex, women with moderate and high levels of physical activity had a significantly reduced risk of Alzheimer's disease, whereas no significant associations were found for men.
Yaffe et al. (2001)	≥65	5,925	Self-reported walking (min/wk)	6-8	Women with higher baseline physical activity levels had reduced odds of experiencing cognitive decline (OR: 0.66; 95% CI: 0.54-0.82).
Verghese et al. (2003)	>75	469	Self-reported participation in cognitive activities and physical activity	5.1	Participants had a reduced risk of dementia following cognitive activities but not following physical activities, although dancing was found to be protective against dementia (HR: 0.24; 95% CI: 0.06-0.99)
Abbott et al. (2004)	71-93	2,257 men	Self-reported walking (min/day)	7	Men who walked 0.4 km/day (<0.25 miles/day) had a 1.8-fold increase in the risk of developing dementia compared with those who walked 3.2 km/day (>2 miles/day) (HR: 1.77; 95% CI: 1.04-3.01)
Weuve et al. (2004)	≥70	16,466 women	Self-reported low, moderate and vigorous physical activity	1.8	Women who engaged in more physical activities had a 20% reduced risk of developing cognitive impairment (OR: 0.80; 95% CI: 0.67-0.95).
Podewils et al. (2005)	≥65	3,375	Self-reported physical activity over the previous 2 wk	6-8	Engagement in ≥4 physical activities was associated with reduced risk of dementia, vascular dementia and Alzheimer's disease for noncarriers of the apolipoprotein E allele 4 gene (HR: 0.44; 95% CI: 0.28-0.69) but no association was found for carriers of the apolipoprotein E allele 4 gene.
Rovio et al. (2005)	65-79	1,449	Frequency of physical activity longer than 20 min that causes breathlessness and sweating	21	2 days/wk of physical activity at midlife had a protective effect against dementia (OR: 0.48; 95% CI: 0.25-0.91), especially among carriers of the apolipoprotein E allele 4 gene.

Source	Age at baseline (yr)	Sample size (n)	Activities examined	Follow-up (yr)	Main findings
Simons et al. (2006)	≥60	2,805	Self-reported physical activity	16	Daily gardening reduces the risk of developing dementia by 36% (HR: 0.64; 95% CI: 0.50-0.83). Daily walking was associated with a 38% lower risk of dementia in men (HR: 0.62; 95% CI: 0.42-0.92), but no significant association was found in women.
Larson et al. (2006)	≥65	1,740	Self-reported days per week engaged in physical activity for at least 15 min	±6.2	Those who participated in any physical activity ≥ 3 times/wk were considered to be regular exercisers and showed a 32% reduction in dementia risk (HR: 0.68; 95% CI: 0.48-0.96).
Verghese et al. (2006)	≥75	437	Self-reported participation in cognitive activities and physical activity	5.6	Cognitive activities were related to decreased risk of developing dementia (HR: 0.95; 95% CI: 0.91-0.99). Physical activity presented no associations (HR: 0.97; 95% CI: 0.93-1.01).
Sumic et al. (2007)	≥85	66 women	Self-reported physical activity	4.73	Women who exercised >4 h/wk had an 88% decreased risk of developing cognitive impairment (95% CI: 0.03-0.41) compared with those who were less active.
Carlson et al. (2008)	Mean: 44.7	147 male twin pairs	Self-reported physical activity	40	Higher midlife cognitive activity was associated with a 26% reduction in risk for dementia, especially among carriers of the apolipoprotein E allele 4 gene, whereas midlife physical activity did not modify dementia risk.
Taaffe et al. (2008)	71-92	2,262	Self-reported average number of hours per day spent basal, sedentary or in slight, moderate or heavy physical activity	±6	High levels of physical activity reduced the risk of dementia by 50% (HR: 0.50; 95% CI: 0.28-0.89) and moderate levels of physical activity showed a protective effect (HR: 0.57; 95% CI: 0.32-0.99), but only in men with low physical function at baseline.
Scarmeas, Luchsinger & Schupf (2009)	Mean: 77.2	1,880	Self-reported vigorous, moderate and light physical activity and diet	5.4	A high score in physical activity was associated with a lower risk of Alzheimer's disease (HR: 0.67; 95% CI: 0.47-0.95). Those with a high score in Mediterranean-type diet and high score in physical activity had a lower risk of developing Alzheimer's disease (HR: 0.65; 95% CI: 0.44-0.96).
Geda et al. (2010)	Mean: 83 for mild cognitive impairment, 80 for normal cognition	1,324 without dementia, 198 with mild cognitive impairment and 1,126 with normal cognition	Self-reported vigorous, moderate and light physical activity	Case-control study (no follow-up)	Any frequency of moderate physical activity in midlife or late life was associated with reduced risk of mild cognitive impairment (OR: 0.61; 95% CI: 0.43-0.88). Light exercise and vigorous exercise did not show any associations.

CI = confidence interval; HR = hazards ratio; OR = odds ratio.

al. (2001), Verghese et al. (2003), Weuve et al. (2004), Sumic et al. (2007) or Geda et al. (2010). In order to avoid this bias, some studies, such as Rovio et al. (2005), Simons et al. (2006) or Carlson et al. (2008), have a long follow-up period.

Among studies, the findings regarding the benefits of physical activity on cognitive function differ for men and women. Differences in hormone metabolism could partially explain these differences (Laurin et al., 2001). Evidence shows that the interaction between estrogen and physical activity has beneficial effects on brain health and plasticity (Taaffe et al., 2008). Laurin and colleagues (2001) reported that regular physical activity clearly reduced dementia and AD risk in women, but this reduction was less clear in men. Conversely, Simons and colleagues (2006) concluded that exercise was associated with a lower risk of dementia in men but that no significant association existed in women. More research is needed to clarify these possible sex differences.

The effects of physical activity on APOE e4 carriers and noncarriers are also controversial. Podewils and colleagues (2005) noted an inverse relationship between physical activity and dementia risk in APOE e4 noncarriers but found no association in APOE e4 carriers. However, Rovio and colleagues (2005) and Carlson and colleagues (2008) concluded that physical activity had a greater effect for protecting against dementia and AD and for delaying the onset of the disease among APOE e4 carriers. In parallel, Larson and colleagues (2006) found that genetic factors did not influence the positive effects of exercise in preventing AD. Again, more research is needed to verify these findings. Although not all studies (e.g., Verghese et al., 2003, 2006) show a protective effect, it seems clear that physical activity reduces the risk of developing dementia and AD.

4   Exercise Conditions Effective at Delaying the Onset of Dementia

The question still remains about the type, duration, frequency and intensity of physical activity required for obtaining the most beneficial effect for protecting against dementia. Despite encouraging indications, it is difficult to compare results and draw robust conclusions because activities have not been assessed consistently among research studies and different interpretive methods have been used. The instrument used for measuring physical activity levels is of key relevance (see chapter 3). All of the studies reviewed in this section use self-reported questionnaires, and some participants may have misreported their activity level. Also, these questionnaires vary significantly among studies and consider factors such as type, duration and intensity in different manners. The use of more objective measures such as pedometers or accelerometers would be desirable. The cost and difficulty of using these measures in studies with large samples would be very high and would require considerable investment, but the benefits of powerful studies that inform behaviour-change policy would be great to an aging society.

Regarding type of physical activity, most research has focussed on aerobic training. Strength training has received less attention and deserves further research. Based on the studies shown in table 10.1, one could argue that some aerobic activities such as walking (Simons et al., 2006), gardening (Simons et al., 2006) or dancing (Verghese et al., 2003) appear to be more beneficial than others, but not enough evidence exists to support this claim. The duration, frequency and intensity of the exercise seem to play a more important role than the type of exercise, but this is not yet fully understood. Podewils and colleagues (2005) suggest that the number of activities may be more important than the frequency and intensity of the activities because total energy expenditure was not shown to be protective against dementia in their study.

Higher levels of physical activity could be more protective against cognitive decline than lower levels (Scarmeas, Luchsinger & Schupf, 2009; Taaffe et al., 2008; Weuve et al., 2004). In addition, the optimum frequency of activity seems to be at least 2 times/wk (Rovio et al.,

2005); 3 or more times/wk is probably more beneficial (Larson et al., 2006; Laurin et al., 2001). The intensity of physical activity may play an important role, but it has been overlooked by researchers such as Friedland et al. (2001), Yaffe et al. (2001), Verguese et al. (2003, 2006), Abbott et al. (2004), Podewils et al. (2005), Rovio et al. (2005), Simons et al. (2006), Larson et al. (2006) and Carlson et al. (2008). One study found that the protective effect of physical activity increased as the intensity of physical activity increased (Laurin et al., 2001). However, a recent study found that any frequency of moderate physical activity showed a protective effect in people with MCI, whereas light and intense physical activity did not show any protective effects (Geda et al., 2010). Physical activity of very low intensity may not be sufficient to cause physiological adaptations. It is also possible that vigorous physical activity may be less protective against cognitive decline because it might increase stress levels (Kudielka, Hellhammer & Wust, 2009), which might result in excessive cortisol levels in the hippocampus (McEwen 2008), thus impairing memory. Furthermore, Green and colleagues (2006) found that high levels of cortisol were associated with increased formation of β-amyloid and tau plaques, which play a key role in the pathology of AD. Nevertheless, based on the current evidence, it is not possible to recommend or refute that vigorous physical activity protects against dementia. More research is needed to shed more light on this issue.

5   Mechanisms By Which Physical Activity May Affect Dementia

The mechanisms responsible for the protective effect of physical activity against dementia and AD are not fully elucidated. However, research has found that aerobic exercise enhances activity in the frontal and parietal regions of the brain (Colcombe et al., 2004). These regions are involved in attentional control and performance on a focussed-attention task (Foster et al., 2011). This enhanced activity is associated with a sig-

nificant increase in gray matter volume, which may be a mechanism through which physical activity affects cognition (Kramer, Erickson & Colcombe, 2006).

In healthy older adults, high fitness levels correlate with larger volumes of hippocampus (Erickson et al., 2009), a brain area that is vital for memory storage and processing as well as spatial orientation (Rothman & Mattson, 2010). As described earlier, the most prevalent subtypes of dementia, including AD, especially affect this area of the brain. Hippocampal atrophy has been shown in patients with MCI (Lupien et al., 1998) and AD (Dickerson et al., 2001). Erickson and colleagues (2011) conducted a randomised controlled trial of 120 older adults and found that aerobic training increased the size of the hippocampus by 2%, thus reversing normal aging loss by 1 to 2 yr and improving spatial learning. This increased size was correlated with an increase in serum levels of BDNF, a mediator of neurogenesis in the hippocampus (Erickson et al., 2011). One explanation of these exercise-induced effects may be that the increase in blood flow in the brain with exercise results in the development of new capillaries (angiogenesis) in the hippocampus (Kramer & Erickson, 2007). The increase of neurotrophic factors with aerobic exercise (Berchtold et al., 2005; Cotman & Berchtold, 2002; Cotman & Engesser-Cesar, 2002; Garza et al., 2004; Kramer & Erickson, 2007; Vaynman et al., 2006) is probably one of the main reasons why physical activity has a protective effect against dementia and AD.

The preventive role of exercise in cardiovascular risk factors (Blair, 1996; Dela et al., 1999; Ivy, Zderic & Fogt, 1999; Mora et al., 2007; Mueller, 2007; Thomas, Elliott & Naughton, 2006) may also be relevant to the increase in blood flow. Furthermore, in animal models physical activity has been shown to improve memory (Nichol et al., 2009; Parachikova, Nichol & Cotman, 2008), decrease the amyloid load in the hippocampus (Adlard et al., 2005) and have a positive impact on inflammatory processes (Cotman, Berchtold & Christie, 2007) and oxidative stress (Radak et al., 2006). Another emerging theory is the role that physical activity plays in the stress neuroendocrine system and its interaction with AD (for a review, see Tortosa-Martínez & Clow, 2012).

6 Physical Activity for Attenuating the Progression and Symptoms of Dementia and Alzheimer's Disease

Although dementia cannot be cured, the symptoms associated with the disease can be influenced (Blankevoort et al., 2010). A therapeutic intervention that delays disease progression by an average of 2 yr would decrease late-stage cases by nearly 7 million and globally decrease the financial, personal and social burdens of the disease (Brookmeyer et al., 2007).

Increasing evidence from clinical trials shows a number of benefits of physical activity interventions in people with dementia and AD. Table 10.2 summarises studies conducted with human populations that have attempted to improve cognition, neuropsychiatric symptoms and physical function in people with MCI, dementia and AD. A review of the literature from the past 10 yr was conducted in Medline, PubMed and PsycINFO to select these articles.

6.1 Exercise and Cognitive Function in Dementia

Cognitive function is the system that is most affected in all types of dementia. Dementia patients usually suffer from memory problems, become disoriented and have difficulty with spatial tasks. In healthy older adults, aerobic training

Table 10.2 Clinical Trial Studies of the Impact of Physical Activity on Dementia and Alzheimer's Disease

Source	Sample size (n)	Age (yr)	Design	Intervention	Measurements	Reported associations
Tappen et al. (2000)	65	87	Randomised controlled trial	3 groups: assisted walking, conversation or combination of walking and conversation. Each performed for 30 min 3 times/wk for 16 wk.	6 min walk test	Assisted walking plus conversation contributed to maintenance of physical function in Alzheimer's disease patients.
Hageman & Thomas (2002)	26	79.2	Case series	Moderate-intensity resistance-exercise training 2-3 sessions/wk for 6 wk.	Gait speed free, gait speed fast, Timed Get-Up-and-Go	The duration and frequency of the resistance-training programme were insufficient to achieve significant gains in gait outcome measures other than fast gait.
Arkin et al. (2003	24	78.8	Clinical trial	Strength, balance, flexibility and aerobic exercises plus memory and language stimulation. 2 40-60 min sessions/wk for 10 wk/semester (2-8 semesters).	6 min. walk test, lower- and upper-body strength	Significant fitness gains in the 6 min walk test and upper- and lower-body strength ($p < .001$) occurred. The rate of cognitive decline was attenuated and mood was improved.

Source	Sample size (n)	Age (yr)	Design	Intervention	Measurements	Reported associations
Heyn (2003)	13	85.7	Clinical trial	Multisensory exercise programme integrating story-telling and imaging strategies. 3 times/wk for 8 wk. Sessions started at 15 min and increased gradually to 70 min.	Resting heart rate, blood pressure and weight; overall mood changes perceived by 8 examiners; Menorah Park Engagement Scale.	Improvement in resting heart rate, overall mood and engagement in physical activity.
Teri et al. (2003)	153	55-93	Randomised clinical trial	Endurance, strength, balance and flexibility training at home. 79% of participants reported exercising 60 min/wk for 3 mo.	36-item Short-Form Health Survey, Sickness Impact Profile's Mobility Subscale, Hamilton Depression Rating Scale, Cornell Scale for Depression in Dementia	Improved physical health and decreased depression.
Thomas & Hageman (2003)	28	80	Clinical trial, pretest–posttest design	Moderate-intensity resistance exercise of the hip extensors and abductors and the knee extensors, flexors and dorsi-flexors using Thera-Bands. 3 sessions/wk for 6 wk.	Gait speed free, gait speed fast, Timed Get-Up-and-Go, knee extensor right and left, STS test	Average improvement of 15.6% in quadriceps strength, 10.1% in handgrip strength, 22.2% in STS time, 9.9% in usual gait time, 5.4% in fast gait time and 14% in the Timed Get-Up-and-Go.
Toulotte et al. (2003)	20	81.4	Randomised clinical trial	Muscular strength, proprioception, static and dynamic balance and flexibility. 2 1 h sessions/wk for 16 wk.	Get-up-and-go test, chair sit-and-reach, walking speed over 10 m, Posturography platform	Walking speed, mobility, flexibility and balance were significantly improved in the intervention group compared with the control group.
Netz, Axelrad & Argov (2007)	29 with dementia	76.9	Randomised controlled trial	Group physical activity versus social activities. 2 45 min sessions/wk for 24 wk.	Timed Get-Up-and-Go, STS, functional reach	Low-intensity physical activity was not associated with any improvements. Moderate-intensity physical activity significantly improved scores on the Timed Get-Up-and-Go but not on the STS or the functional reach tests.
Rolland et al. (2007)	134	83	Randomised controlled trial	Walking, strength, balance and flexibility training. 2 1 h sessions 2 times/wk for 12 mo.	Katz Index of ADL, 6 m walking speed, get-up-and-go test; one-leg balance test	Slower decline in ADL.

(continued)

Table 10.2 *(continued)*

Source	Sample size (n)	Age (yr)	Design	Intervention	Measurements	Reported associations
Williams & Tappen (2007)	90	88	Clinical trial, pre–post design	Supervised walking versus comprehensive exercise (walking plus strength training, balance and flexibility exercises) versus social conversation. 5 days/wk for 16 wk. Sessions progressed up to 30 min long.	Observed Affect Scale, Dementia Mood Assessment Scale, Alzheimer's Mood Scale, MMSE, 3 trial version of the Full Object Memory Evaluation, 6 min walk	Participants in the comprehensive exercise group exhibited higher positive and lower negative affect and mood compared with the other 2 groups.
Christofoletti et al. (2008)	54 with mixed dementia	Mean: 74.3	Controlled trial	Physiotherapy sessions, occupational therapy sessions and physical education sessions versus physiotherapy sessions alone versus control group with no motor intervention. First group: 2 h/day 5 times/wk. Second group: 1 h/day 3 times/wk. Both met for 6 mo.	Mini Mental State Examination, Brief Cognitive Screening Battery, Berg Balance Scale, Timed Get-Up-and-Go	Groups 1 and 2 improved balance compared with the control group. Group 1 improved in 2 specific domains measured by the Brief Cognitive Screening Battery compared with the control group.
Lautenschlager et al. (2008)	138	Exercise: 68.6, control: 68.7	Randomised controlled trial	Home-based programme including 150 min/wk of exercise, mainly walking. Some participants chose strength training in addition to aerobic exercise. 50 min 3 times/wk for 24 wk.	Community Healthy Activities Program for Seniors, Alzheimer Disease Assessment Scale—Cognitive Subscale, Cognitive Battery of the Consortium to Establish a Registry for Alzheimer Disease, Digit-Symbol—Coding Test, Delis-Kaplin Executive Function Battery, Clinical Dementia Rating, Beck Depression Inventory, Medical Outcomes 36-Item Short-Form Health Survey	A 6 mo programme resulted in modest improvement in cognition after an 18 mo follow-up.
Santana-Sosa (2008)	16	Training: 76, control: 73	Randomised controlled trial	Resistance, flexibility, joint mobility and balance or coordination exercises. 3 75 min sessions 3 times/wk for 12 wk.	Timed Get-Up-and-Go, 2 min step test, Tinetti STS test, Katz ADL, Barthel ADL	The programme was effective for improving upper- and lower-body muscle strength and flexibility, agility and dynamic balance, endurance fitness, gait and balance abilities and the ability to perform ADL independently.

Source	Sample size (n)	Age (yr)	Design	Intervention	Measurements	Reported associations
Aman & Thomas (2009)	50 cognitively impaired	79.2	Prospective comparative study	Aerobic and resistance training. 30 min of exercise (15 min of aerobic and 15 min of resistance) 3 days/wk for 3 wk.	Saint Louis Mental Status Examination, 6 m walk time, Cornell Scale for Depression, Pittsburgh Agitation Scale/Cohen-Mansfield Agitation Inventory, Alzheimer's Disease Cooperative Study—Activities of Daily Living	3 wk of exercise led to improvements in the 6 m walk time and a decrease in agitation.
Steinberg at al. (2009)	27	Control: 74.0, exercise: 76.5	Randomised controlled trial	Aerobic exercise (mainly walking), strength training and balance and flexibility training. Control group had a home safety assessment. 12 wk of daily exercise.	Yale Physical Activity Survey, timed 8 foot walk, Jebsen Total Time, chair sit-to-stand test, Mini Mental State Exam, Boston Naming Test, Hopkins Verbal Learning Test, The Alzheimer's Disease Quality Related Life Scale, Neuropsychiatric Inventory, Cornell Scale for Depression in Dementia, Screen for Caregiver Burden	A trend was found for improved functional performance after the intervention.
Baker et al. (2010)	33 with amnestic mild cognitive impairment	Mean: 70	Randomised controlled trial	High-intensity aerobic exercise group (75%-85% of heart rate reserve), stretching control group. 45-60 min sessions 4 days/wk for 6 mo.	Symbol-Digit Modalities, Verbal Fluency, Stroop, Trails B, Task Switching, Story Recall, List Learning, Fasting, plasma levels of insulin, cortisol, brain-derived neurotrophic factor, insulin-like growth factor-I and-beta amyloids 40 and 42	For women, aerobic exercise improvements were correlated with improvements in executive function, increased glucose disposal during the metabolic clamp and reduced fasting plasma levels of insulin, cortisol and brain-derived neurotrophic factor. For men, improvements in aerobic exercise were correlated with increased plasma levels of insulin-like growth factor I.

(continued)

Table 10.2 *(continued)*

Source	Sample size (n)	Age (yr)	Design	Intervention	Measurements	Reported associations
Kemoun et al. (2010)	31 with dementia	Mean: 81.8	Randomised controlled trial	Walking, equilibrium and stamina. 1 h 3 times/wk for 15 wk.	French Rapid Evaluation of Cognitive Function, walking assessment (walking speed, stride length and double-limb support time)	Cognition and walking capacities (through heightened walking speed and stride length and a reduction in double-limb support time) significantly improved in the intervention group compared with the control group. Control group showed a reduction in both walking speed and stride length.
Littbrand et al. (2011)	191 living in residential care facilities	Mean: 85.3 TG, 84.2 CG	Randomised controlled trial	High-intensity strength, balance and gait exercises. At least 2 lower-limb strength exercises and 2 balance exercises/ session. Strength exercises performed at 8- to 12-repetition maximum the comparison group received occupational therapy. 29 sessions over 3 mo.	Berg Balance Scale	The intervention produced improvements in functional stability. People with dementia seemed to obtain functional balance benefits from the high-intensity functional exercise programme that were similar to those obtained by people without dementia.
Yágüez et al. (2011)	27 with Alzheimer's disease living independently	70.5 Target G, 75.7 Control G	Randomised controlled trial	Nonaerobic exercises that included stretching different parts of the body, circular movements of the extremities and isometric tension of muscles groups. 2 h/wk for 6 wk.	The Cambridge Neuropsychological Test Automated Battery—Expedio	The exercise group showed significant improvements in sustained attention and visual memory and a trend in working memory compared with the control group.
Christofoletti et al. (2011)	59 with dementia	Mean: 76	Case-control study	No intervention. Measurement of leisure-time physical activity.	Modified Baecke Questionnaire	Patients who reported engaging in more physical activities had fewer neuropsychiatric symptoms.
Lam et al. (2011)	389 with amnestic mild cognitive impairment or a Clinical Dementia Rating score of 0.5	≥65	Randomised controlled trial	Tai chi programme. At least 30 min/ session 3 times/wk for 12 mo.	Clinical Dementia Rating, Memory Inventory for the Chinese, Alzheimer Disease Assessment Scale—Cognitive Subscale, MMSE, delayed recall, Trail A, verbal fluency test, Berg Balance Scale	The tai chi group showed improvements in balance, visual attention and the Clinical Dementia Rating sum of boxes score.

ADL = activities of daily living; MMSE = Mini Mental State Examination; STS = sit-to-stand.

has several positive associations with cognitive processes, especially executive function (Foster, Rosenblatt & Kuljiš, 2011), which includes planning, organising, scheduling, working memory and multitasking. The effect seems to be most marked when aerobic training is combined with strength and flexibility training (Foster, Rosenblatt & Kuljiš, 2011).

For people with MCI, cognitive benefits of physical activity interventions include improvements in executive function (Baker et al., 2010) and visual attention (Lam et al., 2011). Baker and colleagues (2010) demonstrated that 6 mo of high-intensity aerobic training (4 days/wk for 45 to 60 min/session) resulted in improvements in executive-control abilities (e.g., selective attention, search efficiency, processing speed and cognitive flexibility) of sedentary people with amnestic MCI. The effects were more pronounced in women than in men. These sex differences were correlated with different metabolic effects of exercise, such as improvements in glucoregulation and insulin sensitivity in women but not in men and decreased cortisol levels in women and increased cortisol levels in men. These metabolic effects have important implications for cognition because both insulin sensitivity and high cortisol levels have been linked with impaired memory (Seeman et al., 1997; Wrighten et al., 2009).

Lam and colleagues (2011) conducted an intervention programme for individuals with MCI that consisted of 12 mo of tai chi sessions (3 times/wk for at least 30 min/session). After the intervention, visual attention was improved in the tai chi group compared with the control group. The authors considered that this improvement was related to the specific demands of tai chi in relation to posture and motor sequence. These results could suggest that engaging in physical activities that involve a cognitive component, such as motor sequences in tai chi or step sequences in dancing, could have a greater protective effect (Lautenschlager et al., 2010). The improvements shown in the Clinical Dementia Rating sum of boxes in this study suggest that exercise has a protective effect against dementia.

Studies of people with dementia who undergo physical activity interventions have shown modest improvements in memory and language (Lautenschlager et al., 2008), attenuation of cognitive decline (Arkin, 2003; Christofoletti et al., 2008; Kemoun et al., 2010) and improvements in sustained attention and visual memory (Yágüez et al., 2011). Lautenschlager and colleagues (2008) examined the effects of a physical activity intervention consisting of a 24 wk home-based exercise programme in which participants were encouraged to participate in 150 min/wk of physical activity consisting of 3 sessions of 50 min each. The most common activity was walking, but other types of exercise were acceptable. In contrast to results from a study of individuals with MCI by Baker and colleagues (2010), the benefits on cognitive function were modest and executive function was not improved. However, the researchers considered these benefits potentially important given the relatively modest amount of time participants spent engaged in physical activities.

The study conducted by Arkin and colleagues (2003) showed that a physical activity programme that included aerobic, strength, balance and flexibility training may attenuate the cognitive decline of people with dementia, suggesting that such a programme may slow down the progression of the disease. However, because the programme also included cognitive activities, the positive effect on cognitive function may be at least partially due to cognitive stimulation.

Christofoletti and colleagues (2008) conducted an intervention for people with dementia and divided participants into three groups. Group 1 performed a combination of individual kinesiotherapeutic exercises (stimulating strength, balance and cognition), group occupational therapy (associating motor-coordination exercises with cognition) and group physical education (walking sessions that often included exercises that improved strength, balance, motor coordination, agility, flexibility and aerobic endurance). Group 2 performed only the individual kinesiotherapeutic exercises that group 1 performed. Group 3, the control group, received no motor intervention. After the intervention, group 1 showed attenuation in the decline of some cognitive domains compared with group 3, especially in the clock-drawing test and the semantic verbal fluency test, which require significant activation of executive functions.

Kemoun and colleagues (2010) conducted a randomised controlled trial with people diagnosed with AD who were able to walk 10 m without assistance. The intervention group performed 3 sessions/wk lasting 40 min each for 15 wk. Sessions were divided into objectives of walking, stamina and equilibrium. Walking parameters and equilibrium were worked using motor-route exercises such as striding over a board or zigzagging. The session devoted to stamina consisted primarily of a light to moderate effort on an ergocycle using the arms and legs. A third session included activities that combined walking, equilibrium and stamina such as dancing and stepping. After the intervention, the exercise group improved in cognitive domains, walking speed and walking stride length.

The intervention conducted by Yágüez and colleagues (2011) is the only intervention that showed improvements in cognition that did not include aerobic exercises. This research group implemented a 6 wk intervention of nonaerobic exercises that required fine-motor involvement, balance and eye–hand coordination. The experimental group exhibited significant gains in sustained attention and visual memory and a trend in working memory. Although the experimental group was rather small ($n = 15$), the short period of time that was required to show positive results is noteworthy.

Although the number of studies of the effect of physical activity interventions on cognition in demented populations is still scarce, it seems that physical activity may have a positive impact on cognitive processes in people with MCI and dementia and may attenuate cognitive decline or even lead to small improvements in cognitive function. However, more clinical trials are needed in this area of research.

6.2 Exercise and Depression in Dementia

Depression is often present in demented populations. Depression may be a risk factor for developing dementia and may be a cause for more rapid progression of the disease (Green et al., 2003). In several studies, exercise has been shown to reduce depression in nondemented populations (for a review, see Carek, Laibstain & Carek, 2011). In a study of demented populations by Teri and colleagues (2003), a programme that included aerobic exercises, strength training, balance and flexibility training at least 30 min/wk plus a behavioural training programme for caregivers led to improved physical health and reduced symptoms of depression in participants in the home-based programme compared with those in the control group.

Physical activity programmes, such as those conducted by Arkin (2003), improves the mood of demented individuals. Heyn (2003) evaluated the effects of a multisensory exercise programme offered 3 times/wk for 8 wk. Sessions progressed from 15 to 70 min in duration. The programme comprised a focussed attention task and physical warm-up (using storytelling and imagery), flexibility and aerobic exercises, strength training (using imagery and music) and a cool-down session (using thematic music and storytelling) that focussed on relaxation and breathing techniques. Participants experienced improved resting heart rate, overall mood elevations and higher engagement in physical activities.

Williams and Tappen (2007) examined the effects of three behavioural interventions—comprehensive exercise, walking and social conversation—on affect and mood of residents with AD. The three groups participated in the intervention 5 times/wk, progressing up to 30 min/session, for 16 wk. The comprehensive-exercise programme consisted of 10 min of strength, balance and flexibility training followed by walking. The comprehensive-exercise group showed higher positive and lower negative affect and mood.

6.3 Exercise and Behaviour in Dementia

Behavioural problems, including passivity, agitation and anxiety, are prevalent in demented populations (Heyn, 2003; Putman & Wang, 2007) and are correlated with lower engagement in activities (Heyn, 2003). Lack of physical activity (passivity) is associated with negative changes in the hippocampus, the prefrontal cortex and the amygdala (Scherder et al., 2010), three brain areas that are impaired in the most prevalent subtypes of dementia, including AD. Also, degeneration of the amygdala and the prefrontal cortex is thought to be associated with agitation. Physical activity seems to have a positive impact on these brain structures (Scherder et al., 2010), which could account for the benefits of physical activity for reducing agitation in dementia patients. Another possibility is that those with lower fitness levels show higher stress responses (i.e., increase in cortisol levels) to external stimuli, which could result in agitation (Scherder et al., 2010).

In a case-control study, Christofelletti and colleagues (2011) reported that demented patients who engaged in a higher number of physical activities presented fewer neuropsychiatric symptoms (e.g., anxiety, apathy, delusions, agitation or irritability) compared with those who engaged in fewer physical activities. Aman and Thomas (2009) have shown that a short (3 wk) programme of aerobic and resistance training may be effective in reducing agitation in individuals with high levels of cognitive impairment.

Some evidence shows that physical activity improves depression, mood and agitation in individuals with dementia, but more research is needed to clarify these effects. Good methodological research about the benefits of exercise for improving other important symptoms such as anxiety, apathy and repetitive behaviours is lacking (Thuné-Boyle et al., 2012).

6.4 Exercise and Activities of Daily Living in Dementia

In addition to cognitive and behavioural problems, individuals with dementia experience a decline in physical function that is correlated with deterioration in the performance of activities of daily living (ADL), including both basic ADL (self-care tasks such as personal hygiene or self-feeding) and instrumental ADL (e.g., housework, managing money or shopping) (Blankevoort et al., 2010). It is common to observe losses in muscle mass and strength in people with dementia. These losses are a high risk factor for falls, typically during ambulation, that can result in fractures (Hageman & Thomas, 2002). Dementia has a negative impact on mobility, endurance, lower-extremity strength and balance. As a consequence, dementia patients experience a loss of autonomy and a higher risk of institutionalization (Blankevoort et al., 2010).

Dementia is also characterised by gait deterioration, even in the early stages of the disease, and patients with dementia are at increased risk for falls as a result (Ijmker & Lamoth, 2011). In fact, quantitative gait dysfunction is a predictor of cognitive decline and of higher risk of developing dementia (Verghese et al., 2007). Walking has been associated with cognition, especially executive function (Ijmker & Lamoth, 2011).

In healthy elderly populations, physical activity programmes have successfully improved physical function and ADL significantly (Yokoya, Demura & Sato, 2009). Many studies have proved the efficacy of physical activity programmes for improving physical function in demented populations. These benefits include improvements in endurance (Arkin, 2003; Tappen et al., 2000), strength (Arkin 2003; Thomas & Hageman, 2003), mobility (Netz, Axelrad & Argov, 2007; Thomas & Hageman, 2003; Toulotte et al., 2003), normal gait (Hageman & Thomas, 2002; Thomas & Hageman, 2003), fast-speed gait (Thomas & Hageman, 2003; Toulotte et al., 2003), flexibility (Toulotte et al., 2003) and balance (Christofoletti et al., 2008; Lam et al., 2011; Littbrand et al., 2011; Toulotte et al., 2003). However, only in some studies were these benefits associated with better performance in ADL (Rolland et al., 2007; Santana-Sosa et al., 2008). Physical activity programmes can benefit physical function in patients with different stages of dementia (Blankevoort et al., 2010).

In a systematic review of the benefits of physical activity programmes for improving physical function in people with dementia, Blankevoort and colleagues (2010) concluded that programmes that are at least 12 wk long and consist of 3 sessions/wk (45-60 min/session) confer the largest improvements. This research group also concluded that higher training volumes result in larger improvements in physical functioning.

Physical activity has been used successfully as a strategy for improving a variety of domains of physical function. The existing scientific evidence proves that physical activity programmes need to be included in the care of people with dementia at any stage.

7 Physical Activity Interventions in Dementia and Alzheimer's Disease

Prior to introducing a physical activity programme it is necessary to start by performing an assessment of fitness and physical function. Based on this assessment and the patient's medical record of cognitive decline and behaviour, the practitioner can select appropriate and achievable therapeutic goals. Physical activity programmes should be designed specifically for each patient with the patient's therapeutic goals in mind. The main factors of the exercise programme to consider are the type, duration, frequency and intensity of exercise. The American College of Sports Medicine and the Centers for Disease Control and Prevention suggest that the benefits associated with physical activity are related to the amount of activity performed per day rather than the type of activity (Rolland, van Kan & Vellas, 2008). However, research shows that in people with dementia and AD, activities that include a combination of physical, social and cognitive components achieve the best results via synergistic biological pathways (Fratiglioni, Wang & Putman, 2007). Once the programme of physical activity has been designed and delivered, practitioners should evaluate its out-

comes by recording advantages, disadvantages, successes and failures. This information should inform the creation of future programmes and help disseminate good practice.

7.1 Assessment

Exercise testing in patients with dementia might be difficult, especially during late stages of the disease. Pratitioners should perform several practice sessions before the actual test. All testing should be conducted in the morning because people with AD usually function better during this time of the day (Rimmer & Smith, 2009). Tests of aerobic fitness, muscular strength, gait speed, mobility, balance and flexibility may be conducted.

The most accurate test for assessing aerobic fitness is the effort test for estimating maximal aerobic capacity ($\dot{V}O_2$max). This test is performed on either a stationary bicycle or a treadmill. However, this kind of test is expensive and may not be well tolerated by some individuals, especially those in late stages of disease. The use of measures that are more simple and less expensive, such as the 6 min walk test, is preferable. Several authors, such as Tappen and colleagues (2000), Arkin (2003) and Williams and Tappen (2007), have used this test with demented populations.

Questionnaires can also be used to measure physical activity levels and estimate aerobic fitness. Some questionnaires used by researchers include the Community Healthy Activities Program for Seniors Questionnaire (Lautenschlager et al., 2008), the Yale Physical Activity Survey (Steinberg et al., 2009) and the modified Baecke questionnaire (Christofoletti et al., 2011). None of these questionnaires have yet been validated for use in patients with dementia or MCI. Different methods for assessing muscle strength may be used, such as the 1-repetition maximum test (Arkin, 2003) or more sophisticated measures such as the Microfet2 manual muscle tester (Thomas & Hageman, 2003).

Balance may be assessed to measure the risk of falls. One of the tools most often used is the Berg Balance Scale (Christofoletti et al., 2008;

Littbrand et al., 2011). Other options include the one-leg balance test (Rolland et al., 2007), the Tinetti (Santana-Sosa et al., 2008) and more advanced methods such as the Posturography platform QFP (Toulotte et al., 2003). Balance and stability may also be measured with mobility tests such as the Timed Get-Up-and-Go. Related to stability and risk of falls, gait parameters might be a good measure of physical function (Fitzpatrick et al., 2007). Normal gait and speed gait are commonly assessed using different distances (usually 6-10 m). For discussion on more advanced gait assessment such as variability and stability of gait, see Ijmker and Lamoth (2011).

Finally, flexibility may be assessed with tests such as the chair sit-and-reach test (Toulotte et al., 2003). However, because flexibility varies significantly from one muscle group to another, muscle-specific flexibility tests may have to be performed.

7.2 Therapeutic Goals

Practitioners might target several therapeutic goals when implementing physical activity programmes for demented individuals. These goals can be related to fitness (e.g., improvements in endurance, strength, balance or flexibility) or to behaviour and mood (e.g., improvements in passivity, agitation, mood, stress or depression). It is possible to target different goals in the same programme. Usually, improvements in fitness are associated with improvements in behaviour and mood. The initial fitness assessment combined with the medical record allows professionals to design the best programme possible that includes appropriate and achievable goals.

7.3 Exercise Programmes

Types of exercise include aerobic training, strength and balance training and flexibility training. Programmes that combine different types of physical activity seem to be more effective than programmes that focus on only one component (Blakenvort et al., 2010). In any given exercise programme the main factors to consider are the type, duration, frequency and intensity of exercise. The following sections summarise the considerations for each of these factors.

7.3.1 Aerobic Training

Aerobic training should be implemented in physical activity programmes for people with dementia and AD in order to improve overall health, cardiovascular health, cognition, depression, mood and behaviour. Walking is probably the activity that is most recommended because it is the most feasible (Van Uffelen et al., 2009). Walking speed correlates with performance in psychomotor speed and verbal fluency in the elderly (Soumare et al., 2009). Programmes can also implement the use of treadmills and stationary bikes, as in the programme by Arkin (2003). Depending on the stage of the patient's disease, other aerobic activities such as swimming, biking or dancing may be appropriate. Patients should enjoy the aerobic activities as much as possible; therefore, the type of aerobic training will vary according to both physical function and individual preferences. For example, a woman who used to be a professional dancer is more likely to engage in and enjoy programmes involving music and dancing. Dancing is advantageous because it includes learning and remembering steps and coordinating movements, which involves different brain areas, and musical memory, which is one of the last capacities lost in dementia and AD.

Group-based physical activity games can also be used to build up aerobic capacity and may be an interesting option for day care centres and full-time residences. Fun group activities may result in better adherence and mood of participants. However, it is more difficult to control the intensity and difficulty of physical activity games for each person, and it is probable that some people would enjoy the activities but that others would not.

7.3.2 Strength and Balance Training

The decrease in muscle function associated with aging is related to sarcopenia (loss of muscle mass). Decreased muscle strength leads to a decreased ability to perform ADL, decreased mobility, poor cognitive performance and lower life expectancy. Thus, strength training is very important for any older adult in that it helps prevent frailty and dependence (Hollman et al., 2007). Strength training is related to balance training, which is important for older adults in that it helps prevent falls (Nelson et al., 2007). This is especially important in people with dementia because the pathology affects balance and stability and increases the risk of falls. Falls could lead to head trauma, which is known to be a risk factor for dementia and may worsen the condition (Guo et al., 2000; Magnoni & Brody, 2010). Gait variability and stability also need to be considered in order to reduce the risk of falls. Thus, strength and balance training must be included in physical activity programmes for people with dementia.

The most common form of strength training is the use of resistive bands (Thomas & Hageman, 2003; Toulotte et al., 2003; Steinberg et al., 2009), which are usually color-coded based on level of resistance. Other forms of strength training may include using weight machines (Arkin, 2003) or body weight (Netz, Axelrad & Argov, 2007). The use of free weights is probably not the best option for people in late stages of the disease, and patients should avoid lifting weights above the shoulders in order to prevent injuries (Rimmer & Smith, 2009). Programmes may also include group strength exercises (e.g., two participants hold a ring and pull in opposite directions) (Netz, Axelrad & Argov, 2007).

Balance-training exercises can include shifting the centre of gravity, tandem walks, forward and backward walks and chair sit-to-stands (Steinberg et al., 2009); walking on variety of surfaces and standing on one leg (Toulotte et al., 2003); or walking while changing directions (Netz et al., 2007). The difficulty of the exercises should be increased gradually.

7.3.3   Flexibility Training

Flexibility training should always be part of a fitness programme for any population; it is important to stretch postural muscle groups (Rimmer & Smith, 2009). Because getting down on or up from the floor will be difficult for the patient, the programme should include exercises that can be performed on a mat table, chair or similar surface (Rimmer & Smith, 2009). Emphasising breathing techniques during stretching in order to promote relaxation could reduce stress and agitation.

7.3.4   Duration and Frequency

The World Health Organisation and the American College of Sports Medicine recommend engaging in at least 150 min/wk of moderate physical activity over 5 days, or 75 min of vigorous physical activity over 3 days or any equivalent combination. Short bouts of 10 to 15 min have been found to be just as beneficial when they add up to an optimal total time. Most evidence-based programmes for demented populations show that exercising 3 times/wk is sufficient for the desired outcome. The duration of each session ranges from 15 min to 1 h (Rolland, van Kan & Vellas, 2008). More research is needed to determine the ideal duration and frequency of aerobic programmes.

These guidelines could be applied to aerobic exercise but not to strength and balance training. It has been recommended to perform strength and balance exercises 2 or 3 times/wk. It seems that short-term (e.g., 6 wk) programmes can be effective (Thomas & Hageman, 2003), but it is desirable to increase the length of the programme at least to 12 wk to obtain optimal results (Blankevoort et al., 2010). According to Thomas and Hageman (2003), the majority of gains observed during the 4 to 6 wk of resistance exercise can be attributed to increased coordination or activation of the muscles rather than to hypertrophy, which may not be present in individuals in late stages of dementia.

The minimum frequency of strength training is 2 sessions/wk on nonconsecutive days (48 h of rest between bouts of resistance exercise is necessary), but 3 sessions/wk can be desirable (Thomas & Hageman, 2003). The intensity needs to be at least moderate in order to achieve neuromuscular adaptations. Research has shown that high-intensity resistance training is safe and effective for people with dementia (Littbrand et al., 2011), although further research is needed in this area.

7.3.5 Intensity

Programmes should likely focus on moderate-intensity exercise and activities that the patient enjoys and can successfully perform (Rimmer & Smith, 2009). However, high-intensity physical activity (both aerobic and strength training) is currently recommended for healthy older adults, and it has been proven effective at increasing cognitive function in some studies with MCI and dementia (Baker et al., 2010) (Littbrand et al., 2011). Baker and colleagues (2010) conducted an exercise intervention study with a sample of people with MCI; the results need to be replicated in demented populations. High-intensity aerobic exercise is still controversial because it could result in increased stress (Kudielka, Hellhammer & Wust, 2009) and increased oxidative stress (Ji, 1999). Given the current lack of evidence about the safety of vigorous aerobic exercise for people with dementia, it is probably safer to perform moderate-intensity aerobic exercise rather than high-intensity aerobic exercise. Although further research is needed to support this claim, it is better to first increase duration of exercise rather than intensity.

The two main methods used to monitor the intensity of exercise are percentage of maximal heart rate and the Borg rating of perceived exertion. Heart rate monitors can be used at almost any stage of dementia, although some individuals with behavioural problems may not tolerate them. It is preferable to use the modified 10-point Borg scale of perceived exertion rather than the original version because it is easier for patients with cognitive deficits to use. However, even this easier version may be inaccurate, especially in advanced stages of the disease.

Table 10.3 summarises general guidelines that practitioners should consider when designing

Table 10.3 Physical Activity Programme Guidelines for People With Mild Cognitive Impairment or Dementia

Mode	Goals	Frequency	Duration	Intensity	Progression
Aerobic	Cardiovascular health, physical function, cognitive function, depression and mood, behaviour	2-5 times/wk (at least 3 times/wk on nonconsecutive days is preferred)	Final goal is at least 150 min/wk in sessions of 20-45 min (short bouts of 10-15 min may be used as well)	60%-80% of maximal heart rate (possible to start with as low as 40%); modified rating of perceived exertion 2-4	Increase duration first, then frequency. Increase intensity last, if possible and desirable.
Strength	Physical function, activities of daily living	2-3 times/wk on nonconsecutive days	1 set/major muscle group (10-12 exercises, 10-15 reps/set)	Modified rating of perceived exertion 3-4	Emphasise proper technique, including breathing. Increase weight gradually when neuromuscular adaptations occur. Target postural muscles.
Balance (may be combined with strength training)	Fall prevention, activities of daily living	2-3 times/wk	20 min	Modified rating of perceived exertion 2-4	Increase difficulty gradually (e.g., stand with 2 legs and then 1 leg; eyes open and then eyes closed).
Flexibility	Physical function, activities of daily living	At least 2 times/wk but daily if possible. Include flexibility exercises in the warm-up and cool-down of any aerobic or strength-training session.	10 min for warm-up and cool-down, 25-35 min (or more if tolerated) for a specific flexibility session. Hold the stretch for at least 15 s.	Avoid pain while stretching	Emphasise proper technique first. Then gradually increase range of motion without feeling pain and increase duration of stretch. Target postural muscles.

and implementing a physical activity programme for people with MCI, dementia or AD. Positive results have been demonstrated for different aerobic, strengthening, balance and flexibility exercises, but no optimal overall application exists. The mode, frequency and duration of exercise will depend on the individual's physical and cognitive condition at baseline. With this in mind, including different types of exercise within or among sessions is recommended. If a single session includes strength, balance and aerobic exercise, balance and strength exercises should be performed first.

If a person is very inactive, it is recommended to start with short, low-intensity sessions and to gradually increase duration, frequency and intensity of exercise. In these cases, it is usually easier to start with a walking programme and increase the time and frequency little by little. Other modes of exercise, such as strength, balance or flexibility, can eventually be included as tolerated. Some patients will not tolerate some modes of activities or long periods of activities. These patients should be encouraged but not forced to be active, and pratitioners should assume that for some people the amount of activity tolerated will be well below the recommended guidelines. Nevertheless, a little is always better than nothing, and the first goal of the first physical activity session is having a second session.

Practical Suggestions for Conducting Exercise Programmes for People With Dementia and Alzheimer's Disease

The exercise programme should follow simple strategies in order to achieve the established goals and prevent injuries from falls and other accidents. Some of these strategies are the same as those followed for adults and older adults without cognitive impairment.

- The patient should be under medical supervision and thus get medical clearance before engaging in a physical activity programme. Moderate physical activity programmes are relatively safe, but simple activities such as walking may exacerbate some preexisting cardiovascular conditions.

- Include a warm-up and a cool-down. A few minutes of progressive warm-up exercise should be performed at the beginning of any physical activity session in order to prepare the body physiologically and psychologically for higher levels of effort. This will prevent musculoskeletal injuries. The warm-up may include light aerobic activity, joint mobility and stretching exercises. A few minutes of cool-down exercises consisting of lower-level physical activity should be performed at the end of the physical activity session. Performing a few stretching exercises at the end of the cool-down is recommended. Relaxation exercises may also be incorporated into the cool-down.

- Increase, if possible and desirable, the level of physical activity gradually and slowly. Increase duration and frequency first and intensity last.

- Choose motor tasks that are appropriate for the patient's level of physical and cognitive function. The difficulty of tasks can be gradually built up. Motor-control memory is not altered in many cases of dementia until very late stages, so patients make visible progress in motor skills even when they are not able to remember the instructor from one session to the other.

- Work with the pedagogy of success. This means always choosing feasible motor tasks that provide successful experiences in order to enhance self-esteem and avoid behavioural problems. However, tasks that are too easy may cause boredom and lack of motivation.

- Exercise programmes should have a strong behavioural component.

(continued)

- Participants should wear appropriate footwear and comfortable clothes.

- The programme should incorporate materials that are soft and visible because vision and perception problems may be common among participants. For example, balls used in coordination exercises need to be big enough to be easily manipulated and not be the same color as the floor or walls.

- The exercise programme should preferably be performed in the morning. People with AD usually have a higher level of agitation at the end of the day, and evenings are associated with high levels of fatigue. However, it is desirable for the patient to remain active during various times of the day (Rimmer & Smith, 2009).

- The environment should be safe and free of objects that may cause falls. Excessive visual or auditory stimulation may cause orienteering problems or agitation in some individuals.

- Be able to recognise activities that create behavioural problems in each individual. If an activity causes agitation, it is probably because the patient does not understand instructions or has excessive difficulty and consequent orienteering problems. In these cases, the instructions or the activity need to be adapted. Agitation may also be caused by giving instructions to more than one person at the same time.

- Use simple instructions and give visual examples when possible.

- Involve the caregiver in the programme so that he or she is willing to bring the patient to the exercise programme or to exercise with the patient in home-based programmes.

- It would be better to individualise fitness programmes according to each person through individual planning and monitoring. However, involving patients in group activities has the potential to confer additional positive outcomes because the social component contributes to the possible benefits. The social aspect of the programme also helps patients comply with and adhere to the programme. Group activities have been found to lead to higher adherence rates in healthy populations. Studies that focus on the adherence rate of individual recreation activities compared with group recreation activities in populations with dementia should be conducted. However, group activities may not always be the best option. According to Kolanowski and colleagues (2006), extroverts may benefit the most from social activities, whereas introverts may not benefit as much.

8 Summary

Dementia is a devastating disease and a major problem worldwide. As the population's life expectancy increases, the prevalence of neurodegenerative diseases is increasing at an alarming rate. Because the problem of dementia is so complex, an integrated approach to intervention is most effective. One component of that effort must be physical activity. Physical activity during the life span seems to have a positive effect on cognition and to offer a protective effect against dementia. Increasing the physical activity levels of the population would significantly reduce the number of cases of dementia worldwide, which would have a tremendous positive impact on society. Preventing dementia and AD should be the main focus, but physical activity has also been shown to be effective in delaying and minimizing the damage of dementia by improving cognition or attenuating its deterioration (e.g., executive function or visual attention), improving neuropsychiatric symptoms (e.g., depression or agitation) and improving physical function (e.g., endurance, strength, balance, mobility, gait and flexibility). Thus, physical activity programmes should be included in the treatment of dementia because they have the potential to improve the quality of life of patients with dementia and decrease the burden on their caregivers.

EVIDENCE TO PRACTICE

The following is a sample exercise programme for a dementia patient with these characteristics:

- Age: 78 yr
- Weight: 68 kg
- Height: 170 cm
- Diagnosis of probable AD
- MMSE: Mini Mental State Examination score of 20
- Clinical record of anxiety

Fitness testing revealed a poor cardiovascular condition and a loss of strength in the upper and lower limbs. The client's balance is starting to be altered and the risk of falls is becoming an issue. Flexibility is normal in most muscle groups, although the internal rotators of the shoulder and the abductors of the scapula need to be stretched to improve posture. The client is not very active but reports to enjoy walking and dancing.

A comprehensive programme (aerobic, strength, balance and flexibility training) is required to improve fitness condition, attenuate cognitive impairment and reduce anxiety.

- Aerobic exercise, walking and dancing will be the main activities performed, starting at 20 min 2 times/wk and progressing to 30 min 3 times/wk. The intensity will start at 40% to 50% of maximal heart rate and increase if appropriate. Emphasise enjoyment.

- Include strength training involving the use of resistive bands and body weight 2 times/wk on nonconsecutive days. Target lower limbs to improve stability and external rotators of the shoulder and adductors of the scapula (external deltoid, rhomboids and middle fibres of trapezius) to improve posture. Use a circuit-training format that alternates one lower-limb exercise with one upper-limb exercise and major muscle groups with minor muscle groups. Emphasise proper technique, including proper breathing.

- Include balance exercises (e.g., walking on different surfaces, zigzagging) in the strength-training sessions. Increase difficulty gradually.

- Include flexibility training at least 2 times/wk but daily if possible. Improve flexibility of postural muscles and focus on internal rotators of the shoulder and abductors of the scapula. Emphasise proper breathing and relaxation.

A starting programme would include exercising 2 times/wk on nonconsecutive days. A sample session would include the following:

- 5-10 min of warm-up, including stretching
- 15-20 min of aerobic exercise
- 10 min of strength and balance
- 5 min of stretching as cool-down

Although no convincing evidence shows that physical activity is beneficial for the prevention and treatment of dementia and AD, the literature remains limited in several ways. For example, the length of validated interventions varies from a few weeks up to 1 yr, and the type of physical activity ranges from aerobic activities to strength training to combinations of different types, including flexibility training. More research is needed to determine the exact role that physical activity may play in the progression of the pathology and the mechanisms involved and to determine the exact type and doses of exercise required for optimum results.

9   References

Abbott, R.D., White, R.R., Ross, G.W., Masaki, K.H., Curb, J.D., & Petrovitch, H. (2004). Walking and dementia in physically capable elderly men. *Journal of the American Medical Association, 292,* 1447-1453.

Adlard, P.A., Perreau, V.M., Pop, V., & Cotman, C.W. (2005). Voluntary exercise decreases amyloid load in a transgenic model of Alzheimer's disease. *Journal of Neurosciences*, 25, 4217-4221.

Alzheimer's Association. http://www.alz.org/alzheimers_disease_stages_of_alzheimers.asp Aman, E., & Thomas, D.R. (2009). Supervised exercise to reduce agitation in severely cognitively impaired persons. *Journal of the American Medical Directors Association*, 10, 271-276.

American Psychiatric Association. (2000). *Diagnostic and statistical manual of mental disorders* (4th ed.). Washington, D.C.: American Psychiatric Association.

Arkin, S.M. (2003). Student-led exercise sessions yield significant fitness gains for Alzheimer's patients. *American Journal of Alzheimer's Disease and Other Dementias*, 18(3), 159-170.

Baker, L.D., Frank, L.L., Foster-Schubert, K., Green, P.S., Wilkinson, C.W., McTiernan, A., et al. (2010). Effects of aerobic exercise on mild cognitive impairment. *Archives of Neurology*, 67(1), 71-79.

Berchtold, N.C., Chinn, G., Chou, M., Kesslak, J.P., & Cotman, C.W. (2005). Exercise primes a molecular memory for brain-derived neurotrophic factor protein induction in the rat hippocampus. *Neuroscience*, 133, 853-861.

Blankevoort, C.G., van Heuvelen, M.J.G., Boersma, F., Boersma, F., Luning, H., de Jong, J., et al. (2010). Review of effects of physical activity on strength, balance, mobility and ADL performance in elderly subjects with dementia. *Dementia and Geriatrics Cognitive Disorders*, 30, 392-402.

Brookmeyer, R., Johnson, E., Ziegler-Graham, K., & Arrighi, H.M. (2007). Forecasting the global burden of Alzheimer's disease. *Alzheimer's Dementia*, 3, 186-191.

Carek PJ, Laibstain SE, Carek SM (2011) Exercise for the treatment of depression and anxiety. *International Journal of Psychiatry in Medicine*, 41(1):15-28.

Carlson, M.C., Helms, M.J., Steffens, D.C., Burke, J.R., Potter, G.G., & Plassman, B.L. (2008). Midlife activity predicts risk of dementia in older male twin pairs. *Alzheimer's and Dementia*, 4(5), 324-331.

Christofoletti, G., Oliani, M.M., Gobbi, S., Stella, F., Gobbi, L.T.B., & Canineu, P.R. (2008). A controlled clinical trial on the effects of motor intervention on balance and cognition in institutionalized elderly patients with dementia. *Clinical Rehabilitation*, 22, 618-626.

Christofoletti, G., Oliani, M.M., Bucken-Gobbi, L.T., Gobbi, S., Beinotti, S., & Stella, S. (2011). Physical activity attenuates neuropsychiatric disturbances and caregiver burden in patients with dementia. *Clinics*, 66(4), 613-618.

Colcombe, S.J., Kramer, A.F., Erickson, K.I., Scalf, P., McAuley, E., Cohen, N.J., et al. (2004). Cardiovascular fitness, cortical plasticity, and aging. *Proceedings of the National Academy of Sciences of the United States of America*, 101, 3316-3321.

Cotman, C.W., & Berchtold, N.C. (2002). Exercise: A behavioral intervention to enhance brain health and plasticity. *Trends in Neuroscience*, 25, 295-301.

Cotman, C.W., Berchtold, N.C., & Christie, L.A. (2007). Exercise builds brain health: Key roles of growth factor cascades and inflammation. *Trends in Neuroscience*, 30(9), 464-472.

Cotman, C.W., & Engesser-Cesar, C. (2002). Exercise enhances and protects brain function. *Exercise and Sports Sciences Review*, 30, 75-79.

De Carli, C. (2003). Mild cognitive impairment: Prevalence, prognosis, aetiology, and treatment. *Lancet Neurology*, 2(1), 15-21.

Dela F, Mikines KJ, Larsen JJ, Galbo H. 1999. Glucose clearance in aged trained skeletal muscle during maximal insulin with superimposed exercise. Journal of Applied Physiology 87:2059–2067.

Dickerson, B.C., Goncharova, I., Sullivan, M.P., Forchetti, C., Wilson, R.S., Bennett, D.A., et al. (2001). MRI-derived entorhinal and hippocampal atrophy in incipient and very mild Alzheimer's disease. *Neurobiology of Aging*, 22, 747-754.

Emery, V.O.B. (2011). Alzheimer disease: Are we intervening too late? *Journal of Neural Transmission*, 118, 1361-1378.

Erickson, K.I., Prakash, R.S., Voss, M.W., Chaddock, L., Hu, L., Morris, K.S., et al. (2009). Aerobic fitness is associated with hippocampal volume in elderly humans. *Hippocampus*, 19, 1030-1039.

Erickson, K.I., Voss, M.W., Prakash, R.S., Basak, C., Szabo, A., Chaddock, L., et al. (2011). Exercise training increases size of hippocampus and improves memory. *Proceedings of the National Academy of Sciences of the United States of America*, 108(7), 3017-3022.

Ferri, C.P., Prince, M., Brayne, C., Brodaty, H., Fratiglioni, L., Ganguli, M., et al. (2005). Global prevalence of dementia: A delphi consensus study. *Lancet*, 366, 2112-2117.

Fitzpatrick, A.L., Buchanan, C.K., Nahin, R.L., DeKosky, S.T., Atkinson, H.H., Carlson, M.C., et al. (2007). Associations of gait speed and other measures of physical function with cognition in a healthy cohort of elderly persons. *Journal of Gerontology Series A, 62,* 1244-1251.

Foster, P.P., Rosenblatt, K.P., & Kuljiš, R.O. (2011). Exercise-induced cognitive plasticity, implications for mild cognitive impairment and Alzheimer's disease. *Frontiers of Neurology, 2*(28), 1-15.

Fratiglioni, L., Paillard-Borg, S., & Winblad, B. (2004). An active and socially integrated lifestyle in late life might protect against dementia. *Lancet Neurology, 3,* 343-353.

Friedland, R.P., Fritsch, T., Smyth, K.A., Koss, E., Lerner, A.J., Chen, C.H., et al. (2001). Patients with Alzheimer's disease have reduced activities in midlife compared with healthy control-group members. *Proceedings of the National Academy of Sciences of the United States of America, 98,* 3440-3445.

Garza, A.A., Ha, T.G., Garcia, C., Chen, M.J., & Russo-Neustadt, A.A. (2004). Exercise, antidepressant treatment, and BDNF mRNA expression in the aging brain. *Pharmacology, Biochemistry, and Behavior, 77,* 209-220.

Geda, Y.E., Roberts, R.O., Knopman, D.S., Christianson, T.J.H., Pankrats ,V.S., & Ivnik, R.J. (2010). Physical exercise, aging, and mild cognitive impairment. *Archives of Neurology, 67*(1), 80-86.

Green, K.N., Billings, L.M., Roozendaal, B., McGaugh, J.L., & LaFerla, F.M. (2006). Glucocorticoids increase amyloid-b and tau pathology in a mouse model of Alzheimer's disease. *Journal of Neuroscience, 26,* 9047-9056.

Green, R.C., Cupples, L.A., Kurz, A., Auerbach, S., Go, R., Sadovnick, D., et al. (2003). Depression as a risk factor for Alzheimer disease: The MIRAGE study. *Archives of Neurology, 60,* 753-759.

Guo, Z., Cupples, L.A., Kurz, A., Auerbach, S.H., Volicer, L., Chui, H., et al. (2000). Head injury and the risk of AD in the MIRAGE study. *Neurology, 54,* 1316-1323.

Haan, M.N., & Wallace, R. (2004). Can dementia be prevented? Brain aging in a population-based context. *Annual Review of Public Health, 25,* 1-24.

Hageman, P.A., & Thomas, V.S. (2002). Gait performance in dementia: The effects of a 6-week resistance training program in an adult day-care setting. *International Journal of Geriatric Psychiatry, 17,* 329-334.

Hamer, M., & Chida, Y. (2009). Physical activity and risk of neurodegenerative disease: A systematic review of prospective evidence. *Psychological Medicine, 39,* 3-11.

Haskell, W., Lee, I.-M., Pate, R., Powell, K., Blair, S., Franklin, B., et al. (2007). Physical activity and public health: Updated recommendation for adults from the American College of Sports Medicine and the American Heart Association. *Medicine and Science in Sports Exercise, 39,* 1423-1434.

Helzner, E.P., Luchsinger, J.A., Scarmeas, N., Cosentino, S., Brickman, A.M., Glymour, M.M., et al. (2009). Contribution of vascular risk factors to the progression in Alzheimer disease. *Archives of Neurolology, 66*(3), 343-348.

Heyn, P. (2003). The effect of a multisensory exercise program on engagement, behavior, and selected physiological indexes in persons with dementia. *American Journal of Alzheimer's Disease and Other Dementias, 18,* 247-251.

Hollmann, W., Struder, H.K., Tagarakis, C.V., & King, G. (2007). Physical activity and the elderly. *European Journal of Cardiovascular Prevention and Rehabilitation, 14,* 730-739.

Ijmker, T., & Lamoth, C.J.C. (2012). Gait and cognition: The relationship between gait stability and variability with executive function in persons with and without dementia. *Gait Posture, 35*(1):126-30

Ivy, J.L., Zderic, T.W., & Fogt, D.L. (1999). Prevention and treatment of non-insulin dependent diabetes mellitus. *Exercise and Sport Science Reviews, 27,* 1-35.

Ji, L.L. (1999). Antioxidants and oxidative stress in exercise. *Experimental Biology and Medicine, 222,* 283-292.

Karp, A., Paillard-Borg, S., Wang, H.X., Silverstein, M., Winblad, B., & Fratiglioni, L. (2006). Mental, physical and social components in leisure activities equally contribute to decrease dementia risk. *Dementia and Geriatrics Cognitive Disorders, 21,* 65-67.

Kemoun, G., Thibaud, M., Roumagne, N., Carette, P., Albinet, C., Toussaint, L., et al. (2010). Effects of a physical training programme on cognitive function and walking efficiency in elderly persons with dementia. *Dementia and Geriatric Cognitive Disorders, 29,* 109-114.

Kramer, A.F., & Erickson, K.I. (2007). Capitalizing on cortical plasticity: Influence of physical activity on cognition and brain function. *Trends in Cognitive Science, 11,* 342-348.

Kramer, A.F., Erickson, K.I., & Colcombe, S.J. (2006). Exercise, cognition, and the aging brain. *Journal of Applied Physiology*, 101(4), 1237-1242.

Kudielka, B.M., Hellhammer, D.H., & Wust, S. (2009). Why do we respond so differently? Reviewing determinants of human salivary cortisol responses to challenge. *Psychoneuroendocrinology*, 34, 2-18.

Kuller, L.H., & Lopez, O.L. (2011). Dementia and Alzheimer's disease: A new direction. The 2010 Jay L. Foster Memorial Lecture. *Alzheimer's and Dementia*, 7, 540-550.

Lam, L.C.W., Chau, R.C.M., Wong, B.M.L., Fung, A.W.T., Liu, V.W.C., Tam, C.C.W., et al. (2011). Interim follow-up of a randomized controlled trial comparing Chinese style mind body (tai chi) and stretching exercises on cognitive function in subjects at risk of progressive cognitive decline. *International Journal of Geriatric Psychiatry*, 26, 733-740.

Larson, E.B., Wang, L., Bowen, J.D., McCormick, W.C., Teri, L., Crane, P., et al. (2006). Exercise is associated with reduced risk for incident dementia among persons 65 years of age and older. *Annals of Internal Medicine*, 144, 73-81.

Laurin, D., Verreault, R., Lindsay, J., MacPherson, K., & Rockwood, K. (2001). Physical activity and risk of cognitive impairment and dementia in elderly persons. *Archives of Neurology*, 58(3), 498-504.

Lautenschlager, N.T., Kox, K.L., Flicker, L., Foster, J.K., van Bockxmeer, F.M., Xiao, J., et al. (2008). Effect of physical activity on cognitive function in older adults at risk for Alzheimer's disease: A randomized controlled trial. *Journal of the American Medical Association*, 300(9), 1027-1037.

Lautenschlager NT, Cox K, Kurz AF. (2010) Physical activity and mild cognitive impairment and Alzheimer's disease. *Current Neurology and Neuroscience Reports*. 10(5):352-8.

Lautenschlager, N.T., Cox, K., & Ciarto, E.V. (2012). The influence of exercise on brain aging and dementia. *Biochimica et Biophysica Acta*, 1822(3):474-81.

Littbrand, H., Carlsson, M., Lundin-Olsson, L., Lindelof, N., Lena Haglin, L., Gustafson, Y., et al. (2011). Effect of a high-intensity functional exercise program on functional balance: Preplanned subgroup analyses of a randomized controlled trial in residential care facilities. *Journal of the American Geriatrics Society*, 59, 1274-1282.

Lupien, S.J., de Leon, M., de Santi, S., Convit, A., Tarshish, C., Nair, N.P., et al. (1998). Cortisol levels during human aging predict hippocampal atrophy and memory deficits. *Nature Neuroscience*, 1, 69-73.

Magnoni, S., & Brody, D.L. (2010). New perspectives on amyloid-b dynamics after acute brain injury. *Archives of Neurology*, 67, 1068-1073.

McEwen, B.S. (2008). Central effects of stress hormones in health and disease: Understanding the protective and damaging effects of stress and stress mediators. *European Journal Pharmacology*, 583, 174-185.

Middleton, L., & Yaffe, K. (2009). Promising strategies for the prevention of dementia. *Archives of Neurology*, 66(10), 1210-1215.

Mora, S., Cook, N., Buring, J.E., Ridker, P.M., & Lee, I-M. (2007). Physical activity and reduced risk of cardiovascular events: Potential mediating mechanisms *Circulation*, 116, 2110-2118.

Mueller, P.J. (2007). Exercise training and sympathetic nervous system activity: Evidence for physical activity dependent neural plasticity. *Clinical and Experimental Pharmacology and Physiology*, 34, 377-384.

Nelson, M., Rejeski, W., Blair, S., Duncan, P., Judge, J., King, A., et al. (2007). Physical and public health in older adults. Recommendations from the American College of Sports Medicine and the American Heart Association. *Medicine and Science in Sports and Exercise*, 39(8), 1435-1445.

Netz, Y., Axelrad, S., & Argov, E. (2007). Group physical activity for demented older adults feasibility and effectiveness. *Clinical Rehabilitation*, 21, 977-986.

Nichol, K.E., Deeny, S.P., Seif, J., Camaclang, K., & Cotman, C.W. (2009). Exercise improves cognition and hippocampal plasticity in APOE 34 mice. *Alzheimer's and Dementia*, 5, 287-294.

O'Brien, J.T., Erkinjuntti, T., Reisberg, B., Roman, G., Sawada, T., Pantoni, L., et al. (2003). Vascular cognitive impairment. *Lancet Neurology*, 2, 89-98.

Parachikova, A., Agadjanyan, M.G., Cribbs, D.H., Blurton-Jones, M., Perreau, V., Rogers, J., et al. (2007). Inflammatory changes parallel the early stages of Alzheimer disease. *Neurobiology of Aging*, 28(12), 1821-1833.

Parachikova, A., Nichol, K.E., & Cotman, C.W. (2008). Short-term exercise in aged Tg2576 mice alters neuroinflammation and improves cognition. *Neurobiology of Disease*, 30, 121-129.

Petersen, R.C., Smith, G.E., Waring, S.C., Ivnik, R.J., Tangalos, E.G., & Kokmen, E. (1999). Mild cognitive impairment: Clinical characterization and outcome. *Archives of Neurology*, 56, 303-308.

Podewils, L.J., Guallar, E., Kuller, L.H., Fried, L.P., Lopez, O.L., Carlson, M., et al. (2005). Physical activity, APOE genotype, and dementia risk: Findings from the cardiovascular health cognition study. *American Journal of Epidemiology*, 161, 639-651.

Putman L, Wang JT. (2007) The Closing Group: Therapeutic recreation for nursing home residents with dementia and accompanying agitation and/or anxiety. *American Journal of Alzheimer's Disease and Other Dementias.* 22(3):167-75.

Querfurth, H.W., & LaFerla, F.M. (2010). Mechanisms of disease: Alzheimer's disease. *The New England Journal of Medicine*, 362, 329-344.

Radak, Z., Toldy, A., Szabo, Z., Siamilis, S., Nyakas, C., Silye, G., et al. (2006). The effects of training and detraining on memory, neurotrophins and oxidative stress markers in rat brain. *Neurochemistry International*, 49, 387-392.

Rimmer JH, Smith DL. 2009. Alzheimer's disease. In: Durstine JL, Moore GE, Painter PL, Roberts SD, editors. *ACSM's management for persons with chronic diseases and disabilities*. Champaign, IL: Human Kinetics. p 368–374.

Rolland, Y., Pillard, F., Klapouszczak, A., Reynish, E., Thomas, D., Andrieu, S., et al. (2007). Exercise program for nursing home residents with Alzheimer's disease: A 1-year randomized, controlled trial. *Journal of the American Geriatrics Society*, 55, 158-165.

Rolland, Y., van Kan, G.A., & Vellas, B. (2008). Physical activity and Alzheimer's disease: From prevention to therapeutic perspectives. *Journal of the American Medical Directors Association*, 9(6), 390-405.

Rothman, S.M., & Mattson, M.P. (2010). Adverse stress, hippocampal networks, and Alzheimer's disease. *Neuromolecular Medicine*, 12(1), 56-70.

Rovio, S., Kåreholt, I., Helkala, E.L., Viitanen, M., Winblad, B., Tuomilehto, J., et al. (2005). Leisure-time physical activity at midlife and the risk of dementia and Alzheimer's disease. *Lancet Neurolology*, 4(11), 690-691.

Rovio S, Spulber G, Nieminen LJ, Niskanen E, Winblad B, Tuomilehto J, Nissinen A, Kivipelto M. 2010. The effect of midlife physical activity on structural brain changes in the elderly. *Neurobiology of Aging* 31:927–936.

Santana-Sosa, A., Barriopedro, M.I., Lopez-Mojares, L.M., Perez, M., & Lucia, A. (2008). Exercise training is beneficial for Alzheimer's patients. *International Journal of Sports Medicine*, 29, 845-850.

Scarmeas, N., Luchsinger, J.A., & Schupf, N. (2009). Physical activity, diet, and risk of Alzheimer disease. *Journal of the American Medical Association*, 302(6), 627-637.

Scherder, E.J.A., Bogen, T., Eggermont, L.H.P., Hamers, J.P.H., & Swaab, D.F. (2010). The more physical inactivity, the more agitation in dementia. *International Psychogeriatrics*, 22(8), 1203-1208.

Seeman, T.E., McEwen, B.S., Singer, B.K., Albert, M.S., & Rowe, J.W. (1997). Increase in urinary cortisol excretion and memory declines: MacArthur studies of successful aging. *Journal of Clinical Endocrinology and Metabolism*, 82(8), 2458-2465.

Simons, L.A., Simons, J., McCallum, J., & Friedlander, Y. (2006). Lifestyle factors and risk of dementia: Dubbo Study of the elderly. *Medical Journal of Australia*, 184, 68-70.

Smith, A.D., & Zigmond, M.J. (2003). Can the brain be protected through exercise? Lessons from an animal model of parkinsonism. *Experimental Neurology*, 184(1), 31-39.

Solfrizzi, V., Capurso, C., D'Introno, A., Colacicco, A.M., Santamato, A., Ranieri, M., et al. (2008). Lifestyle-related factors in predementia and dementia syndromes. *Expert Review of Neurotherapeutics*, 8, 133-158.

Soumare, A., Tavernier, B., Alperovitch, A., Tzourio, C., & Elbaz, A. (2009). A cross-sectional and longitudinal study of the relationship between walking speed and cognitive function in community-dwelling elderly people. *Journal of Gerontology Series A*, 64, 1058-1065.

Steinberg, M., Leoutsakos, J.M.S., Podewils, L.J., & Luketsos, C.G. (2009). Evaluation of a home-based exercise program in the treatment of Alzheimer's disease: The Maximizing Independence in Dementia (MIND) study. *International Journal of Geriatric Psychiatry*, 24, 680-685.

Sumic, A., Michael, Y.L., Carlson, N.E., Howieson, D.B., & Kaye, J.A. (2007). Physical activity and the risk of dementia in oldest old. *Journal of Aging and Health*, 19, 242.

Sun, Q., Townsend, M.K., Okercke, O.I., Franco, O.H., Hu, F.B., & Grodstein, F. (2010). Physical activity at midlife in relation to successful survival in women at age 70 years or older. *Archives of Internal Medicine*, 170, 194-201.

Taaffe, D.R., Irie, F., Masaki, K.H., Abbot, R., Petrovitch, H., Ross, W., et al. (2008). Physical activity, physical function, and incident dementia in elderly men: The Honolulu-Asia aging study. *Journals of Gerontology Series A*, 63(5), 529-535.

Tappen, R.M., Roach, K.E., Applegate, E.B., & Stowell, P. (2000). Effect of a combined walking and conversation intervention on functional mobility of nursing home residents with Alzheimer disease. *Alzheimer Disease and Associated Disorders*, 14, 196-201.

Teri, L., Gibbons, L.E., McCurry, S.M., Logsdon, R.G., Buchner, D.M., Barlow, W.E., et al. (2003). Exercise plus behavioral management in patients with Alzheimer disease. A randomized controlled trial. *Journal of the American Medical Association*, 290(15), 2015-2022.

Thomas, D.E., Elliott, E.J., & Naughton, G.A. (2006). Exercise for type 2 diabetes mellitus. *Cochrane Database Systems Review*, 3, 1-41.

Thomas, V.S., & Hageman, P.A. (2003). Can neuromuscular strength and functioning people with dementia be rehabilitated using resistance exercise training? Results from a preliminary intervention study. *Journal of Gerontology Series A*, 58A, 746-751.

Thuné-Boyle, I.C.V., Iliffe, S., Cerga-Pashoja, A., Lowery, D., & Warner, J. (2012). The effect of exercise on behavioral and psychological symptoms of dementia: Towards a research agenda. *International Psychogeriatrics*, 24(7), 1046-1057.

Tortosa-Martínez, J., & Clow, A. (2012). Does physical activity reduce risk for Alzheimer's disease through interaction with the stress neuroendocrine system? *Stress*, 15(3), 243-261.

Toulotte, C., Fabre, C., Dangremont, B., Lensel, G., & Thevenon, A. (2003). Effects of physical training on the physical capacity of frail, demented patients with a history of falling: A randomized controlled trial. *Age and Ageing*, 32, 67-73.

Van Uffelen, J.G., ChinaPaw, M.J.M., Hopman-Rock, M., & van Mechelen, W. (2009). Feasibility and effectiveness of a walking program for community-dwelling older adults with mild cognitive impairment. *Journal of Aging and Physical Activity*, 17, 398-415.

Vaynman, S.S., Ying, Z., Yin, D., & Gomez-Pinilla, F. (2006). Exercise differentially regulates synaptic proteins associated to the function of BDNF. *Brain Research*, 1070, 124-130.

Verghese, J., LeValley, A., Derby, C., Kuslansky, G., Katz, M., Hall, C., et al. (2006). Leisure activities and the risk of amnestic mild cognitive impairment in the elderly. *Neurology*, 66, 821-827.

Verghese, J., Lipton, R.B., Katz, M.J., Hall, C.B., Derby, C.A., Kuslansky, G., et al. (2003). Leisure activities and the risk of dementia in the elderly. *New England Journal of Medicine*, 348, 2508-2516.

Verghese, J., Wang, C., Holtzer, R., Lipton, R., & Xue, X. (2007). Quantitative gait dysfunction and risk of cognitive decline and dementia. *Journal of Neurology, Neurosurgery, and Psychiatry*, 78, 929-935.

Weuve, J., Kang, J.H., Manson, J.E., Breteler, M.M., Ware, J.H., & Grodstein, F. (2004). Physical activity, including walking, and cognitive function in older women. *Journal of the American Medical Association*, 292, 1454-1461.

Williams, C. L., & Tappen, R.M. (2007). Effect of exercise on mood in nursing home residents with Alzheimer's disease. *American Journal of Alzheimer's Disease and Other Dementias*, 22, 389-397.

Wilson, R.S., Scherr, P.A., Schneider, J.A., Tang, Y., & Bennett, D.A. (2007). Relation of cognitive activity to risk of developing Alzheimer disease. *Neurology*, 69, 1911-1920.

Wrighten, S.A., Piroli, G.G., Grillo, C.A, & Reagan, L.P. (2009). A look inside the diabetic brain: Contributors to diabetes-induced brain aging. *Biochimica et Biophysica Acta*, 1792, 444-453.

Yaffe, K., Barnes, D., Nevitt, M., Lui, L.Y., & Covinsky, K. (2001). A prospective study of physical activity and cognitive decline in elderly women: Women who walk. *Archives of Internal Medicine*, 161, 1703-1708.

Yágüez, L., Shaw, K., Morris, R., & Matthews, D. (2010). The effects on cognitive functions of a movement-based intervention in patients with Alzheimer's type dementia: A pilot study. *International Journal of Geriatric Psychiatry*, 26, 173-181.

Yokoya, T., Demura, S., & Sato, S. (2009). Three-year follow-up of the fall risk and physical function characteristics of the elderly participating in a community exercise class. *Journal of Physiological Anthropology*, 28, 55-62.

Schizophrenia

Guy Faulkner, PhD
University of Toronto, Toronto, Ontario, Canada

Paul Gorczynski, MA
University of Toronto, Toronto, Ontario, Canada

Chapter Outline

1. Schizophrenia and Physical Health
2. Self-Report Physical Activity Measures in Schizophrenic Populations
3. Factors That Influence Physical Activity in Schizophrenic Populations
4. Physical Activity Interventions in Schizophrenic Populations
5. Promoting Exercise in the Treatment of Schizophrenia
6. Summary
7. References

Editors' Introduction

This chapter addresses the role of physical activity in attenuating the signs and side effects of schizophrenia. Understanding the predictors of and barriers to physical activity in this population can help illuminate theory and practice. This chapter also evaluates evidence that physical activity interventions can be effective in alleviating both psychopathology and physical ill-being in this population. Practical advice points to the need for social support and development of self-efficacy and discusses ways of achieving these goals in this population. This chapter highlights the role of physical activity in motivating and managing patients with this severe mental health condition

Schizophrenia is a serious mental illness that is characterised by psychotic symptoms (e.g., hallucinations, delusions), disorganised speech and behaviour, negative symptoms and serious neurocognitive and social cognitive deficits (American Psychiatric Association, 1994). The range and nature of symptoms in schizophrenia vary widely among individuals but can be divided into positive and negative symptoms (United States Department of Health and Human Services, 1999). Positive symptoms, which reflect an excess or distortion of normal functions, include delusions, hallucinations and thought disorder. Negative symptoms, which reflect a reduction or loss of normal functions, include affective flattening, apathy, avolition, alogia, social withdrawal and cognitive impairments. Antipsychotic medication is the standard treatment for schizophrenia. Although such medication can be effective for controlling the positive symptoms of the disease, it is typically less effective in alleviating negative symptoms and cognitive deficits (Tandon, Nasrallah & Keshavan, 2010).

The leading journal *Nature* has described schizophrenia as the "worst disease affecting mankind" (Editorial, 1988, p. 95) given the extent of disability associated with the disease. Schizophrenia is usually experienced by people first at a young age and then throughout life. Individuals who live with schizophrenia experience distortions of reality, changes in thinking and perceptions, difficulties in social situations and problems with daily functioning. Based on current estimates from epidemiological studies, approximately 15.2 in 100,000 individuals develop schizophrenia annually, and the lifetime prevalence is 4 in 1,000 individuals (McGrath et al., 2008).

A key objective of this chapter is to provide an overview of the behavioural epidemiological framework in schizophrenia. First, the chapter highlights the physical health needs of this population and briefly describes several validation studies of self-report physical activity measures. The chapter also describes the factors that influence physical activity in individuals with schizophrenia and reviews existing randomised controlled trials that examine the effect of exercise on mental health outcomes in individuals with schizophrenia. Finally, the chapter suggests some implications for practice.

1 Schizophrenia and Physical Health

The life expectancy of individuals with schizophrenia is approximately 20 to 25 yr less than that of the general population (Dixon et al., 1999; Hennekens et al., 2005; McGrath et al., 2008). Recent data suggest that this mortality gap is widening (Saha, Chant & McGrath, 2007). Reviews have concluded that patients with schizophrenia die from suicide at increased rates compared with the general population (Hor & Taylor, 2010). However, excess mortality from disease (i.e., death from natural causes) accounts for even more years of life lost in these patients than does suicide (Colton & Manderscheid, 2006). This increased rate of mortality is reflected in higher rates of morbidity. Reviews confirm that 35% to 70% of individuals with schizophrenia have an additional morbidity (Casey & Hansen, 2009). Almost all disorders occur at rates that are higher than expected, but the prevalence of cardiovascular disease and diabetes is particularly elevated in this population (Bresee et al., 2010).

Potential causes of this excess mortality and morbidity are varied but can be broadly categorised in terms of changes in treatment (e.g., metabolic side effects of atypical antipsychotic medication), greater prevalence of engagement in unhealthy behaviours (e.g., smoking, physical inactivity and poor nutritional habits) and limited access to health care (Casey & Hansen, 2009). Because health behaviours are potentially modifiable and because empirically based interventions that address the increased risk of obesity, cardiovascular disease and metabolic disease in these patients are lacking, attention has turned to the health behaviours of individuals with schizophrenia (Allison et al., 2009). Research is urgently required in developing evidence-based behavioural interventions for preventing and treating premature morbidity that are specific to this population. One component of such efforts—reducing the high prevalence of physical inactivity—is a priority given the well-documented physical health benefits of physical activity. To advance knowledge about physical activity in schizophrenia, we recommend adopting a behavioural epidemiological framework (Sallis & Owen, 1999) that advocates five stages of investigation and culminates in the translation of research into practice:

1. Establish the links between physical activity and physical (and mental) health.
2. Develop methods for accurately measuring physical activity.
3. Identify factors that influence physical activity.
4. Evaluate interventions that promote physical activity.
5. Translate research into practice.

Physical inactivity is itself a major cause of morbidity and mortality and merits the same level of concern as other risk factors for cardiovascular disease (e.g., Wei et al., 1999). Individuals with schizophrenia are less active than individuals in the general population (Brown et al., 1999; Daumit et al., 2005; Lindamer et al., 2008), and the majority of individuals with schizophrenia have lower cardiorespiratory fitness and physical functional capacity compared with population standards (Strassnig, Brar & Ganguli, 2011). Clinical samples show that the prevalence of smoking is high (58%-88%) in patients with schizophrenia and that the prevalence of physical inactivity can be even greater than that of smoking. For example, in the most comprehensive study of physical activity using accelerometry in a clinical population, 96% of the sample did not perform at least 150 min/wk of moderate- to vigorous-intensity physical activity in bouts of at least 10 min (Jerome et al., 2009). In a validation study, 74% did not meet physical activity guidelines of at least 150 min/wk of moderate- to vigorous-intensity physical activity (Faulkner, Cohn & Remington, 2006). Therefore, physical inactivity should be considered a risk factor that is comparable with smoking, particularly in terms of prevalence, for individuals with schizophrenia.

Incontrovertible evidence shows that regular exercise is an effective strategy for preventing premature mortality, cardiovascular disease, stroke, hypertension, colon cancer, breast cancer and type 2 diabetes in the general population

KEY CONCEPTS

- The risk of premature mortality and morbidity is elevated among individuals with schizophrenia, who experience increased rates of death from natural causes such as cardiovascular disease. The majority of individuals with schizophrenia have lower cardiorespiratory fitness and physical functional capacity compared with population standards.

- The adoption of a behavioural epidemiological framework can advance knowledge about physical activity in schizophrenia.

- Further work is needed in validating suitable measures of physical activity in this population, and more prospective, theo-ry-driven research is needed to identify physical activity determinants for persons with schizophrenia.

- Existing intervention research demonstrates that exercise interventions are feasible and that they can have a modest impact on some components of mental health.

- Theoretically driven research and practice are required to examine how to reliably help individuals with schizophrenia adopt and maintain physical activity in the face of significant motivational and cognitive deficits that are inherent to schizophrenia.

(Warburton et al., 2010). Nothing suggests that such evidence would not apply to individuals with schizophrenia (see also Vancampfort et al., 2010). The current Canadian and U.S. physical activity guidelines for adults (i.e., 150 min/wk of moderate- to vigorous-intensity physical activity) are sufficient for reducing the risk for multiple chronic diseases simultaneously. Sedentary individuals can markedly reduce their risk for all-cause mortality with relatively minor increases in physical activity; this might be a starting point for individuals with schizophrenia. A systematic review showed that the effect of interventions on self-reported physical activity in sedentary, nonclinical adults was positive and moderate (pooled standardized mean difference, or SMD = 0.28; 95% confidence interval (CI) = 0.15-0.41, as was the effect of interventions on cardiorespiratory fitness (pooled SMD of random effects model = 0.52; 95% CI = 0.14-0.90) (Hillsdon, Foster & Thorogood, 2005). According to Greaves and colleagues (2011), these are "significant and clinically meaningful changes in physical activity (typically equivalent to 30 to 60 minutes of walking per week)" (p. 8).

Overall, evidence from both nonclinical and clinical populations demonstrates the deleterious implications of physical inactivity for premature morbidity and mortality, and evidence from mostly nonclinical populations demonstrates that physical activity interventions can be effective and have a meaningful impact on health parameters. For these reasons, physical activity programmes for individuals with schizophrenia should be integrated into mental health services (Richardson et al., 2005). Irrespective of weight and fitness outcomes, reviews have concluded that increased physical activity may also improve psychological health and social well-being in this population (Faulkner, 2005).

2   Self-Report Physical Activity Measures in Schizophrenic Populations

Chapter 3 discusses the measurement of physical activity. Measurement must be accurate in order to determine the prevalence of physical activity (or inactivity) in a population, assess intervention effects and identify the relationships between physical activity and health. Given the cognitive disability (e.g., impaired performance of routine tasks or activities) common to individuals with schizophrenia, it is necessary to identify a self-report instrument that is easy to administer and relatively nondemanding.

Faulkner, Cohn and Remington (2006) examined the reliability and validity of the International Physical Activity Questionnaire (IPAQ; Craig et al., 2003), a self-report physical activity measure that is commonly used in adults and is available in multiple languages. This study found adequate 1 wk test–retest reliability (Spearman's rho = .68) and concurrent validity of .37 between total minutes of physical activity as assessed on the IPAQ and accelerometry among 35 outpatients with a *Diagnostic and Statistical Manual of Mental Disorders (DSM) -IV* diagnosis of schizophrenia. Validity and reliability improved for individuals who had first been treated for schizophrenia within the past 5 yr. This may reflect declines in cognitive functioning that are part of the aging process and that are exacerbated by medical illness, medication side effects and environmental understimulation (Brenner & Cohen, 2009).

In contrast, Lindamer and colleagues (2008) examined the test–retest reliability and concurrent validity of the Yale Physical Activity Scale (YPAS; DiPietro et al., 1993) among 55 outpatients with schizophrenia. They reported that the YPAS was a reliable measure of physical activity in individuals with schizophrenia for some indices. Although the YPAS demonstrated concurrent validity with other self-report measures, it did not demonstrate concurrent validity when compared with physical activity as measured by accelerometry. Both validation studies caution that self-report measures might be useful as a surveillance tool for assessing levels of physical activity in populations but that these measures need to be complemented by objective measures of physical activity, particularly when assessing the impact of interventions at a group level.

3 Factors That Influence Physical Activity in Schizophrenic Populations

To reliably affect physical and psychological health through physical activity, one must first understand how to help individuals with schizophrenia initiate and maintain physical activity. Identifying the factors that influence physical activity is critical to designing effective interventions. Interventions can target modifiable factors for change. This is not to suggest that new and unique factors influence physical activity in this population; rather, it is necessary to identify the determinants that appear to be most strongly related to physical activity behaviour in those with schizophrenia. These determinants may be similar to those in the general population. Specific knowledge would provide a framework on which to build interventions and develop measures that would confidently assess how well interventions are influencing variables that potentially mediate behaviour change. The authors conducted a review to identify the correlates and determinants of physical activity or exercise that have been examined in individuals living with schizophrenia.

The framework used for this review followed the approach described by Trost and colleagues (2002) in their review and update of the evidence relating to the personal, social and environmental factors associated with physical activity in adults. Studies were included in the current review if they met the following inclusion criteria: At least 50% of participants had a diagnosis of schizophrenia; the dependent variable was physical activity, exercise or exercise adherence and the study included participants aged 18 yr or older; and the study was written in English. Qualitative studies, conference proceedings and case reports were not included in this review. Two search strategies were used to identify relevant studies. First, the literature was searched up to July 2011 using the electronic databases PsychINFO, PubMed, Medline, SPORTDiscus and Google Scholar. The key words used in this search included *determinants*, *correlates*, *predictors*, *physical activity*, *physical inactivity*, *exercise*, *schizophrenia* and *serious mental illness*. After identifying relevant studies, a manual search of reference lists was conducted.

A total of 16 studies met the inclusion criteria and were included in this review. All included studies had a cross-sectional research design. Sample sizes ranged from 55 to 1,704 participants. Studies relied mainly on nonvalidated questionnaires to assess physical activity. The majority of studies were constructed to investigate a range of correlates or determinants without referring to a specific theoretical framework. One study investigated the strength of factors pertaining to the transtheoretical model (Archie, Goldberg, Akhtar-Danesh, Landeen, et al., 2007), and one study evaluated the utility of protection motivation theory in explaining physical activity and other behaviours among people with schizophrenia and depression (Leas & Mccabe, 2007). Table 11.1 presents study characteristics. Table 11.2 presents correlates of physical activity, exercise or exercise adherence, which are categorised as demographic factors; psychosocial, cognitive or emotional factors; behavioural factors; and physical activity factors. We also highlight the findings reported by Trost and colleagues (2002) concerning the strength of findings in the general literature examining physical activity correlates among adults. Salient factors that influenced physical activity in this population were identified when two or more studies provided the same positive or negative association.

3.1 Demographic Factors

A total of 10 studies examined demographic factors and their association with physical activity. Age and sex status appeared to be consistent correlates of physical activity (Jerome et al., 2009; McCreadie, 2003; McLeod, Jaques & Deane, 2009; Roick et al., 2007; Vancampfort et al., 2011b). Studies showed that males were more physically active than females and that levels of activity were negatively correlated with increased age. Individuals who were free of physical health problems, including metabolic

Table 11.1 Correlate Study Descriptives

Study	Participants (n)	Age (yr)	Female	Nonwhite	Outpatient	Length of illness (yr)	Method	Physical activity measure
Arango et al. (2008) [1]	1,452	40.7 ± 12.2	555 (39.1%)	Unclear	1,452 (100%)	15.5 ± 10.8	Cross-sectional	Unclear; measure of moderate to intense physical exercise
Arbour-Nicitopoulos, Faulkner & Cohn (2010) [2]	92	37.8 ± 11.1	32 (34.8%)	27 (29.3%)	92 (100%)	Unclear	Cross-sectional	International Physical Activity Questionnaire Short Form
Archie et al. (2007) [3]	101	35.0 ± 10.5	37 (36.6%)	16 (15.8%)	101 (100%)	<1 = 21 2-5 = 19 6-10 = 16 >10 = 55	Cross-sectional	Godin Leisure Time Exercise Questionnaire
Martín-Sierra et al. [4]	1,704	40.2 ± 12.3	688 (40.4%)	Unclear	1,704 (100%)	15.0 ± 10.9	Cross-sectional	Patient self-reported exercise at least 2-3/wk
Jerome et al. (2009) [5]	55	44	28 (50.9%)	26 (47.3%)	Unclear	Unclear	Cross-sectional	Accelerometer
Leas & Mccabe (2007) [6]	83	39.3 ± 10.3	33 (40%)	Unclear	74 (89%)	Unclear	Cross-sectional	Patient self-reported exercise 20 minutes of vigorous exercise 3/wk
McCreadie (2003) [7]	102	45 ± 13	30 (29.4%)	Unclear	102 (100%)	21 ± 13	Cross-sectional	Scottish Physical Activity Questionnaire
McLeod, Jaques & Deane (2009) [8]	125	40.3 ± 12.4	44 (35.2%)	Unclear	Unclear	<5 = 34 >5 = 91	Cross-sectional	Active Australian Survey
Osborn, Nazareth & King (2007) [9]	74	47.2	32 (43.2%)	26 (35.1%)	Unclear	Unclear	Cross-sectional	Godin Leisure Time Exercise Questionnaire
Roick et al. (2007) [10]	194	44.7 ± 13.6	Unclear	Unclear	194 (100%)	16 ± 12	Cross-sectional	Amount of time individuals spent being active in the last 3 mo
Sharpe et al. (2006) [11]	8	28.0 ± 6.7	0 (0%)	Unclear	8 (100%)	Unclear	Cross-sectional	Doubly labelled water
Vancampfort et al. (2011a) [12]	38	35.4	9 (23.7%)	38 (100%)	0 (0%)	Unclear	Cross-sectional	Baecke Leisure Time Physical Activity
Vancampfort et al. (2011b) [13]	60	38.1 ± 10.4	22 (36.7%)	38 (100%)	0 (0%)	Unclear	Cross-sectional	Baecke Leisure Time Physical Activity

Study	Participants (n)	Age (yr)	Female	Nonwhite	Outpatient	Length of illness (yr)	Method	Physical activity measure
Vancampfort et al. (2011c) [14]	60	38.1 ± 10.4	22 (36.7%)	38 (100%)	0 (0%)	Unclear	Cross-sectional	Baecke Leisure Time Physical Activity
Vancampfort et al. (2011d) [15]	106	35.4	37 (34.9%)	106 (100%)	0 (0%)	Unclear	Cross-sectional	Baecke Leisure Time Physical Activity
Wichniak et al. (2011) [16]	73	29.2 ± 10.2	27 (37%)	Unclear	0 (0%)	Unclear	Cross-sectional	Actigraphic recordings

Study number indicated in square brackets.

Table 11.2 Correlate Study Results

Correlate	Positive	Negative	Null	Trost et al. (2002)
DEMOGRAPHIC FACTORS				
Age		[5, 10]	[8, 13]	– –
Sex (male)	[5, 10]		[7, 8, 13, 16]	++
Sex (female)		[5, 10]	[7, 8, 13, 16]	– –
Race or ethnicity (white)			[5]	++
Race or ethnicity (nonwhite)			[5]	– –
Employment	[10]			++
Education	[10]			++
Single status			[10]	–
Low income	[9]			++
Home ownership	[9]			++
Receipt of state benefits	[9]			
Physical health status	[3]			+
Presence of metabolic syndrome		[1, 13, 15]		–
Body mass index			[3, 5, 8, 11]	– –
Number of mental health hospitalisations in past 3 yr		[8]		
Admitted within past 5 yr			[9]	
Weeks since hospitalisation			[8]	
Duration of hospitalisation			[8]	
More than 3 general practitioner consults in 1 yr			[9]	
Taking atypical antipsychotic medication			[9]	
Taking depot antipsychotic medication			[9]	
Higher British National Formulary antipsychotic maximum dose			[9]	

(continued)

Table 11.2 (continued)

Correlate	Positive	Negative	Null	Trost et al. (2002)
Higher chlorpromazine equivalent antipsychotic dose			[9]	
PSYCHOSOCIAL, COGNITIVE AND EMOTIONAL FACTORS				
Body image			[2, 3, 14]	–
Perceived sport competence or condition	[12]		[14]	0
Intentions to participate	[6]			
Self-efficacy	[6]			
Social support			[6]	
Perceived physical strength			[14]	
Perceived physical self-worth	[14]			
Negative symptoms		[13, 15, 16]		
Anxiety			[8]	
Psychological distress			[5, 8]	
Depression			[5, 8]	
Neuropsychological status			[5]	
Mental health	[9]		[6]	
Social problems		[8]		
Knowledge of coronary heart disease	[9]			
BEHAVIOURAL FACTORS				
Smoking		[4]		–
Diet (fat intake)			[3]	– –
Diet (fruit and vegetable intake)	[3]			++
Overreaction or aggression	[8]			+
PHYSICAL ACTIVITY FACTORS				
Mild intensity			[3]	+
Moderate intensity	[3]			–
Vigorous intensity	[3]			–

++ = repeatedly documented positive association with physical activity; + = weak or mixed evidence of positive association with physical activity; 0 = weak or mixed evidence of no association with physical activity; – – = repeatedly documented negative association with physical activity; – = weak or mixed evidence of negative association with physical activity.

Study number described in table 11.1 indicated in square brackets in table 11.2

Trost et al. 2002.

syndrome, were more active as well (Arango et al., 2008; Archie et al., 2007; Vancampfort et al., 2011b,d). In contrast to results found in the general population (Trost et al., 2002), body mass index and body weight were not related to physical activity in the schizophrenic population (Archie et al., 2007; Jerome et al., 2009; McLeod, Jaques & Deane, 2009; Sharpe et al., 2006).

3.2 Psychosocial, Cognitive and Emotional Factors

Nine studies examined the association between psychosocial, cognitive and emotional factors and physical activity (Arbour-Nicotopoulos et al., 2010; Archie et al., 2007; Jerome et al., 2009; Leas & Mccabe, 2007; McLeod, Jaques & Deane, 2009; Osborn, Nazareth & King, 2007; Vancampfort et al., 2011a,c; Wichniak et al., 2011). Mixed results were found for perceived sport competence and fitness levels (Vancampfort et al., 2011a,c). Five studies indicated that other psychosocial, cognitive and emotional factors were not related to physical activity. These included body image (Arbour-Nicitopoulos et al., 2010; Archie et al., 2007; Vancampfort et al., 2011c), psychological distress (Jerome et al., 2009; McLeod, Jaques & Deane, 2009) and depression (Jerome et al., 2009; McLeod, Jaques & Deane, 2009). Leas and Mccabe (2007) reported that self-efficacy and response efficacy were the strongest predictors of intention to increase levels of physical activity in individuals with a psychiatric diagnosis (schizophrenia or major depression). One consistent correlate was the presence of negative symptoms, which was inversely related to physical activity in three studies (Vancampfort et al., 2011b,d; Wichniak et al., 2011).

Although this review addressed many factors, most factors were supported by evidence from only one study. Salient factors that influenced physical activity—those for which two or more studies showed a positive or negative relationship—included age, sex, presence of metabolic syndrome and presence of negative symptoms. Being younger, male and free of metabolic

syndrome was positively associated with being active; Trost and colleagues (2002) previously documented these factors and associations in the general population. Studies included in this review found that body mass index was not associated with levels of physical activity. The lack of association in our review may be explained by limiting factors found in each of the studies, including small sample size, a lack of diversity in body mass index (i.e., a high prevalence of obesity) or levels of physical activity in the sample or a lack of valid and reliable self-report measures. The finding regarding negative symptomatology is not surprising. Some researchers have suggested that motivational deficits are the central link between negative symptoms and functional impairment in schizophrenia (Foussias et al., 2009)—a clear challenge for developing and implementing physical activity interventions in this population.

Overall, the limited understanding of modifiable, theory-based determinants of physical activity in persons with schizophrenia inhibits the ability to develop, implement and evaluate interventions for increasing physical activity. Hence, more prospective, theory-driven research is needed to identify determinants of physical activity for persons with schizophrenia using valid and appropriate measures. Greater diversity in sampling may also be informative. Samples have been dominated by male, white and middle-aged participants.

4 Physical Activity Interventions in Schizophrenic Populations

Given the inherent physical health benefits of regular physical activity, interventions for promoting physical activity should be integrated into mental health services. An added benefit of participation may be improvements in mental health—important in its own right but possibly critical for continued participation in the physical activity that is necessary for physical health benefits to accrue. Faulkner (2005) reviewed the evidence on the effects of physical activity on the mental health of individuals with schizophrenia. Although he noted the methodological flaws in the literature, he concluded that some preliminary support shows that participating in exercise is associated with the alleviation of negative symptoms associated with schizophrenia such as depression, low self-esteem and social withdrawal. These conclusions are drawn primarily from studies of pre-experimental design. This chapter focusses specifically on methodologically rigorous trials (randomised controlled trials) in updating current consensus concerning the potential role of exercise in improving the mental health of individuals with schizophrenia.

Using the same search strategy described by Faulkner (2005), the literature was searched from 2005 to 2011 using PsychINFO, PubMed, Medline, SPORTDiscus and Google Scholar. The authors supplemented the search by examining the references of the retrieved papers. Only experimental studies (randomised controlled

trials) were included in this update. Studies were excluded if exercise or physical activity was not the specific intervention examined, if mental health outcomes were not reported or if the sample used did not specifically consist of individuals with a diagnosis of schizophrenia. In the last review of exercise interventions for mental health in schizophrenia, two randomised controlled trials existed (Faulkner, 2005). Seven randomised controlled trials now exist. This growth may indicate that greater attention is being focussed on the physical health needs of this population (Acil, Dogan & Dogan, 2008; Beebe et al., 2005; Behere et al., 2011; Duraiswamy et al., 2007; Lukoff et al., 1986; Marzolini, Jensen & Melville, 2009; Pelham et al., 1993) (see table 11.3).

Participants (n = 198) were predominantly adult males and outpatients. Common psychological assessment instruments used included the Brief Symptom Inventory (Derogatis &

Table 11.3   Randomised Controlled Trials Examining Psychological Effects of Exercise for Individuals With Schizophrenia

Study	Participants	Design	Treatment	Psychological instruments	Outcome
Acil, Dogan & Dogan (2008)	30 outpatients (18 male, 12 female; M = 32.4 yr)	Participants randomly assigned to a treatment group (n = 15) or a control group (n = 15)	10 wk group-based aerobic exercise programme consisting of 40 min sessions 3 days/wk. Sessions consisted of 10 min of warm-up, 25 min of aerobic exercises and 5 min of cool-down.	SANS, SAPS, BSI, WHOQOL-BREF-TR	Significant improvements (p < .05) on SANS, SAPS and BSI in the exercise group. Significant improvements in physical and mental domains (p < .05) of the WHOQOL in the exercise group.
Beebe et al. (2005)	10 outpatients (8 male, 2 female; M = 52 yr)	Participants randomly assigned to an experimental group (n = 4) or a waitlist control group (n = 6)	16 wk group-based treadmill exercise programme 3 days/wk, building to 30 min/session.	PANSS	Improvements on the PANSS and 6-Minute Walking Distance in the exercise group, but not statistically significant.
Behere et al. (2011)	66 outpatients (47 male, 19 female; M = 31.8 yr)	Participants randomly assigned to an experimental yoga group (n = 27), exercise group (n = 17) or waitlist control group (n = 22)	Participants in both yoga and exercise groups received 1 mo of instruction and were then asked to practise yoga or exercises (brisk walking, jogging and aerobic and stretching exercises) at home for 2 mo. Patients' caregivers maintained a log.	PANSS, SOFS, TRENDS, TRACS	Significant improvement in positive and negative symptoms, socio-occupational functioning and performance on TRENDS (p < .05) in the yoga group only.

Study	Participants	Design	Treatment	Psychological instruments	Outcome
Duraiswamy et al. (2007)	41 outpatients (28 male, 13 female; M = 30.4 ± 7.9 yr)	Participants randomly assigned to an experimental yoga group (n = 21) or a physical-training group (n = 20)	Participants in both yoga and physical-training groups received 3 wk of instruction and were then asked to participate in a 3 mo programme (5 days/wk for 1 h/day). The 1 h module of exercises consisted of brisk walking, jogging and stretching exercises. Therapist recorded attendance.	PANSS, SOFS, SAS, AIMS, WHOQOL-BREF	Participants in the yoga group had significantly less psychopathology than those in the training group at the end of 4 mo. They also had significantly greater social and occupational functioning and quality of life.
Lukoff et al. (1986)	28 male inpatients	Participants randomly assigned to a social skills treatment (n = 14) or a holistic treatment (n = 14) intervention that included exercise and stress-management education	Holistic intervention included 30 min of walking or running each weekday for 9 wk. Adherence not clearly described.	Symptom Checklist-90, PAS, NGI, TSC	Significant increase in fitness in the holistic group. Significant improvement from baseline to the end of the 9 wk intervention in both groups on psychopathology measures, but no differences between groups. No change in self-concept for either group.
Marzolini, Jensen & Melville (2009)	13 outpatients (8 male, 5 female; M = 44.6 ± 2.6 yr)	Participants randomly assigned to the exercise group (n = 7) or standard care group (n = 6)	Supervised exercise group met for 90 min 2 times/wk for 12 wk. Each session included 20 min of resistance training and 60 min of walking and flexibility exercises. Adherence measured by attendance.	MHI	Significant improvement in total MHI score (p < .03) for the exercise group; no change in the control group. Nonsignificant increase on the 6-Minute Walk Test in the exercise group.
Pelham et al. (1993)	10 outpatients (18-45 yr)	Fitness assessed; participants randomly assigned to an aerobic (n = 5) or nonaerobic (n = 5) condition	Aerobic: 30 min of bike ergometry (65%-75% of heart rate reserve) 4 times/wk for 8 wk. Nonaerobic: muscle tone and strengthening exercises 30 min 4 times/wk for 8 wk. Adherence not described.	Predicted $\dot{V}O_2$max tests, BDI	Aerobic group: Significant increase (20.9%) in $\dot{V}O_2$max and reduction (61%) in BDI (p < .05) from baseline to the end of wk 12. Nonaerobic group: No change in $\dot{V}O_2$max and insignificant reductions in BDI.

AIMS = Abnormal Involuntary Movements Scale; BDI = beck depression Inventory; BSI = Brief Symptom Inventory; MHI = Mental Health Inventory; NGI = Nurses Global Impressions; PANSS = Positive and Negative Symptom Scale; PAS = Premorbid Adjustment Scale; SANS = Scale for the Assessment of Negative Symptoms; SAPS = Scale for the Assessment of Positive Symptoms; SAS = self-rating anxiety scale; SOFS = Socio-Occupational Functioning Scale; TRACS = TRENDS Accuracy Score; TRENDS = Tool for Recognition of Emotions in Neuropsychiatric Disorders; TSC = Tennessee Self-Concept Test; WHOQOL-BREF-TR = World Health Organisation Quality of Life Scale—Turkish Version.

Melisaratos, 1983), the Positive and Negative Symptom Scale (Kay, Fiszbein & Opler, 1987), the Scale for the Assessment of Negative Symptoms (Derogatis, 1993), the Scale for the Assessment of Positive Symptoms (Andreasen, 1990), the World Health Organisation Quality of Life Scale—Turkish Version (Fidaner et al., 1999), the Mental Health Inventory (Veit & Ware, 1983) and the Socio-Occupational Functioning Scale (Saraswat et al., 2006).

Exercise programmes lasted from 8 to 16 wk. Frequency ranged from 2 to 5 sessions/wk and session duration ranged from 30 min to 1 h. The study by Acil, Dogan and Dogan (2008) examined a 10 wk group-based exercise programme that consisted of 40 min sessions 3 times/wk. The programme was led by physical education experts and involved outpatients at a psychiatric clinic in a university hospital located in the Central Anatolia region of Turkey. It is not clear whether participant attendance was tracked. A pre- and postexperimental design was used that evaluated the effects of exercise on both the experimental and control groups. Participants were matched for inclusion criteria and then randomly assigned to either the experimental or control condition. It is not clear from the study what treatment, if any, the control group received. Significant reductions occurred in negative and positive symptoms in the patient group as measured by the Scale for the Assessment of Negative Symptoms, Scale for the Assessment of Positive Symptoms and Brief Symptom Inventory. Additionally, self-reported ratings of physical and mental health and quality of life improved significantly, but social and environmental ratings did not change in the patient group.

In the study by Marzolini, Jensen and Melville (2009), participants were randomised to either a combined aerobic and strength-training group or a standard-care group. Participants in the combined exercise group met 2 times/wk for 12 wk. Sessions, led by a cardiac rehabilitation exercise specialist, were 90 min in length and consisted of a brief warm-up, resistance training, aerobic training and short cool-down. The Mental Health Inventory showed improvements in participant ratings for depression, positive affect, behaviour and anxiety, but changes were not significantly different from the control group. Similarly, fitness improvements were found for the exercise group, but no significant differences were found between the treatment and control groups.

Several recent studies in India have compared yoga with aerobic exercise and stretching (Behere et al., 2011; Duraiswamy et al., 2007). Improvements were generally found for both groups, but improvements were greatest for the yoga groups. For example, Duraiswamy and colleagues (2007) reported that participants took part in a 3 mo programme of either yoga

or aerobic and stretching exercises 5 days/wk for 1 h/day. Scores on the Positive and Negative Symptom Scale and the Socio-Occupational Functioning Scale decreased significantly in both groups, and greater decreases were found in the yoga group. In a study by Behere and colleagues (2011), 66 outpatients were randomised into an experimental yoga group, an aerobic and stretching exercise group or a waitlist control group. Participants in the yoga and exercise groups received 1 mo of instruction and then were asked to practise yoga or aerobic and stretching exercises at home. Participants' caregivers were asked to monitor yoga therapy and keep a log. After 2 mo of home-based yoga or aerobic and stretching exercises, ratings on the Positive and Negative Symptom Scale and Socio-Occupational Functioning Scale decreased from baseline in both groups, but changes were significant only in the yoga group. Whether these findings are generalisable to Western settings is not known.

Overall, these studies show that exercise therapy can have a modest positive impact and no adverse effects on some components of mental health and a limited effect on physical health outcomes such as weight. Heterogeneity in study designs, interventions (exercise frequency, intensity, type and time) and outcome measures makes it difficult to draw clear conclusions. The included studies illustrate that it is possible to conduct randomised controlled trials that examine the mental health effects of physical activity with individuals with schizophrenia, although the studies are short term and include only small samples. Importantly, attrition rates were similar among the trials, and no significant differences between groups were found. Gorczynski and Faulkner (2010) describe a range of limitations in the existing research that need to be addressed in the future. The exact nature of the exercise programme must be clearly defined, and the duration, frequency and intensity of exercise must be reported. Adherence, changes in fitness levels and the incorporation of follow-up measures in research designs should all be documented. The study should clearly describe participants in terms of age, sex, diagnosis, duration of illness and medication regimen. Outcome measures should include measures relevant to schizophrenia-related symptomatology, particularly the negative symptoms, and consider broader clinical outcomes such as use of health services, medication compliance and rate of relapse.

One critical limitation in this existing body of research is a lack of theory used to structure physical activity or exercise interventions. Previous research has shown that physical activity interventions are more effective when they are structured theoretically (Kahn et al., 2002). Because these interventions are not structured theoretically, researchers and clinicians do not fully understand how behaviour change occurs and how physical activity interventions may be enhanced in the future.

5 Promoting Exercise in the Treatment of Schizophrenia

The results of this review indicate that individuals with schizophrenia can improve components of mental health by participating in exercise. However, clear guidance regarding the dose of exercise that works best for improving mental health is limited by the small number of studies and the variability of the interventions themselves as well as their intensity and duration. People with schizophrenia should be encouraged to ask their clinicians for support and advice regarding becoming more physically active. Similarly, clinicians should educate patients, family and caregivers about the metabolic risks associated with antipsychotic medications and provide lifestyle advice regarding diet and physical activity (Faulkner, Cohn & Remington, 2007). The common physical activity guidelines for adults (i.e., 150 min/wk of moderate- to vigorous-intensity physical activity) appear to be applicable and relevant to individuals with schizophrenia in terms of potential benefit for mental and physical health. However, theoretically driven research and practice are required to examine how to reliably help individuals with schizophrenia adopt and maintain physical activity in the face of the

significant motivational and cognitive deficits that are inherent to schizophrenia. Such work will be needed before specific types of exercise interventions are more broadly disseminated to this population.

Some suggestions for practice can be gleaned from the literature and clinical experience. Richardson and colleagues (2005) describe examples of structured, supervised, facility-based exercise programs as well as lifestyle physical activity interventions that encourage participants to incorporate walking into everyday life and discuss a range of practical issues related to promoting physical activity in this population. More broadly, grounding physical activity intervention in the tenets of social–cognitive theory (Bandura, 1997) seems to be a reasonable basis for developing interventions in the absence of compelling theory-based intervention work (see figure 11.1).

In self-efficacy theory, participation in physical activity could be viewed as being influenced by both cognitions (e.g., values, beliefs, attitudes) and external stimuli (e.g., social norms, access to facilities). Self-efficacy, a situation-specific form of self-confidence, is integral to social–cognitive theory and is a robust predictor of behaviour change in a variety of situations (Bandura, 1986). Additionally, self-efficacy has been found to be a significant predictor of physical activity among individuals with schizophrenia (Leas & Mccabe, 2007) and in broader samples of individuals with serious mental illness (Gorczynski et al., 2010; Ussher et al., 2007). Bandura (1997) describes four sources of self-efficacy: past performance, vicarious experiences, social persuasion and physiological factors. Each can be considered in the context of physical activity promotion in this population.

5.1 Past Performance

Past performance is considered the most important source of an individual's self-efficacy. Given that many individuals with schizophrenia have low initial fitness levels and that drowsiness and fatigue may be side effects of some medications, a very gradual approach to increasing physical

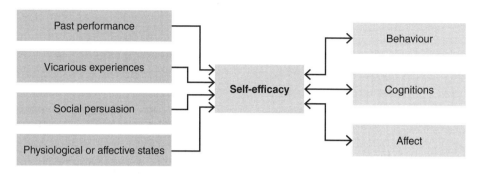

Figure 11.1   Sources of self-efficacy.

Adapted, by permission, from A. Bandura, 1977, "Self-efficacy: Toward a unifying theory of behavioral change," *Psychological Review* 84(2): 191-215.

activity is necessary (Mutrie & Faulkner, 2003). Determining an individual's activity history and interests maximizes the potential for success by ensuring that a match exists between those interests and the type of activity being promoted (e.g., group versus individual, structured exercise versus lifestyle physical activity). Participants need assistance from practitioners in setting appropriate, realistic goals for increasing physical activity and in developing the skills to self-monitor achievement. Attending group sessions or using pedometers to track physical activity (i.e., step counts) might be useful.

Reviews of the literature on mediators of interventions indicate that self-regulatory constructs (e.g., planning, contingency strategies, self-monitoring) are the most consistent agents of change (Lewis et al., 2002; Rhodes & Pfaeffli, 2009). In general, programmes for changing health behaviour that teach behavioural skills for self-management are recommended because they are effective in promoting physical activity (Kahn et al., 2002). Regulatory skills are required to link positive intentions to subsequent behaviour. These regulatory skills include, for example, the specifics of a behavioural plan (e.g., what, when, where, with whom), problem solving and monitoring of action. Success can then be defined in terms of learning and applying these new self-regulatory skills in the context of increasing physical activity. Practitioners may use weekly calendars to help patients plan for physical activity in the coming week and to brainstorm solutions to the barriers they may face.

5.2   Modelling

Seeing others succeed, particularly those who are similar to oneself, can be another source of self-efficacy. Individuals with serious mental illness such as schizophrenia are more likely to be socially excluded, poor and unemployed, live in substandard housing and have reduced social networks (Sainsbury Centre for Mental Health, 2002). Previous research shows that the social networks of people with schizophrenia are significantly poorer than those of a control group in both quantity and quality and that most want more social contact (Bengtsson-Tops & Hansson, 2001). Strength of social support may be a key determinant of quality of life in people with schizophrenia (Hansson, 2006), and it has been recommended that interventions in mental health care target increased social interaction as an outcome (Eklund & Hansson, 2007).

Accordingly, it may be that group-based physical activity programming for patients is essential only when a patient first becomes physically active at first in order to provide opportunities for increasing social interaction and social support. Furthermore, many people with schizophrenia are often involved in few meaningful activities. It may be that the process of participating in physical activity in a group is secondary to the sense of purpose and socialisation that participation brings (Faulkner & Carless, 2006; Hodgson, McCulloch & Fox, 2011). Carter-Morris and Faulkner (2003) describe a case study of a football project for individuals with schizophrenia. One notable finding was that participation made opportunities for social interaction accessible within a context of a normalizing activity. The caregiver of Larry, one of the service users in the football project, describes the benefits for Larry most eloquently.

He speaks to a lot of his friends now who he was at school with who are working and they can talk about what they did at work and interact with people. Sometimes you think I don't want to meet these people because all I'm going to talk to them about is "I took 2 pink pills in the morning and 4 green ones in the afternoon" sort of thing. It's all "down" conversation. But if you can tell them you went to play football, they beat us 4-0 and then it's what are you playing football for? It makes him feel as though he's part of a group and not estranged from the "normal" population.

5.3 Social Persuasion

Social persuasion concerns verbal and nonverbal tactics used by others to promote a person's self-efficacy. The opportunity for consistent and structured physical activity experiences needs to be integrated into the delivery of mental health services. This requires interdisciplinary and collaborative coordination of appropriate personnel, resources and facilities [Faulkner, 2005; see Marzolini, Jensen & Melville (2009) as an example]. Intensive support will likely be required over a long period of time to help people with schizophrenia initiate and maintain physical activity. Carless (2007) describes three possible components of this support: awareness raising, to help the patient consider the potential benefits of physical activity; engagement, involving close interaction (usually one to one) between a health professional and each individual in order to capture interest and generate enthusiasm; and practical facilitation, where health professionals take care of organisational aspects of the exercise sessions on a day-to-day basis and may include attending each exercise session in person to provide verbal encouragement, reassurance and support. Overall, long-term engagement with a supported programme may be necessary for some individuals with schizophrenia (Hodg-

son, McCulloch & Fox, 2011). The need for such intensive support has clear implications for the sustainability of such interventions. Barry, a participant in an exercise-intervention case study reported by Faulkner and Sparkes (1999), found that exercise provided him a range of mental health benefits but he stopped exercising as soon as formal support was withdrawn. Barry stated, "I need someone to push me, I don't think I could ever do it on my own bat, I think I need somebody to give me that little push, to make sure that I do it ... it's just having that person there to say, a member of staff or someone saying, go out and do it."

5.4 Physiological Factors

An individual's physiological and affective states can also be a source of, or threat to, self-efficacy. In these circumstances, the threat could be taken into account in understanding behavior and also the affective response to the bout of exercise. Providing a supportive, nonthreatening environment and no-pressure sessions that allow people to go at their own pace (Hodgson, McCulloch & Fox, 2011) can help reduce anxiety about participating in physical activity.

More speculatively, a person's perception of physiological responses to exercise might alter that person's self-efficacy. That is, the extent to which a bout of exercise makes someone feel bad rather than good may be associated with nonadherence and, ultimately, dropout. In their review, Ekkekakis, Parfitt and Petruzzello (2011) summarise data that demonstrate that most adults who are sedentary and overweight or obese (likely characteristics of many with schizophrenia) experience reduced pleasure over most of the range of exercise intensity. Yet a relationship of medium effect size exists between enjoyment (or affective judgement) and physical activity (Rhodes, Fiala & Conner, 2009). In a mixed sample of psychiatric patients, Sorenson (2006) found that the odds for being active rather than inactive were 20 times greater if intrinsic motivation was present compared with if intrinsic motivation was not present. That is, although physical activity offers instrumental benefits, greater priority might be placed on ensuring that individuals enjoy the experience of exercise. Such experiences were important for Joanne (in Faulkner & Sparkes, 1999), who recalled her feelings during exercise as follows: "Just the pleasure really, just it being a pleasure, just it being a big pleasure cos it was a change from the routine, and it was a change of scenery, and using my muscles again so it's alright."

Focussing on the affective experience of physical activity may be an approach for directly addressing the negative symptoms of schizophrenia—possibly the greatest challenge for successful physical activity intervention. Practically, this means recommending that participants exercise in a way that maintains a constant or improving (but not diminishing) level of pleasure (Ekkekakis, Parfitt & Petruzzello, 2011). Encouraging individuals to monitor how they feel before, during and after bouts of physical activity might help them develop the skills to reliably do this as well as encourage awareness of how physical activity might positively regulate other moods, emotions or feelings such as fatigue, poor concentration or sleepiness. Research to assess this possibility

is required and presents an exciting opportunity for moving the field forward.

6   Summary

Given the physical health benefits inherent to physical activity and the possibility of significant effects on psychological well-being, the consideration of physical activity and exercise is a win–win situation for many clinical populations such as those with schizophrenia (Mutrie & Faulkner, 2003). Certainly, the potential for benefit far outweighs any risk. Patients should seek medical clearance before participating in exercise. Meyer and Broocks (2000) suggest that almost no contraindications to participating in exercise programmes exist for psychiatric patients if they are free from cardiovascular disease. Additionally, the combination of exercise and psychotropic medication presents no known serious complications (Martinsen & Stanghelle, 1997). Systematic research should focus on developing, assessing and disseminating physical activity interventions in this population. Theoretically informed approaches [e.g., self-efficacy theory as proposed here; see also Williams & French

EVIDENCE TO PRACTICE

- Given the inherent physical health benefits of regular physical activity, interventions that promote physical activity should be integrated into the delivery of mental health services. In addition to physical health benefits, preliminary evidence shows that participating in exercise is associated with the alleviation of negative symptoms associated with schizophrenia such as depression, low self-esteem and social withdrawal.
- Practitioners should seek to educate patients, family and caregivers about physical activity.
- Common physical activity guidelines for adults (i.e., 150 min/wk of moderate- to vigorous-intensity physical activity)

appear to be applicable and relevant to individuals with schizophrenia in terms of potential mental and physical health benefits. Physical activity should be increased very gradually.
- Practitioners should help patients be physically active in ways that promote self-efficacy. Practitioners can help patients build mastery through goal setting and developing specific, detailed plans for behaviour change; by developing opportunities for social support; by providing ongoing feedback and reinforcing patients' efforts to become more physically active; and by structuring opportunities so that patients enjoy the process of being physically active.

(2011)] should be prioritised over atheoretical approaches in any population. Although balanced with an attitude of hopeful scepticism, it is necessary to adopt a rigorous hypothesis-testing approach in order to advance this area both theoretically and clinically (Tandon, Nasrallah & Keshavan, 2010).

Consideration must be given to how the research reported here can be disseminated to mental health professionals through training or continuing professional development. The support of these professionals is essential in legitimizing the inclusion of exercise in an individual's care plan, helping patients overcome barriers specific to mental illness and providing the ongoing reinforcement necessary for the long-term adoption of regular physical activity (Richardson et al., 2005). However, it is important to acknowledge that behavioural interventions may not be appropriate for individuals with schizophrenia who have significant impairment in functioning and insight. Attention also needs to be directed toward how the environment that many people with schizophrenia inhabit (e.g., psychiatric facilities, community care homes) can be modified to promote habitual physical activity and reduced energy intake (Faulkner, Gorczynski & Cohn, 2009). For example, such settings may facilitate increased energy intake (e.g., overeating, easy access to high-calorie snacks and beverages, skipping breakfast) and reduce opportunities for energy expenditure (e.g., lack of access to staircases, availability of screen time). Cohn, Grant and Faulkner (2010) reported some success in changing how meals are delivered in one psychiatric unit; these changes were associated in reductions in weight.

Future research is required to examine how environments may be structured in psychiatric group homes, inpatient units and community clinics to encourage consistent reductions in sitting time rather than increase physical activity per se. Such an approach would complement the development of interventions targeting those individuals who can access or are interested in accessing traditional exercise interventions and contribute to a healthier workplace that makes it easier for both patients and staff to be physically active throughout the day.

7 References

Acil, A.A., Dogan, S., & Dogan, O. (2008). The effects of physical exercises to mental state and quality of life in patients with schizophrenia. *Journal of Psychiatric and Mental Health Nursing*, 15, 808-815.

Allison, D.B., Newcomer, J.W., Dunn, A.L., Blumenthal, J.A., Fabricatore, A.N., Daumit, G.L., et al. (2009). Obesity among those with mental disorders: A National Institute of Mental Health meeting report. *American Journal of Preventive Medicine*, 36, 341-350.

American Psychiatric Association. (1994). *Diagnostic and statistical manual of mental disorders* (4th ed.). Washington, D.C.: American Psychiatric Association.

Andreasen, N.C. (1990). Methods for assessing positive and negative symptoms. *Modern Problems of Pharmacopsychiatry*, 24, 73-88.

Arango, C., Bobes, J., Randa, P., Carmena, R., Garcia-Garcia, M., Rejas, J., et al. (2008). A comparison of schizophrenia outpatients treated with antipsychotics with and without metabolic syndrome: Findings from the Clamors study. *Schizophrenia Research*, 104, 1-12.

Arbour-Nicitopoulos, K.P., Faulkner, G., & Cohn, T. (2010). Body image in individuals with schizophrenia: Examination of the B-Wise questionnaire. *Schizophrenia Research*, 118, 307-308.

Archie, S., Wilson, J.H., Osborne, S., Hobbs, H., & McNiven, J. (2003). Pilot study: Access to fitness facility and exercise levels in olanzapine-treated patients. *Canadian Journal of Psychiatry*, 48, 628-632.

Archie SM, Goldberg JO, Akhtar-Danesh N, Landeen J, McColl L, McNiven J. (2007) Psychotic disorders, eating habits, and physical activity: who is ready for lifestyle changes? *Psychiatric Services*. 2007 Feb;58(2):233-9.

Bandura, A. (1986). *Social foundations of thought and action: A social cognitive theory.* Englewood Cliffs, NJ: Prentice-Hall.

Bandura, A. (1997). *Self-efficacy: The exercise of control.* New York: Freeman.

Beebe, L.H., Tian, L., Morris, N., Goodwin, A., Swant Allen, S., & Kuldau, J. (2005). Effects of exercise on mental and physical health parameters of person with schizophrenia. *Issues in Mental Health Nursing*, 26, 661-676.

Behere, R.V., Arasappa, R., Jagannathan, A., Varambally, S., Venkatasubramanian, G., Thirthalli, J., et al. (2011). Effect of yoga therapy on facial emotion recognition deficits, symptoms and functioning in patients with schizophrenia. *Acta Psychiatricia Scandinavica*, 123, 147-153.

Bengtsson-Tops, A., & Hansson, L. (2001). Quantitative and qualitative aspects of the social network in schizophrenic patients living in the community. Relationship to sociodemographic characteristics and clinical factors and subjective quality of life. *International Journal of Social Psychiatry*, 47, 67-77.

Brenner, S., & Cohen, C.I. (2009). Medical health in aging persons with schizophrenia. In J.M. Meyer & H.A. Nasrallah (Eds.), *Medical illness and schizophrenia* (2nd ed.) (pp. 377-413). Washington, D.C.: American Psychiatric.

Bresee, L.C., Majumdar, S.R., Patten, S.B., & Johnson, J.A. (2010). Prevalence of cardiovascular risk factors and disease in people with schizophrenia: A population-based study. *Schizophrenia Research*, 117, 75-82.

Brown, S., Birtwistle, J., Roe, L., & Thompson, C. (1999). The unhealthy lifestyle of people with schizophrenia. *Psychological Medicine*, 29, 697-701.

Carless, D. (2007). Phases in physical activity initiation and maintenance among men with serious mental illness. *International Journal of Mental Health Promotion*, 9, 17-27.

Carter-Morris, P., & Faulkner, G. (2003). A football project for service users: The role of football in reducing social exclusion. *Journal of Mental Health Promotion*, 2, 24-31.

Casey, D.E., & Hansen, T.E. (2009). Excessive mortality and morbidity associated with schizophrenia. In J.M. Meyer & H.A. Nasrallah (Eds.), *Medical illness and schizophrenia* (2nd ed.) (pp. 17-35). Washington, D.C.: American Psychiatric.

Cohn, T., Grant, S., & Faulkner, G.E. (2010). Schizophrenia and obesity: Addressing obesogenic environments in mental health settings. *Schizophrenia Research*, 121, 277-278.

Colton, C.W., & Manderscheid, R.W. (2006). Congruencies in increased mortality rates, years of potential life lost, and causes of death among public mental health clients in eight states. *Preventing Chronic Disease*, 3(2), A42.

Craig, C.L., Marshall, A.L., Sjöström, M., Baumanm A.E., Booth, M.L., Ainsworth, B.E., et al. (2003). International physical activity questionnaire: 12-country reliability and validity. *Medicine and Science in Sports and Exercise*, 35, 1381-1395.

Daumit, G.L., Goldberg, R.W., Anthony, C., Dickerson, F., Brown, C.H., Kreyenbuhl, J., et al. (2005). Physical activity patterns in adults with severe mental illness. *Journal of Nervous and Mental Diseases*, 193, 641-646.

Derogatis, L.R. (1993). *BSI Brief Symptom Inventory. Administration, scoring, and procedures manual*. Minneapolis: National Computer Systems.

Derogatis, L.R., & Melisaratos, N. (1983). The brief symptom inventory: An introduction report. *Psychological Medicine*, 13, 595-605.

DiPietro, L., Caspersen, C.J., Ostfeld, A.M., & Nadel, E.R. (1993). A survey for assessing physical activity among older adults. *Medicine and Science in Sports and Exercise*, 25, 628-642.

Dixon, L., Postrado, L., Delahanty, J., Fischer, P.J., & Lehman, A. (1999). The association of medical comorbidity in schizophrenia with poor physical and mental health. *The Journal of Nervous and Mental Disease*, 187, 496-502.

Duraiswamy, G., Thirthalli, J., Nagendra, H.R., & Gangadhar, B.N. (2007). Yoga therapy as an add-on treatment in the management of patients with schizophrenia—A randomized controlled trial. *Acta Psychiatrica Scandinavica*, 116, 226-232.

Editorial. (1988). Where next with psychiatric illness? *Nature*, 336, 95-96.

Ekkekakis, P., Parfitt, G., & Petruzzello, S.J. (2011). The pleasure and displeasure people feel when they exercise at different intensities: Decennial update and progress towards a tripartite rationale for exercise intensity prescription. *Sports Medicine*, 41, 641-671.

Eklund, M., & Hansson, L. (2007). Social network among people with persistent mental illness: Associations with sociodemographic, clinical and health-related factors. *International Journal of Social Psychiatry*, 53, 293-305.

Faulkner, G. (2005). Exercise as an adjunct treatment for schizophrenia. In G. Faulkner & A. Taylor (Eds.), *Exercise, health and mental health: Emerging relationships* (pp. 27-47). London: Routledge.

Faulkner, G., & Carless, D. (2006). Physical activity and the process of psychiatric rehabilitation: Theoretical and methodological issues. *Psychiatric Rehabilitation Journal*, 29, 258-266.

Faulkner, G., Cohn, T., & Remington, G. (2006). Validation of a physical assessment tool for individuals with schizophrenia. *Schizophrenia Research*, 82, 225-231.

Faulkner, G., Cohn, T., & Remington, G. (2007). Interventions to reduce weight gain in schizophrenia. *Cochrane Database of Systematic Reviews*, 24(1), CD005148.

Faulkner, G., Gorczynski, P., & Cohn, T. (2009). Dissecting the obesogenic nature of psychiatric settings. *Psychiatric Services*, 60, 538-541.

Faulkner, G., & Sparkes, A. (1999). Exercise as therapy for schizophrenia: An ethnographic study. *Journal of Sport and Exercise Psychology*, 21, 39-51.

Fidaner, H., Elbi, H., Fidaner, C., Eser, S.Y., Eser, E., & Göker, E. (1999). The measurement of quality of life, WHOQOL-100 and WHOQOL-TR-BREF [in Turkish]. *3P Dergisi*, 7(Suppl. 2), 5-13.

Foussias, G., Mann, S., Zakzanis, K.K., van Reekum, R., & Remington, G. (2009). Motivational deficits as the central link to functioning in schizophrenia: A pilot study. *Schizophrenia Research*, 115, 333-337.

Gorczynski, P., & Faulkner, G. (2010). Exercise therapy for schizophrenia. *Cochrane Database of Systematic Reviews*, 5, CD004412.

Gorczynski, P., Faulkner, G., Greening, S., & Cohn, T. (2010). Exploring the construct validity of the transtheoretical model to structure physical activity interventions for individuals with serious mental illnesses. *Psychiatric Rehabilitation Journal*, 34, 61-64.

Greaves, C.J., Sheppard, K.E., Abraham, C., Hardeman, W., Roden, M., Evans, P.H., et al. (2011). Systematic review of reviews of intervention components associated with increased effectiveness in dietary and physical activity interventions. *BMC Public Health*, 11, 119.

Hansson, L. (2006). Determinants of quality of life in people with severe mental illness. *Acta Psychiatrica Scandinavica*, 429, 46-50.

Hennekens, C.H., Hennekens, A.R., Hollar, D., & Casey, D.E. (2005). Schizophrenia and increased risks of cardiovascular disease. *American Heart Journal*, 150, 1115-1121.

Hillsdon, M., Foster, C., & Thorogood, M. (2005). Interventions for promoting physical activity. *Cochrane Database of Systematic Reviews*, 1, CD003180.

Hodgson, M.H., McCulloch, H.P., & Fox, K.R. (2011). The experiences of people with severe and enduring mental illness engaged in a physical activity programme integrated into the mental health service. *Mental Health and Physical Activity*, 4, 23-29.

Hor, K., & Taylor, M. (2010). Suicide and schizophrenia: A systematic review of rates and risk factors. *Journal of Psychopharmacology*, 24(4 Suppl.), 81-90.

Jerome, G.J., Young, D.R., Dalcin, A., Charleston, J., Anthony, C., Hayes, J., et al. (2009). Physical activity levels of persons with mental illness attending psychiatric rehabilitation programs. *Schizophrenia Research*, 108, 252-257.

Kahn, E.B., Ramsey, L.T., Brownson, R.C., Heath, G.W., Howze, E.H., Powell, K.E., et al. (2002). The effectiveness of interventions to increase physical activity: A systematic review. *American Journal of Preventative Medicine*, 22, 73-107.

Kay, S.R., Fiszbein, A., & Opler, L.A. (1987). The positive and negative syndrome scale (PANSS) for schizophrenia. *Schizophrenia Bulletin*, 13, 261-276.

Leas, L., & Mccabe, M. (2007). Health behaviors among individuals with schizophrenia and depression. *Journal of Health Psychology*, 12, 563-579.

Lewis, B.A., Marcus, B., Pate, R.R., & Dunn, A.L. (2002). Psychosocial mediators of physical activity behavior among adults and children. *American Journal of Preventive Medicine*, 23, 26-35.

Lindamer, L.A., McKibbin, C., Norman, G.J., Jordan, L., Harrison, K., Abeyesinhe, S., et al. (2008). Assessment of physical activity in middle-aged and older adults with schizophrenia. *Schizophrenia Research*, 104, 294-301.

Lukoff, D., Wallace, C.J., Liberman, R.P., & Burke, K. (1986). A holistic program for chronic schizophrenic patients. *Schizophrenia Bulletin*, 12, 274-282.

Martín-Sierra, A., Vancampfort, D., Probst, M., Bobes, J., Maurissen, K., Sweers, K., De Schepper, E., De Hert, M. (2011) Walking capacity is associated with health related quality of life and physical activity level in patients with schizophrenia: a preliminary report. Actas Espanolas de Psiquiatria. 39(4):211-6. Epub 2011 Jul 1.

Martinsen, E.W., & Stanghelle, J.K. (1997). Drug therapy and physical activity. In W.P. Morgan (Ed.), *Physical activity and mental health* (pp. 81-90). Washington, D.C.: Taylor & Francis.

Marzolini, S., Jensen, B., & Melville, P. (2009). Feasibility and effects of a group-based resistance and aerobic exercise programme for individuals with severe schizophrenia: A multidisciplinary approach. *Mental Health and Physical Activity*, 2, 29-36.

McCreadie, R.G. (2003). Diet, smoking and cardiovascular risk in people with schizophrenia: Descriptive study. *British Journal of Psychiatry*, 183, 534-539.

McGrath, J., Saha, S., Chant, D., & Welham, J. (2008). Schizophrenia: A concise overview of incidence, prevalence, and mortality. *Epidemiological Reviews*, 30, 67-76.

McLeod, H.J., Jaques, S., & Deane, F.P. (2009). Base rates of physical activity in Australians with schizophrenia. *Psychiatric Rehabilitation Journal*, 32, 269-275.

Meyer, T., & Broocks, A. (2000). Therapeutic impact of exercise on psychiatric diseases: Guidelines for exercise testing and prescription. *Sports Medicine*, 30, 269-279.

Mutrie, N., & Faulkner, G. (2003). Physical activity and mental health. In T. Everett, M. Donaghy, & S. Fever (Eds.), *Physiotherapy and occupational therapy in mental health: An evidence based approach* (pp. 82-97). Oxford: Butterworth Heinemann.

Osborn, D.P.J., Nazareth, I., & King, M.B. (2007). Physical activity, dietary habits and coronary heart disease risk factor knowledge amongst people with severe mental illness: A cross sectional comparative study in primary care. *Social Psychiatry and Psychiatric Epidemiology*, 42, 787-793.

Pelham, T.W., Campagna, P.D., Ritvo, P.G., & Birnie, W.A. (1993). The effects of exercise therapy on clients in a psychiatric rehabilitation program. *Psychosocial Rehabilitation Journal*, 16, 75-84.

Rhodes, R.E., Fiala, B., & Conner, M. (2009). A review and meta-analysis of affective judgments and physical activity in adult populations. *Annals of Behavioral Medicine*, 38, 180-204.

Rhodes, R.E., & Pfaeffli, L.A. (2009). Mediators of physical activity behaviour change among adult non-clinical populations: A review update. *International Journal of Behavioral Nutrition and Physical Activity*, 7, 37.

Richardson, C., Faulkner, G., McDevitt, J., Skrinar, G.S., Hutchison, D.S., & Piette, J.D. (2005). Integrating physical activity into mental health services for individuals with serious mental illness. *Psychiatric Services*, 56, 324-331.

Roick, C., Fritz-Wieacker, A., Matschinger, H., Heider, D., Schindler, J., Riedel-Heller, S., et al. (2007). Health habits of patients with schizophrenia. *Social Psychiatry and Psychiatric Epidemiology*, 42, 268-276.

Saha, S., Chant, D., & McGrath, J. (2007). A systematic review of mortality in schizophrenia: Is the differential mortality gap worsening over time? *Archives of General Psychiatry*, 64, 1123-1131.

Sainsbury Centre for Mental Health. (2002). *Working for inclusion*. London: Sainsbury Centre for Mental Health.

Sallis, J., & Owen, N. (1999). *Physical activity and behavioral medicine*. Thousand Oaks, CA: Sage.

Saraswat, N., Rao, K., Subbakrishna, D.K., & Gangadhar, B.N. (2006). The Social Occupational Functioning Scale (SOFS): A brief measure of functional status in persons with schizophrenia. *Schizophrenia Research*, 81, 301-309.

Sharpe, J.K., Stedman, T.J., Byrne, N.M., & Hills, A.P. (2006). Energy expenditure and physical activity in clozopine use: Implications for weight management. *Australian and New Zealand Journal of Psychiatry*, 40, 810-814.

Sorenson, M. (2006). Motivation for physical activity of psychiatric patients when physical activity was offered as part of treatment. *Scandinavian Journal of Medicine and Science in Sports*, 16, 391-398.

Strassnig, M., Brar, J.S., & Ganguli, R. (2011). Low cardiorespiratory fitness and physical functional capacity in obese patients with schizophrenia. *Schizophrenia Research*, 126, 103-109.

Tandon, R., Nasrallah, H.A., & Keshavan, M.S. (2010). Schizophrenia, "just the facts" 5. Treatment and prevention. Past, present, and future, *Schizophrenia Research*, 122, 1-23.

Trost, S.G., Owen, N., Bauman, A.E., Sallis, J.F., & Brown, W. (2002). Correlates of adults' participation in physical activity: Review and update. *Medicine and Science in Sports and Exercise*, 34, 1996-2001.

United States Department of Health and Human Services. (1999). *Mental health: A report of the Surgeon General*. Atlanta: U.S. Department of Health and Human Services.

Ussher, M., Stanbury, L., Cheeseman, V., & Faulkner, G. (2007). Physical activity preferences and perceived barriers to activity among persons with severe mental illness in the United Kingdom. *Psychiatric Services*, 58, 405-408.

Vancampfort, D., De Hert, M., Maurissen, K., Sweers, K., Knapen, J., Raepsaet, J., et al. (2011a). Physical activity participation, functional exercise capacity and self-esteem in patients with schizophrenia with high and low physical self perception. *International Journal of Therapy and Rehabilitation*, 18, 222-230.

Vancampfort, D., Knapen, J., Probst, M., van Winkel, R., Deckx, S., Maurissen, K., et al. (2010). Considering a frame of reference for physical activity research related to the cardiometabolic risk profile in schizophrenia. *Psychiatry Research*, 177, 271-279.

Vancampfort, D., Probst, M., Scheewe, T., Maurissen, K., Sweers, K., Knapen, J., et al. (2011b). Lack of physical activity during leisure time contributes to an impaired health related quality of life in patients with schizophrenia. *Schizophrenia Research*, 129, 122-127.

Vancampfort, D., Probst, M., Sweers, K., Maurissen, K., Knapen, J., & De Hert, M. (2011c). Relationships between obesity, functional exercise capacity, physical activity participation and physical self perception in people with schizophrenia. *Acta Psychiatrica Scandinavica*, 123, 423-430.

Vancampfort, D., Sweers, K., Probst, M., Maurissen, K., Knapen, J., Minguet, P., et al. (2011d). The association of metabolic syndrome with physical activity performance in patients with schizophrenia. *Diabetes and Metabolism*, 37(4):318-23.

Veit, C.T., & Ware, J.E. (1983). The structure of psychological distress and well-being in general populations. *Journal of Consulting and Clinical Psychology*, 51, 730-742.

Warburton, D.E.R., Charlesworth, S., Ivey, A., Nettlefold, L., & Bredin, S.S.D. (2010). A systematic review of the evidence for Canada's Physical Activity Guidelines for Adults. *International Journal of Behavioral Nutrition and Physical Activity*, 7, 39.

Wei, M., Kampert, J.B., Barlow, C.E., Nichaman, M.Z., Gibbons, L.W., Paffenbarger, R.S. Jr., et al. (1999). Relationship between low cardiorespiratory fitness and mortality in normal weight, overweight and obese men. *Journal of the American Medical Association*, 282, 1547-1553.

Wichniak, A., Skowerska, A., Chojnacka-Wojtowicz, J., Taflinski, T., Wierzbicka, A., Jernajczyk, W., et al. (2011). Actigraphic monitoring of activity and rest in schizophrenic patients treated with olanzapine or risperidone. *Journal of Psychiatric Research* 45(10):1381-6

Williams, S.L., & French, D.P. (2011). What are the most effective intervention techniques for changing physical activity self-efficacy and physical activity behaviour—And are they the same? *Health Education Research*, 26, 308-322.

Addictive Behaviour

Michael Ussher, PhD
St. George's University of London, London, United Kingdom

Chapter Outline

Editors' Introduction

This chapter reviews evidence from epidemiological studies showing that physical activity is generally associated with fewer addictive behaviours and explores the neurobiological and psychosocial mechanisms linking exercise and addictive behaviours. It also discusses the impact of physical activity interventions on individuals with addiction to alcohol, drugs or tobacco. Finally, it addresses implications for practice and provides valuable advice on designing interventions for those with addictions.

Addiction to alcohol, drugs and tobacco is a global public health problem. In the United States, 9% of those aged 12 yr or older are classed as having drug or alcohol dependence and 23% are smokers (Substance Abuse and Mental Health Services Administration, 2010). In England and Wales, 21% of the population are smokers and 13% of females and 22% of males consume more than double the recommended limit of alcohol each week (Health Survey for England, 2011). In the United Kingdom, 36.3% of people aged 16 to 59 yr report having tried an illegal drug at least once, and the reported prevalence of problem illegal-drug use is approximately 1% (Eaton et al, 2008). This has serious health consequences. For example, 4% of deaths globally are attributed to alcohol (Rehm et al., 2009) and, despite the dramatic decline in smoking rates in the past 50 yr, smoking remains the leading cause of death in industrialised nations (Doll et al., 2004). Consequently, smoking, alcohol dependence and drug dependence are the mental disorders that create the highest economic burden on society (Eaton et al., 2008). Treating addiction with cognitive–behavioural and pharmaceutical therapies is effective in the short term, but at least 80% of patients commonly relapse within 12 mo (Marlatt & Donovan, 2005). Effective adjuncts to these treatments are needed. Participation in physical activity has been proposed as an intervention for preventing and treating addiction. This chapter builds on two previous reviews, one relating to exercise and smoking cessation (Ussher, Taylor & Faulkner, 2012) and the other concerning exercise for alcohol and drug rehabilitation (Donaghy & Ussher, 2005). In this chapter, the terms *physical activity* and *exercise* are used interchangeably.

1 Links Between Physical Activity and Addictive Behaviours

Evidence consistently and overwhelmingly shows that levels of physical activity are lower among smokers. However, the findings related to physical activity levels among those who misuse alcohol or illicit substances are less consistent and vary according to sex, age and type of physical activity. More studies are needed to fully examine the relationship between physical activity and drug use in adults. The following sections summarise the current state of knowledge.

1.1 Smoking and Physical Activity

In general, cross-sectional surveys show that adults and adolescents who are more physically active are less likely to smoke (Kaczynski et al., 2008). Some exceptions to these findings exist when taking into account different types of exercise and sex. For instance, when examining only leisure-time activity, exercise is associated with less prevalence of smoking in men but not in women (Schroder, Elosua & Marrugat, 2003). Similarly, participation in sport has been correlated with reduced chances of smoking in men but not in women (Helmert, Herman & Shea, 1994). Children who have higher levels of physical activity are less likely to start smoking (Audrain-McGovern, Rodriguez & Moss, 2003). In addition, smokers who are more physically active are more likely to attempt to quit (deRuiter et al., 2008), to be confident about abstaining (King et al., 1996) and to successfully quit (Abrantes et al., 2009).

1.2 Alcohol Abuse and Physical Activity

Adults who are more active are generally more likely to drink more alcohol, usually in social situations (French, Popovici & Maclean, 2009), and to binge drink (Vickers et al., 2004). However, adults with sustained hazardous levels of drinking are less active (Liangpunsakul, Crabb & Qi, 2010). The findings diverge when considering sex, age and type of exercise. For example, among women only, higher alcohol use at baseline predicts increased physical activity at follow-up (Laaksonen et al., 2002). Regarding age, higher levels of vigorous physical activity have been associated with increased alcohol use in individuals under 50 yr but not in those over 50 yr (Lisha, Martens & Leventhal, 2011). Lisha, Martens and Leventhal postulate that this may be because older adults are less likely to exercise with others and consume alcohol socially. In the same study, the association between higher levels of moderate physical activity in the past year and increased alcohol use was stronger for men than for women. The authors reason that this might be because men are more likely than women to take part in recreational sports in which drinking might be culturally accepted as the norm.

The findings for adolescents contrast with those for adults. Higher overall levels of activity are associated with lower rates of alcohol use (Tur et al., 2003) and predict lower rates of alcohol use as adults (Korhonen et al., 2009). In some surveys, however, findings vary according to type of exercise and sex. For instance, sport participants report higher levels of alcohol consumption compared with nonparticipants in some studies (Peretti-Watel, Beck & Legleye, 2002) and lower levels of alcohol consumption in other studies (Ferron at al., 1999). These inconsistent reports reflect the complexity of the relationship between alcohol use and physical activity during adolescence and may be related to different patterns for males and females across the adolescent period. Interestingly, Moore and Werch (2005) observed that girls in school-sponsored dance, cheerleading or gymnastics were at decreased risk of alcohol use, whereas those in out-of-school dance, cheerleading or gymnastics,

skateboarding or surfing were at increased risk of using alcohol, cigarettes or marijuana. Boys in out-of-school swimming were at decreased risk of heavy alcohol use, whereas boys in school football, swimming, wrestling or out-of-school tennis were at increased risk of using alcohol, cigarettes or marijuana. Again, these findings point to the complexity of the relationship between alcohol use and physical activity during adolescence.

1.3   Substance Abuse and Physical Activity

Studies have generally found that adolescents who are more active report less use of illicit substances (e.g., Field, Diego & Sanders, 2001). Yet again, type of exercise and sex must be considered. For instance, some studies observe this association only for females (Kulig, Brener & McManus, 2003) or only for males (Winnail et al., 1995). Additionally, sport participation has been associated with less use of these substances in boys but not in girls (Pate et al., 2000). Also, adolescents who are more active are less likely to use illicit drugs as young adults (Terry-McElrath & O'Malley, 2011) and are less likely to develop substance-use disorders (Strohle et al., 2007). No cross-sectional surveys of adults could be identified, although one study showed that those engaging in physical activity or related behaviours (e.g., planning physical activity) during treatment for substance use report lower rates of substance use than those not engaged in these activities (Weinstock, Barry & Petry, 2008).

KEY CONCEPTS

- One well-conducted randomised controlled trial has shown that exercise is beneficial in the long term for helping smokers quit.
- One well-designed randomised controlled trial observed that participating in

an exercise programme increased long-term rates of alcohol abstinence.
- No well-conducted trials have shown that exercise is beneficial in the long term for treating substance misuse.

2 Mechanisms Underlying the Role of Physical Activity in Treatments for Addiction

Physical activity has many benefits for physical health in the general population, particularly in terms of maintaining fitness levels and protecting against cardiovascular disease and cancer (Garber et al., 2011). Among smokers, physical activity improves cardiovascular health and fitness (Hedblad et al., 1997; Ussher, Taylor & Faulkner, 2012), reduces cancer incidence (Leitzmann et al., 2009) and lessens weight gain after quitting (Farley et al., 2012; Kawachi et al., 1996). For those with alcohol or drug dependence, regular physical activity can improve cardiovascular health and fitness and can reduce body weight or body fat (Donaghy & Ussher, 2005; Peterson & Johnstone, 1995). Figure 12.1 summarises the proposed mechanisms by which physical activity can be used to treat addiction.

2.1 Neurobiological Influence

The influence of exercise on opioids, dopamine, cortisol and other neurotransmitters largely supports the idea that exercise can positively influence addiction. First, alcohol, drug and tobacco addictions are associated with disruption of the opioid system (neurotransmitters have a powerful analgesic effect) and a decrease in circulating opioids during drug withdrawal (Gianoulakis, 2009; Hadjiconstantinou & Neff, 2011). These addictions also lead to dysregulation of brain-reward pathways, which is reflected in a decreased production of dopamine and a potential limit on the capacity to experience pleasure during recovery (Koob, 2013; Koob & Kreek, 2007; Shoaib, 1998). Strenuous aerobic exercise can increase plasma levels of both dopamine (Meeusen, 2005) and the opioid β-endorphin (Leelarungrayub et al., 2010). Thus, exercise could provide a healthy avenue for stimulating opioids and dopamine and, as observed in animal studies, could act as an alternative reward (Cosgrove, Hunter & Carroll, 2002).

Second, smoking withdrawal is characterised by a decline to subnormal levels of the glucocorticoid cortisol (Steptoe & Ussher, 2006). This is important because low cortisol during withdrawal is associated with elevated cravings, tobacco withdrawal symptoms and perceived stress (Steptoe & Ussher, 2006). Also, a greater decline in cortisol at this time predicts relapse to smoking (Steptoe & Ussher, 2006). Exercise, particularly vigorous exercise, acutely increases cortisol (Jacks et al., 2002) and may restore cortisol to normal levels during withdrawal.

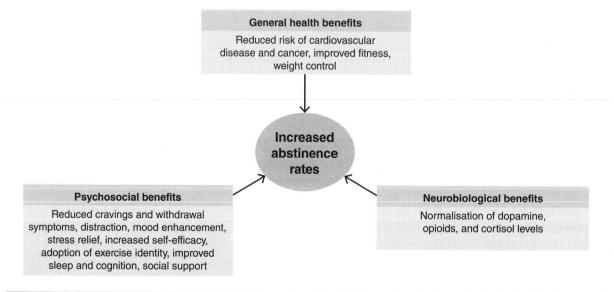

Figure 12.1   Possible mechanisms by which physical activity can be used to treat addiction.

One study showed that vigorous-intensity (i.e., running) but not moderate-intensity (i.e., walking) exercise increased cortisol during smoking abstinence, although cortisol was not related to cravings in this study (Scerbo et al., 2010). However, the smokers were abstinent for only 3 h, which provided little potential to investigate withdrawal-related changes in cortisol. Alcoholism and substance misuse also interfere with cortisol production (Lovallo et al., 2000), and exercise may normalise cortisol in populations with these disorders. In addition, high levels of stress are associated with dysregulated patterns of cortisol secretion and with relapse to smoking and alcohol or drug use. Exercise may also help restore more normative patterns of cortisol secretion. More work is needed in this area to clarify the relationships between levels of cortisol, physical activity and relapse to smoking. Animal studies indicate that physical activity might contribute to other neurobiological mechanisms related to addiction, including effects on norepinephrine, glutamate and synaptic plasticity.

2.2 Psychosocial Influence

This section discusses plausible psychosocial benefits of exercise for addicted individuals, including distraction, mood enhancement, stress management, enhanced self-efficacy, adoption of an exercise identity, social support and improved sleep and cognition. At its simplest level, it has been suggested that paying attention to physical cues during exercise (e.g., movement, breathing) is a strategy for distraction. Exercise has been shown to reduce attention to images of smoking (Van Rensburg, Taylor & Hodgson, 2009), although other work concluded that exercise is unlikely to play a major role as a distractor during smoking withdrawal (Daniel, Cropley & Fife-Schaw, 2006). It is unlikely that exercise reduces cravings by distraction alone because the effects do not dissipate quickly after exercise stops (Taylor, Ussher & Faulker, 2007).

Those with depression are at increased risk of developing addictions and of failing in addiction-treatment programmes (Berlin & Covey, 2006;

Brown et al., 1998). Exercise is likely to be beneficial for managing depression among those with addictions (Palmer et al., 1995; Vickers et al., 2003). Perceived stress also exacerbates addictive behaviour (e.g., Shiffman et al., 1996). Exercise is effective for acutely relieving stress among abstaining smokers (Taylor, Ussher & Faulkner, 2007) and may be beneficial for managing stress in those with other addictions.

Individuals who are dependent on illicit substances or alcohol tend to have lower self-esteem, perceived coping ability and self-efficacy, all of which might be positively influenced by exercise. For example, Medina and colleagues (2011) observed that among adults exposed to trauma, higher levels of vigorous exercise were related to reduced motivation to use alcohol for coping. Participating in physical activity also encourages individuals to adopt an identity as an exerciser, defined by having high aspirations for health and fitness. If an individual behaves in a manner that is inconsistent with this identity (e.g., takes drugs), the mismatch may motivate the person to confront their addiction (Strachan et al., 2011). For instance, the finding that more active individuals are less likely to smoke is said to partly depend on the extent to which these individuals have adopted an identity of being physically active (Verkooijen, Nielsen & Kremers, 2008).

Sleep disturbance is common during recovery from addictions and is a predictor of relapse to drug or alcohol use (Brower, Aldrich & Hall, 1998; Liu et al., 2000). Exercise has been shown to benefit sleep in the general population (Youngstedt, 2005) as well as in withdrawing smokers (Grove et al., 2006), and this benefit may extend to other addictions. The early stage of abstinence from smoking or drug use is also characterised by impaired cognition, including attention and memory deficits (Heishman, 1999; Tomasi et al., 2007). Exercise enhances cognition in the general population (Kramer & Erickson, 2007) and may combat cognitive decrements experienced during abstinence from drug use or smoking. For example, exercise has been shown to improve concentration among withdrawing smokers

(Taylor et al., 2007). Finally, exercise provides social support from exercise leaders and fellow exercisers, which fosters an environment for successful behaviour change.

2.3 Managing Withdrawal Symptoms and Cravings

Smokers who experience strong cravings and depression when they try to quit are more likely to fail (West, Hajek & Belcher, 1989). Other withdrawal symptoms, such as irritability and restlessness, are also a serious discomfort to smokers. Pharmacological interventions for smoking cessation, such as nicotine-replacement therapy (NRT), manage cravings and withdrawal symptoms; exercise may similarly help. A recent review presented evidence from 18 studies that tobacco-withdrawal symptoms and cravings are acutely reduced in exercise groups compared with passive control groups (Ussher, Taylor & Faulkner, 2012). Moreover, the magnitude of the reduction in cravings is comparable with, or in many cases exceeds, the reduction found with the use of NRT. Of the 18 studies reviewed, 17 included smokers who were temporarily abstinent and 1 included smokers who were attempting to quit. Reductions in cravings were evident for both moderate- and vigorous-intensity aerobic exercise, for hatha yoga and for seated isometric exercise, and lasted 5 to 30 min in duration. The evidence that exercise acutely ameliorates cigarette cravings and withdrawal symptoms provides the most compelling argument that exercise might be an effective adjunctive treatment for smoking cessation (see figure 12.2). More studies of smokers who are attempting to quit are needed.

Cravings also likely play an important role in alcohol and drug dependence (e.g., Monti, Rohsenow & Hutchison, 2000). Four studies have assessed the impact of exercise on alcohol or drug cravings and withdrawal. Li, Chen and Mo (2002) showed that, among abstinent heroin addicts, a programme of qigong exercise reduced withdrawal and craving relative to detoxification medication or minimal treat-

ment. Ussher and colleagues (2004) reported that, among individuals recruited after 10 days of alcohol detoxification, 10 min of moderate-intensity exercise (stationary cycling) reduced withdrawal and craving significantly more than did a 10 min bout of light-intensity exercise. In an uncontrolled study by Roessler (2010), those with substance dependence participated in aerobic exercise and sport at least 3 times/wk for 2 to 6 mo. After the exercise programme, the percentage of participants reporting an urge to take the substance was reduced from 65% to 47%. However, the latter findings may have been biased because only about one half of those recruited completed the assessments. Finally, in an uncontrolled study by Buchowski and colleagues (2011), cannabis users participated in 10 sessions of aerobic exercise over 2 wk. On average, cravings during treatment were significantly reduced relative to baseline. Overall, these findings are promising, and further studies of the effects of exercise on alcohol and drug cravings and withdrawal are needed. Studies of exercise interventions targeting addictions need to routinely include measures of these symptoms.

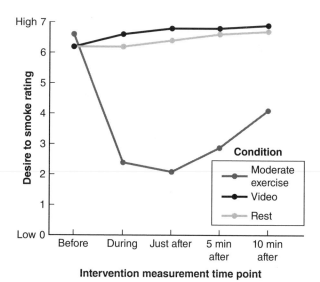

Figure 12.2. Acute (i.e., immediate) effect of 10 min of stationary cycling on the strength of the desire to smoke in abstinent smokers.

Adapted, by permission, from M. Ussher et al., 2001, "Effect of a short bout of exercise on tobacco withdrawal symptoms and desire to smoke," *Psychopharmacology* 158(1): 66-72.

3 Physical Activity Interventions for Addictive Behaviours

Given the prevalence of addictive behaviours and their cost to physical and mental health, every effort should be made to introduce effective interventions in order to reduce the cost to individuals and society. Physical activity is an inexpensive but effective intervention. The following section summarises studies that have evaluated the benefits of physical activity on addictive behaviours.

3.1 Impact of Physical Activity Interventions on Smoking Cessation

A recent review examined 15 trials that tested whether exercise interventions are effective in helping people quit smoking (Ussher, Taylor & Faulkner, 2012). The review included only randomised controlled trials (RCTs) that compared an exercise programme alone, or combined with a standard smoking-cessation programme, with a cessation programme alone. All the trials recruited smokers or recent quitters and included a follow-up at least 6 mo after the study ended. One study delivered the interventions online and the interventions in the remaining studies were delivered in person. Seven studies included NRT in the cessation programme, and this may have reduced the potential for exercise to aid smoking cessation. However, NRT is a standard treatment, and studies need to examine whether exercise has an effect when added to standard pharmaceutical treatments. Most of the trials employed supervised, group-based, cardiovascular-type exercise supplemented with a home-based (i.e., independent) programme. One study used only brief one-to-one counselling to promote exercise, and another focussed exclusively on resistance exercise (i.e., weight training).

3.1.1 Effects of Interventions

Three studies showed significantly higher quit rates in the exercise group compared with a control group at the end of treatment (Marcus et al., 1991, 1999; Martin, Kalfas & Patten, 1997). One of these studies also showed an exercise benefit at the 3 mo follow-up and a benefit of borderline significance ($p = .05$) at the 12 mo follow-up (Marcus et al., 1999). In the study by Martin, Kalfas and Patten (1997), the abstinence rates at 12 mo were 12% for the exercise group and 5% for the control group. One study showed significantly higher abstinence rates for the exercise group compared with the control group at the 3 mo follow-up but not at the end of treatment or at 12 mo (Marcus et al., 2005). This study also found that those who were more active were significantly more likely to be abstinent from smoking at the end of treatment. The other studies showed no significant effect of exercise on quit rates. However, as discussed later, methodological explanations for these negative findings exist.

3.1.2 Limitations of Studies

In only six studies (Bize et al., 2010; Marcus et al., 1999, 2005; Martin et al., 1997; McKay et al., 2008; Ussher et al., 2007) was the sample size sufficiently large to have a realistic prospect of detecting a significant difference in quit rates between the groups. The positive findings for one of the studies (Martin et al., 1997) may have been confounded by the exercise group receiving a different cessation programme than the control group. In two studies (Marcus et al., 1991; Martin et al., 1997) reporting benefits of exercise, the exercise group had more contact with staff than did the control group, bringing into question whether the outcomes for abstinence were attributable to exercise alone or to additional support. Only one study (Ussher et al., 2003, 2007) described an intervention in which the smoking-cessation and exercise components were integrated in order to reinforce exercise as a coping strategy for reducing cigarette cravings and withdrawal symptoms.

In studies in which the exercise programme commenced on or after the quit date, the impact of exercise on smoking cessation may have been hampered by the demand to cope with two major changes in health behaviour (i.e., exercise and smoking cessation) simultaneously. Also, in studies in which the exercise programme started after a period of smoking abstinence, the potential for exercise to help with withdrawal symptoms during this period after stopping smoking was lost. In two studies the exercise programmes lasted for less than 6 wk; this duration may have been insufficient to encourage long-term adherence to exercise. Most studies promoted home-based exercise, but in studies in which home programmes were not offered, participants' dependence on supervised exercise may have reduced their level of postintervention physical activity. In all the adequately powered trials that did not show a consistent effect of exercise on smoking abstinence (i.e., Bize et al., 2010; Marcus et al., 2005; McKay et al., 2008; Ussher et al., 2007) the interventions were low intensity in that they promoted moderate-intensity rather than vigorous-intensity exercise, relied solely on exercise counselling, provided supervised exercise only 1 time/wk or used only a web-based programme. In these studies the exercise intervention may have been insufficiently intense to benefit smoking abstinence. Only two studies provided further exercise programming after the initial exercise intervention; this may have reduced postintervention adherence to exercise. When studies offered supervised exercise, attendance at these sessions was high, and when studies emphasised home-based exercise, only a minority of the participants achieved the criterion level of exercise. For example, in one study that combined home-based exercise with 1 supervised session of exercise/wk, 50% of those in the exercise group were still classified as sedentary at the end of treatment (Bize et al., 2010).

3.1.3 Summary

Of the 15 RCT studies described, only one study showed a long-term effect of exercise on smoking cessation (Marcus et al., 2005). This study combined a supervised programme of vigorous-intensity exercise 3 times/wk with cognitive–behavioural support. It has yet to be determined whether a less-intensive exercise intervention can aid smoking cessation. The trials that did not

show a significant effect of exercise on smoking abstinence were too small to reliably exclude an effect of the intervention, had numerous methodological limitations or included an intervention that was not intense enough to produce the required change in exercise levels. Consequently, evidence is insufficient to recommend exercise as a specific aid to smoking cessation. However, good evidence exists to recommend exercise as an aid for reducing tobacco withdrawal and cravings. Further trials with larger sample sizes and sufficiently intense exercise interventions are needed. Further work is also needed to unravel the relationship between different intensities and timings of exercise intervention, different types of exercise and the effect on smoking abstinence.

3.2 Impact of Physical Activity Interventions on Alcohol Use

Eight studies investigating physical activity interventions with outcomes related to alcohol consumption have been identified. Four were RCTs that compared a vigorous- or moderate-intensity aerobic-exercise intervention with a passive control condition (Antiss, 1991; Donaghy, 1997; Murphy, Pagano & Marlatt, 1986; Scott & Myers, 1988), one compared a brief sport intervention with a brief wellness programme (Werch et al., 2005), another compared three physical activity interventions (Werch et al., 2003), one was a pilot study that did not include a control group (Brown et al., 2009) and the final study was quasiexperimental and compared an aerobic-exercise treatment programme with standard treatment at a rehabilitation centre (Sinyor et al., 1982). Four studies recruited patients undergoing treatment for alcohol dependence and the others targeted heavy drinkers (Murphy et al., 1986) or adolescent students (Scott & Myers, 1988; Werch et al., 2003, 2005). All but two of the studies (Werch et al., 2003, 2005) entailed supervised exercise; the programmes ranged from 3 to 24 wk in duration.

3.2.1 Effects of Interventions

When compared with a control group, three of the eight studies showed significant benefits on alcohol-related outcomes for the physically active group. One study that targeted those with alcohol dependence showed significantly higher abstinence rates for the exercise group compared with the control group at posttreatment and at the 3 and 18 mo follow-ups (Sinyor et al., 1982). In another study of heavy drinkers (Murphy et al., 1986), alcohol consumption was significantly lower after 8 wk of exercise compared with the control condition. Among adolescents, Werch and colleagues (2005) observed significantly lower alcohol consumption in the sport group compared with the control group at 3 mo pos-tintervention. In the two studies without a control group (Brown et al., 2009; Werch et al., 2003), abstinence rates were significantly higher relative to baseline at postintervention in both studies and higher at the 3 mo follow-up for Brown and colleagues (2009). Other studies examining the effect of an exercise intervention on those with alcohol dependence have not assessed alcohol consumption, although in general these studies show benefits for the exercise intervention (e.g., improved fitness and self-esteem and reduced anxiety and depression) (Donaghy, Ralston & Mutrie, 1991; Ermalinski et al., 1997; Frankel & Murphy, 1974; Gary & Guthrie, 1972; Palmer, Vacc & Epstein, 1988; Tsukue & Shohoji, 1981; Ussher et al., 2000).

3.2.2 Limitations of Studies

Two of the studies that did not find a significant effect of exercise on alcohol consumption were limited in that they had a high dropout rate, and their full findings have not been published (Antiss, 1991; Donaghy, 1997). Self-report has been found to be a poor outcome measure for alcohol abstinence (Stibler, 1991), and only one study (Donaghy, 1997) included a biochemical marker of alcohol consumption. Finally, only one of the studies (Brown et al., 2009) included cognitive–behavioural counseling in order to encourage home-based exercise.

3.2.3 Summary

Compared with a passive control group, only one RCT found that exercising significantly increased rates of alcohol abstinence (Sinyor et al., 1982).

Evidence is insufficient to recommend exercise as an aid for reducing alcohol intake, and more large RCTs that biochemically validate drinking levels are needed. One rigorous study shows that a short bout of exercise can reduce cravings for alcohol (Ussher et al., 2004); this benefit needs to be explored using different doses of exercise and longer follow-ups.

3.3 Impact of Physical Activity Interventions on Substance Use

Nine studies have been identified that reported the effect of an exercise intervention on the use of illicit substances; only two of these studies were RCTs. One study (Li, Chen & Mo, 2002) compared qigong exercise with no treatment. Another study (Werch et al., 2005) compared a brief sport intervention with a brief well-ness programme. The remaining seven studies (Brown et al., 2010; Buchowski et al., 2011; Burling et al., 1992; Collingwood et al., 1991, 2000; Collingwood, Sunderlin & Kohl, 1994; Roessler, 2010) did not include a control group. Three studies by Collingwood and colleagues (1991, 1994, 2000) plus one by Werch and colleagues (2005) targeted adolescents. Three studies recruited patients with various types of dependence (Brown et al., 2010; Burling et al., 1992; Roessler, 2010), Buchowski and colleagues (2011) included cannabis users and Li and colleagues (2011) focussed on those with heroin dependence. Except for the work by Collingwood (1994 and 2000) and by Werch and colleagues (2005), adults were recruited. Most studies promoted supervised moderate- or vigorous-intensity cardiovascular exercise or sport, and the duration of the programmes ranged from 2 wk to 6 mo.

3.3.1 Effects of Interventions

Six of nine studies reported significantly lower rates of substance use in either the exercise group alone or the exercise group compared with the control group. Li, Chen and Mo (2002) observed lower morphine use in the exercise group compared with the control group after 5 days of treatment. Burling and colleagues (1992) reported higher rates of abstinence from drugs and alcohol in the exercise group compared with the control group 3 mo after the intervention. At 3 mo postintervention, Werch (2005) and colleagues observed lower rates of substance use for the exercise group compared with the control group. Brown and colleagues (2010) found an increase relative to baseline in the percentage of days abstinent from drug use at the end of the exercise intervention. Buchowski and colleagues (2011) reported lower average cannabis use compared with baseline during a 2 wk exercise intervention and at 2 wk postintervention. At 12 mo posttreatment, Roessler (2010) found a tendency for less substance use; however, this was not analysed statistically. Of the three studies by Collingwood and colleagues (1991, 1994, 2000), only the 1994 study reported a significant reduction in substance use at the end of the intervention. In addition to the studies with substance-use outcomes, a further RCT showed that participation in a strength-training programme reduced depression scores (Palmer et al., 1995).

3.3.2 Limitations of Studies

Only one of the studies employed biochemical validation of substance use (Li, Chen & Mo, 2002). Also, the outcome in the study by Werch and colleagues (2005) specified marijuana or smoking; therefore, it was not possible to distinguish whether the effects were specific for either drug use. In the study by Collingwood and colleagues (2000), only a very small percentage of the sample reported substance use at the outset; therefore, the chances of detecting any influence of the exercise intervention on the use of illicit substances were minimal. The findings of Burling and colleagues (1992) were confounded by the physical activity group remaining in treatment longer than the control group. Finally, the intervention by Li, Chen and Mo (2002) combined traditional Chinese physical exercises with meditation, relaxation, guided imagery and breathing exercises; therefore, it was not possible to distinguish the effect of exercise from the effect of the other treatment components.

3.3.3 Summary

Evidence from two RCTs suggests that an exercise intervention might be effective for reducing use of illicit substances. One of these studies (Li, Chen & Mo, 2002) has various methodological flaws as described previously. The other study (Werch et al., 2005) was more rigorous, but the findings are specific to a general population of adolescents rather than to those undergoing treatment for substance dependence, and benefits observed at 3 mo postintervention were not maintained at 12 mo.

4 Designing a Physical Activity Programme for Individuals With Addictions

The evidence points to the efficacy of physical activity interventions for use in treating addictive behaviours. However, implementation of behavior change in this population can present practitioners with specific challenges. This section discusses the suggestions for designing effective interventions for those with addictions based on the evidence reviewed so far as well as practical considerations.

4.1 Exercise Type, Frequency and Intensity

Most studies have promoted moderate-intensity cardiovascular-type exercise such as brisk walking for use in those with addictive behaviours. Some work also incorporates more vigorous activities such as running. Because individuals with addictions are often extremely sedentary, a programme of moderate-intensity activity is likely to be acceptable and safe. However, a progression to more vigorous exercise may be beneficial. For example, the only study that found a long-term benefit of exercise for smoking cessation entailed 30 to 40 min of vigorous exercise 3 times/wk for 12 wk (Marcus et al., 1999). Similarly, the single study that showed a long-term impact of exercise on alcohol abstinence involved 1 h of progressively vigorous exercise 5 days/wk for 6 wk (Sinyor et al., 1982).

None of the trials reviewed compared the effects of vigorous-intensity and moderate-intensity exercise on abstinence rates. Experimental studies have compared the effects of bouts of moderate-intensity and vigorous-intensity exercise and have shown that both intensities are effective in the short term for reducing tobacco-withdrawal symptoms (Taylor et al., 2007).

The intensity of activity that an individual is capable of depends on initial level of fitness, medical condition and stage of recovery from addiction. Careful medical screening is vital. For example, those addicted to amphetamine or cocaine are often undernourished, and problem drinkers often have weak muscles. Such individuals may require nutrition advice. Ultimately, individuals will have preferences regarding types of exercise, and programmes should be tailored to these preferences (Abrantes et al., 2011; Everson-Hock et al., 2010). Some individuals may prefer noncardiovascular types of exercise, which may also be beneficial. Resistance (i.e., weight) training, yoga and isometric exercise have all been successfully piloted as aids for smoking cessation and need to be tested in larger trials (Ussher, Taylor & Faulkner, 2012).

Regarding frequency and volume of exercise, the findings from Marcus and colleagues (2005) suggest that abstaining smokers need to accumulate at least 110 min/wk of moderate-intensity activity to maintain abstinence; supervised exercise on 2 or 3 days/wk may be necessary in order to achieve this. Shorter bouts of exercise can be used on an as-needed basis in response to cravings, and longer scheduled bouts can be used to maintain positive mood, manage stress and prevent cravings from arising. Research has not yet addressed the optimum dose of exercise for assisting alcohol and drug rehabilitation.

4.2 Exercise Supervision

The majority of intervention studies have employed group-based supervised exercise. In smokers, exercise counselling alone did not increase exercise levels sufficiently (Ussher et al., 2003), and all the interventions that showed a significant impact on long-term abstinence from alcohol or smoking entailed supervised exercise. Among novice exercisers, an element of supervised exercise may be useful to ensure initial adoption of regular exercise and to provide information about safe exercise (e.g., warm-up) and exercise intensities (e.g., using heart rate monitors). Counselling toward pursuing home-based exercise is also likely to be important for encouraging patients to maintain exercise levels after the initial exercise programme ends.

4.3 Stages of Addiction Treatment

Early recovery from drug and alcohol dependence is a major transition that affects close relationships and employment and involves numerous treatment sessions. An exercise programme needs to complement these changes. Most exercise interventions discussed in this chapter have required patients to alter their substance- or alcohol-misuse behaviour and exercise behaviour simultaneously, yet it is not clear whether this is optimal. For some individuals the challenge of changing two health behaviours simultaneously may be too demanding. Also, it is not clear whether involvement in physical activity increases the motivation to manage substance intake or vice versa.

Among smokers, exercise has often been introduced in the studies discussed several weeks before an attempt to quit, thereby allowing people to adjust to the demands of increased exercise before starting to quit. This also allows exercise to play a role in managing cravings during the crucial early days of abstinence, when relapse rates are highest. Empirical work is required to determine the relative benefits of initiating exercise at different points in the addiction-treatment process. During later stages of treatment exercise may be useful for preventing relapse (e.g., by promoting an exercise identity that is incompatible with drug use). Studies are also needed to determine whether exercise can be used to increase substance abstinence among those who are not motivated to attempt abstinence.

4.4   Integrating Exercise With Standard Addiction Treatments

Greater integration of addiction and exercise programmes may enhance abstinence rates. For instance, rather than just proposing exercise as a means for getting fitter and managing weight, the practitioner could present exercise more as a self-control strategy for managing withdrawal symptoms and a way to address psychological and physical harms caused by addiction. Exercise could be used more in combination with pharmaceutical interventions. Whereas pharmaceutical interventions focus on reducing withdrawal symptoms (e.g., NRT), exercise could ideally be used to provide an added effect in client-led management of addictive symptoms.

4.5   Perceived Barriers to Exercise

Individuals with addictions are likely to have specific barriers to exercise, and these need to be determined. In the general population, use of cognitive–behavioural techniques is effective for overcoming perceived barriers and increasing exercise adherence. Few addiction studies have included cognitive–behavioural counseling. Techniques such as self-monitoring (e.g., diaries), goal-setting and relapse-prevention planning are commonly used. Also, pedometers are now commonly used as a motivational tool. These and other motivational aids (e.g., financial incentives) need to be tested with exercise interventions in addicted populations.

4.6   Interventions for Different Subgroups

Exercise interventions need to be tested among addicted populations who might especially benefit from such interventions. Given the high prevalence of addictions among people with mental illness and the established benefits of regular physical activity for mental health, research that examines the role that

---

EVIDENCE TO PRACTICE

- Both moderate- and vigorous-intensity exercise have been shown to be effective for reducing tobacco-withdrawal symptoms and cravings.
- Progressing from light- and moderate-intensity exercise (e.g., brisk walking) to more vigorous-intensity exercise is advisable.
- Careful medical screening is required, especially among those with long-term alcohol or drug dependence (e.g., for malnutrition).
- Exercise interventions should be tailored to individual preferences.
- Abstaining smokers should accumulate at least 110 min/wk of moderate-intensity exercise.
- Interventions involving supervised exercise on 2 or 3 days/wk are likely to be necessary to be effective in treating addictive behaviours.
- Exercise can be performed on an as-needed basis for managing cravings or in scheduled bouts.
- If the exercise programme is to assist with early withdrawal symptoms, it ideally needs to begin before abstinence is attempted.
- Participating in physical activity encourages individuals to adopt an identity as an exerciser, which is incompatible with using addictive substances.
- Perceived barriers to exercise need to be identified and addressed using cognitive–behavioural techniques.
- The intervention needs to be adapted to various subgroups (e.g., according to sex, body weight and mental health).

physical activity may play in this population is needed (Arbour-Nicitopoulos et al., 2011).

Exercise interventions might be particularly appealing to adolescents, and controlled trials with young people are needed. Addicted individuals who are overweight may have a need for weight-control interventions such as exercise; no trial has yet focussed on this population. Additionally, surveys suggest that a nonpharmaceutical intervention such as exercise is likely to appeal to pregnant smokers (Ussher at al., 2008). Finally, sex needs to be considered when planning an appropriate intervention. Some evidence shows that women often prefer walking and aerobics, whereas men have more interest in sport, running and strength training.

5 Summary

Drug, alcohol and tobacco addictions are growing global problems. Exercise has many benefits for physical and psychological health, and evidence convincingly shows that exercise is effective for managing cravings and withdrawal symptoms, particularly in smokers. Regular exercise fosters a healthy lifestyle and exercise identity that is largely incompatible with addiction, and individuals undergoing rehabilitation for addiction express interest in exercising more. Exercise interventions are inexpensive, can be easily integrated with existing addiction treatments and have minimal side effects compared with pharmacological treatments. This chapter demonstrates that exercise is a highly plausible adjunctive treatment for addictive behaviour and that exercise programmes can be readily disseminated. However, limited evidence currently supports the benefits of exercise for helping smokers quit or helping those with drug or alcohol dependence abstain. This lack of evidence can partly be explained by the small number of large RCTs that have been conducted, lack of knowledge about effective doses of exercise and limited attention to methods for maximizing exercise adherence. This area of research is in its infancy, and further well-designed trials are needed.

6 References

Abrantes, A.M., Battle, C.L., Strong, D.R., Ing, E., Dubreuil, M.E., Gordon, A., & Brown, R.A. (2011). Exercise preferences of patients in substance abuse treatment. *Mental Health and Physical Activity*, 4(2), 79-87.

Abrantes, A.M., Strong, D.R., Lloyd-Richardson, E.E., Niaura, R., Kahler, C.W., & Brown, R.A. (2009). Regular exercise as a protective factor in relapse following smoking cessation treatment. *American Journal on Addictions*, 18(1), 100-101.

Antiss, T.J. (1991). A randomized controlled trial of aerobic exercise in the treatment of the alcohol dependent. *Medicine and Science in Sports and Exercise*, 23, S118.

Arbour-Nicitopoulos, K.P., Faulkner, G.E., Cohn, T.A., & Selby P. (2011). Smoking cessation in women with severe mental illness: Exploring the role of exercise as an adjunct treatment. *Archives of Psychiatric Nurs*ing, 25(1), 43-52.

Audrain-McGovern, J., Rodriguez, D., & Moss, H.B. (2003). Smoking progression and physical activity. *Cancer Epidemiology, Biomarkers and Prevention*, 12(11), 1121-1129.

Berlin, I., & Covey, L.S. (2006). Pre-cessation depressive mood predicts failure to quit smoking: The role of coping and personality traits. *Addiction*, 101(12), 1814-1821.

Bize, R., Willi, C., Chiolero, A., Stoianov, R., Payot, S., Locatelli, I., et al. (2010). Participation in a population-based physical activity programme as an aid for smoking cessation: A randomised trial. *Tobacco Control*, 19(6), 488-494.

Brower, K.J., Aldrich, M.S., & Hall, J.M. (1998). Polysomnographic and subjective sleep predictors of alcoholic relapse. *Alcoholism, Clinical and Experimental Research*, 22(8), 1864-1871.

Brown, R.A., Abrantes, A.M., Read, J.P., Marcus, B.H., Jakicic, J., Strong, D.R., et al. (2009). Aerobic exercise for alcohol recovery: Rationale, program description, and preliminary findings. *Behavior Modification*, 33(2), 220-249.

Brown, R.A., Abrantes, A.M., Read, J.P., Marcus, B.H., Jakicic, J., Strong, D.R., et al. (2010). A pilot study of aerobic exercise as an adjunctive treatment for drug dependence. *Mental Health and Physical Activity*, 3(1), 27-34.

Brown, R.A., Monti, P.M., Myers, M.G., Martin, R.A., Rivinus, T., Dubreuil, M.E., et al. (1998). Depression among cocaine abusers in treatment:

Relation to cocaine and alcohol use and treatment outcome. *American Journal of Psychiatry*, 155(2), 220-225.

Buchowski, M.S., Meade, N.N., Charboneau, E., Park, S., Dietrich, M.S., Cowan, R.L., et al. (2011). Aerobic exercise training reduces cannabis craving and use in non-treatment seeking cannabis-dependent adults. *PLoS One*, 6, e17465.

Burling, T.A., Seidner, A.L., Robbins-Sisco, D., Krinsky, A., & Hanser, B.B. (1992). Batter up! Relapse prevention for homeless veteran substance abusers via softball team participation. *Journal of Substance Abuse*, 4(4), 407.

Collingwood, T.R., Reynolds, R., Kohl, H.W., Smith, W., & Sloan, S. (1991). Physical fitness effects on substance abuse risk factors and use patterns. *Journal of Drug Education*, 21(1), 73-84.

Collingwood, T.R., Sunderlin, J., & Kohl, H.W. III. (1994). The use of a staff training model for implementing fitness programming to prevent substance abuse with at-risk youth. *American Journal of Health Promotion*, 9(1), 20-23.

Collingwood, T.R., Sunderlin, J., Reynolds, R., & Kohl, H.W. III. (2000). Physical training as a substance abuse prevention intervention for youth. *Journal of Drug Education*, 30(4), 435-451.

Cosgrove, K.P., Hunter, R.G., & Carroll, M.E. (2002). Wheel-running attenuates intravenous cocaine self-administration in rats: Sex differences. *Pharmacology Biochemistry and Behavior*, 73(3), 663-671.

Daniel, J.Z., Cropley, M., & Fife-Schaw, C. (2006). The effect of exercise in reducing desire to smoke and cigarette withdrawal symptoms is not caused by distraction. *Addiction*, 101(8), 1187-1192.

deRuiter, W.K., Faulkner, G., Cairney, J., & Veldhuizen, S. (2008). Characteristics of physically active smokers and implications for harm reduction. *American Journal of Public Health*, 98(5), 925-931.

Doll, R., Peto, R., Boreham, J., & Sutherland, I. (2004). Mortality in relation to smoking: 50 years' observations on male British doctors. *British Medical Journal*, 328, 1519.

Donaghy, M. (1997). *An investigation into the effects of exercise as an adjunct to the treatment and rehabilitation of the problem drinker* (Unpublished doctoral dissertation). Glasgow: University of Glasgow.

Donaghy, M., Ralston, G., & Mutrie, N. (1991). Exercise as a therapeutic adjunct for problem drinkers. *Journal of Sports Sciences*, 9(4), 440.

Donaghy, M., & Ussher, M. (2005). Exercise interventions in drug and alcohol rehabilitation. In G. Faulkner & A. Taylor (Eds.), *Exercise, health and mental health: Emerging relationships* (pp. 48-69). London: Routledge.

Eaton, W.W., Martins, S.S., Nestadt, G., Bienvenu, O.J., Clarke, D., & Alexandre, P. (2008). The burden of mental disorders. *Epidemiologic Reviews*, 30, 1-14.

Ermalinski, R., Hanson, P.G., Lubin, B., Thornby, J.I., & Nahormek, P.A. (1997). Impact of a body-mind treatment component on alcohol inpatients. *Journal of Psychosocial Nursing*, 35(7), 39-45.

Everson-Hock, E.S., Taylor, A.H., Ussher, M., & Faulkner, G. (2010). A qualitative perspective on multiple health behaviour change: Views of smoking cessation advisors who promote physical activity. *Journal of Smoking Cessation*, 5(1), 7-14.

Farley, A.C., Hajek, P., Lycett, D., & Aveyard, P. (2012). Interventions for preventing weight gain after smoking cessation. *Cochrane Database of Systematic Reviews*, 1, CD006219.

Ferron, C., Narring, F., Cauderay, M., & Michaud, P.A. (1999). Sport activity in adolescence: Associations with health perceptions and experimental behaviours. *Health Education Research*, 14(2), 225-233.

Field, T., Diego, M., & Sanders, C.E. (2001). Exercise is positively related to adolescents' relationships and academics. *Adolescence*, 36(141), 105-110.

Frankel, A., & Murphy, J. (1974). Physical fitness and personality in alcoholism. Canonical analysis of measures before and after treatment. *Quarterly Journal on the Studies of Alcohol*, 35(4), 1272-1278.

French, M.T., Popovici, I., & Maclean, J.C. (2009). Do alcohol consumers exercise more? Findings from a national survey. *American Journal of Health Promotion*, 24(1), 2-10.

Garber, C.E., Blissmer, B., Deschenes, M.R., Franklin, B.A., Lamonte, M.J., Lee, I.M., et al. (2011). Quantity and quality of exercise for developing and maintaining cardiorespiratory, musculoskeletal, and neuromotor fitness in apparently healthy adults: Guidance for prescribing exercise. *Medicine and Science in Sports and Exercise*, 43(7), 1334-1359.

Gary, V., & Guthrie, D. (1972). The effect of jogging on physical fitness and self concept on hospitalized alcoholics. *Quarterly Journal of Studies in Alcohol*, 33(4), 1073-1078.

Gianoulakis, C. (2009). Endogenous opioids and addiction to alcohol and other drugs of abuse. *Current Topics in Medicinal Chemistry*, 9(11), 999-1015.

Grove, J.R., Wilkinson, A., Dawson, B., Eastwood, P., & Heard, P. (2006). Effects of exercise on subjective aspects of sleep during tobacco withdrawal. *Australian Psychologist*, 41(1), 69-76.

Hadjiconstantinou, M., & Neff, N.H. (2011). Nicotine and endogenous opioids: Neurochemical and pharmacological evidence. *Neuropharmacology*, 60(7-8), 1209-1220.

Hedblad, B., Ogren, M., Isacsson, S.O., & Janzo, L. (1997). Reduced cardiovascular mortality risk in male smokers who are physically active. *Archives of Internal Medicine*, 157(8), 893-899.

Health Survey for England (2011) Volume 1 Chapter 6: Drinking Patterns https://catalogue.ic.nhs.uk/publications/public-health/surveys/heal-surv-eng-2011/HSE2011-Ch6-Drinking-Patterns.pdf

Heishman, S.J. (1999). Behavioral and cognitive effects of smoking: Relationship to nicotine addiction. *Nicotine and Tobacco Research,* 1(Suppl. 2), 143-147.

Helmert, U., Herman, B., & Shea, S. (1994). Moderate and vigorous leisure-time physical activity and cardiovascular disease risk factors in West Germany, 1984-1991. *International Journal of Epidemiology*, 23(2), 285-292.

Jacks, D.E., Sowash, J., Anning, J., McGloughlin, T., & Andres, F. (2002). Effect of exercise at three exercise intensities on salivary cortisol. *Journal of Strength and Conditioning Research*, 16(2), 286-289.

Kaczynski, A.T., Manske, S.R., Mannell, R.C., & Grewal, K. (2008). Smoking and physical activity: A systematic review. *American Journal of Health Behavior*, 32(1), 93-110.

Kawachi, I., Troisi, R.J., Rotnitzky, A.G., Coakley, E.H., Colditz, M.S., & Colditz, M.D. (1996). Can exercise minimise weight gain in women after smoking cessation? *American Journal of Public Health*, 86(7), 999-1004.

King, T.K., Marcus, B.H., Pinto, B.M., Emmon, K.M., & Abrams, D.B. (1996). Cognitive behavioural mediators of changing multiple behaviours: Smoking and a sedentary lifestyle. *Preventive Medicine*, 25(6), 684-691.

Koob, G.F. (2013). Theoretical frameworks and mechanistic aspects of alcohol addiction: Alcohol addiction as a reward deficit disorder. *Current Topics in Behavioural Neurosciences*, 13, 3-30.

Koob, G., & Kreek, M.J. (2007). Stress, dysregulation of drug reward pathways, and the transition to drug dependence. *American Journal of Psychiatry*, 164(8), 1149-1159.

Korhonen, T., Kujala, U.M., Rose, R.J., & Kaprio, J. (2009). Physical activity in adolescence as a predictor of alcohol and illicit drug use in early adulthood: A longitudinal population-based twin study. *Twin Research and Human Genetics*, 12(3), 261-268.

Kramer, A.F., & Erickson, K.I. (2007). Capitalizing on cortical plasticity: Influence of physical activity on cognition and brain function. *Trends in Cognitive Sciences*, 11(8), 342-348.

Kulig, K., Brener, N.D., & McManus, T. (2003). Sexual activity and substance use among adolescents by category of physical activity plus team sports participation. *Archives of Pediatric and Adolescent Medicine*, 157, 905-912.

Laaksonen, M., Luoto, R., Helakorpi, S., & Uutela, A. (2002). Associations between health-related behaviors: A 7-year follow-up of adults. *Preventive Medicine*, 34(2), 162-170.

Leelarungrayub, D., Pratanaphon, S., Pothongsunun, P., Sriboonreung, T., Yankai, A., & Bloomer, R.J. (2010). Vernonia cinerea Less. supplementation and strenuous exercise reduce smoking rate: Relation to oxidative stress status and beta-endorphin release in active smokers. *Journal of the International Society of Sports Nutrition*, 7, 21.

Leitzmann, M.F., Koebnick, C., Abnet, C.C., Freedman, N.D., Park, Y., Hollenbeck, A., et al. (2009). Prospective study of physical activity and lung cancer by histologic type in current, former, and never smokers. *American Journal of Epidemiology*, 169(5), 542-553.

Li, M., Chen, K., & Mo, Z. (2002). Use of qigong therapy in the detoxification of heroin exercise. *Alternative Therapies in Health and Medicine*, 8, 50-59.

Liangpunsakul, S., Crabb, D.W., & Qi, R. (2010). Relationship among alcohol intake, body fat, and physical activity: A population-based study. *Annals of Epidemiology*, 20(9), 670-675.

Lisha, N.E., Martens, M., & Leventhal, A.M. (2011). Age and gender as moderators of the relationship between physical activity and alcohol use. *Addictive Behaviors*, 36(9), 933-936.

Liu, T., Xiaoping, W., Wei, H., & Zeng, W. (2000). Frequency of withdrawal symptoms of natural detoxification in heroin addicts. *Chinese Mental Health Journal*, 14(2), 114-116.

Lovallo, W.R., Dickensheets, S.L., Myers, D.A., Thomas, T.L., & Nixon, S.J. (2000). Blunted stress cortisol response in abstinent alcoholic and polysubstance-abusing men. *Alcoholism, Clinical and Experimental Research, 24*(5), 651-658.

Marcus, B.H., Albrecht, A.E., King, T.K., Parisi, A.F., Pinto, B.M., Roberts, M., et al. (1999). The efficacy of exercise as an aid for smoking cessation in women: A randomised controlled trial. *Archives of Internal Medicine, 159*(11), 1229-1234.

Marcus, B.H., Albrecht, A.E., Niaura, R.S., Abrams, D.B., & Thompson, P.D. (1991). Usefulness of physical exercise for maintaining smoking cessation in women. *American Journal of Cardiology, 68*(4), 406-407.

Marcus, B.H., Lewis, B.A., Hogan, J., King, T.K., Albrecht, A.E., Bock, B., et al. (2005). The efficacy of moderate-intensity exercise as an aid for smoking cessation in women: A randomized controlled trial. *Nicotine and Tobacco Research, 7*(6), 871-880.

Marlatt, G.A., & Donovan, D.M. (2005). *Relapse prevention: Maintenance strategies in the treatment of addictive behaviours* (2nd ed.). New York: Guilford Press.

Martin, J.E., Kalfas, K.J., & Patten, C.A. (1997). Prospective evaluation of three smoking interventions in 205 recovering alcoholics: One-year results of project SCRAP-Tobacco. *Journal of Consulting and Clinical Psychology, 65*(1), 190-194.

McKay, H.G., Danaher, B.G., Seeley, J.R., Lichtenstein, E., & Gau, J.M. (2008). Comparing two web-based smoking cessation programs: Randomized controlled trial. *Journal of Medical Internet Research, 10*(5), e40.

Medina, J.L., Vujanovic, A.A., Smits, J.A., Irons, J.G., Zvolensky, M.J., & Bonn-Miller, M.O. (2011). Exercise and coping-oriented alcohol use among a trauma-exposed sample. *Addictive Behaviors, 36*(3), 274-277.

Meeusen, R. (2005). Exercise and the brain: Insight in new therapeutic modalities. *Annals of Transplantation, 10*(4), 49-51.

Monti, P.M., Rohsenow, D.J., & Hutchison, K.E. (2000). Toward bridging the gap between biological, psychobiological and psychosocial models of alcohol craving. *Addiction, 95*(Suppl. 2), S229-S236.

Moore, M.J., & Werch, C.E. (2005). Sport and physical activity participation and substance use among adolescents. *Journal of Adolescent Health, 36*(6), 486-493.

Murphy, T.J., Pagano, R.R., & Marlatt, G.A. (1986). Lifestyle modification with heavy alcohol drinkers: Effects of aerobic exercise and meditation. *Addictive Behaviors, 11*(2), 175-186.

Palmer, J.A., Palmer, L.K., Michiels, K., & Thigpen, B. (1995). Effects of type of exercise on depression in recovering substance abusers. *Perceptual and Motor Skills, 80*(2), 523-530.

Palmer, J., Vacc, N., & Epstein, J. (1988). Adult inpatient alcoholics: Physical exercise as a treatment intervention. *Journal of Studies on Alcohol, 49*(5), 418-421.

Pate, R.R., Trost, S.G., Levin, S., & Dowda, M. (2000). Sports participation and health-related behaviors among U.S. youth. *Archives of Pediatrics and Adolescent Medicine, 154*(9), 904-911.

Peretti-Watel, P., Beck, F., & Legleye, S. (2002). Beyond the U-curve: The relationship between sport and alcohol, cigarette and cannabis use in adolescents. *Addiction, 97*(6), 707-716.

Peterson, M., & Johnstone, B.M. (1995). The Atwood Hall Health Promotion Program, Federal Medical Center, Lexington, KY. Effects on drug-involved federal offenders. *Journal of Substance Abuse Treatment, 12*(1), 43-48.

Rehm, J., Mathers, C., Popova, S., Thavorncharoensap, M., Teerawattananon, Y., & Patra, J. (2009). Global burden of disease and injury and economic cost attributable to alcohol use and alcohol-use disorders. *Lancet, 373*(9682), 2223-2233.

Roessler, K.K. (2010). Exercise treatment for drug abuse—A Danish pilot study. *Scandinavian Journal of Public Health, 38*(6), 664-669.

Scerbo, F., Faulkner, G., Taylor, A., & Thomas, S. (2010). Effects of exercise on cravings to smoke: The role of exercise intensity and cortisol. *Journal of Sports Sciences, 28*(1), 11-19.

Schroder, H., Elosua, R., & Marrugat, J. (2003). The relationship of physical activity with dietary cancer-protective nutrients and cancer-related biological and lifestyle factors. *European Journal of Cancer Prevention, 12*(4), 339-346.

Scott, K.A., & Myers, A.M. (1988). Impact of fitness training on native adolescents' self-evaluations and substance use. *Canadian Journal of Public Health, 79*(6), 424-429.

Shiffman, S., Hickcox, M., Paty, J.A., Gnys, M., Kassel, J.D., & Richards, T.J. (1996). Progression from a smoking lapse to relapse: Prediction from abstinence violation effects, nicotine dependence, and lapse characteristics. *Journal of Consulting and Clinical Psychology*, 64(5), 993-1002.

Shoaib, M. (1998). Is dopamine important in nicotine dependence? *Journal of Physiology*, 92(3-4), 229-233.

Sinyor, D., Brown, T., Rostant, L., & Seraganian, P. (1982). The role of a physical fitness program in the treatment of alcoholism. *Journal of Studies on Alcohol*, 43(3), 380-386.

Steptoe, A., & Ussher, M. (2006). Smoking, cortisol and nicotine. *International Journal of Psychophysiology*, 59(3), 228-235.

Stibler, H. (1991). Carbohydrate-deficient transferrin in serum: A new marker of potentially harmful alcohol consumption reviewed. *Clinical Chemistry*, 37(12), 2029-2037.

Strachan, S.M., Flora, P.K., Brawley, L.R., & Spink, K.S. (2011). Varying the cause of a challenge to exercise identity behaviour: Reactions of individuals of differing identity strength. *Journal of Health Psychology*, 16(4), 572-583.

Strohle, A., Hofler, M., Pfister, H., Muller, A.G., Hoyer, J., Wittchen, H.U., et al. (2007). Physical activity and prevalence and incidence of mental disorders in adolescents and young adults. *Psychological Medicine*, 37(11), 1657-1666.

Substance Abuse and Mental Health Services Administration. (2010). *Results from the 2009 National Survey on Drug Use and Health: Volume I. Summary of national findings.* Rockville, MD: Substance Abuse and Mental Health Services Administration.

Taylor, A.H., Ussher, M.H., & Faulkner, G. (2007). The acute effects of exercise on cigarette cravings, withdrawal symptoms, affect and smoking behaviour: A systematic review. *Addiction*, 102(4), 534-543.

Terry-McElrath, Y.M., & O'Malley, P.M. (2011). Substance use and exercise participation among young adults: Parallel trajectories in a national cohort-sequential study. *Addiction*, 106(10), 1855-1865.

Tomasi, D., Goldstein, R.Z., Telang, F., Maloney, T., Alia-Klein, N., Caparelli, E.C., et al. (2007). Widespread disruption in brain activation patterns to a working memory task during cocaine abstinence. *Brain Research*, 1171, 83-92.

Tsukue, I., & Shohoji, T. (1981). Movement therapy for alcoholic patients. *Journal of Studies on Alcohol*, 42(1), 144-149.

Tur, J.A., Puig, M.S., Pons, A., & Benito, E. (2003). Alcohol consumption among school adolescents in Palma de Mallorca. *Alcohol*, 38(3), 243-248.

Eaton G, Davies C, English L, Lodwick A, McVeigh J, Bellis M. (2008) United Kingdom drug situation: annual report to the European Monitoring Centre for Drugs and Drug Addiction (EMCDDA) http://www.emcdda.europa.eu/attachements. cfm/att_86785_EN_NR_2008_UK.pdf

Ussher, M., Aveyard, P., Coleman, T., Straus, L., West, R., & Marcus, B. (2008). Physical activity as an aid to smoking cessation during pregnancy: Two feasibility studies. *BMC Public Health*, 8(1), 328.

Ussher, M., McCusker, M., Morrow, V., & Donaghy, M. (2000). A physical activity intervention in a community alcohol service. *British Journal of Occupational Therapy*, 63(12), 598-604.

Ussher, M., Nunziata, P., Cropley, M., & West, R. (2001). Effect of a short bout of exercise on tobacco withdrawal symptoms and desire to smoke. *Psychopharmacology*, 158(1), 66-72.

Ussher, M., Sampuran, A.K., Doshi, R., West, R., & Drummond, D.C. (2004). Acute effect of a brief bout of exercise on alcohol urges. *Addiction*, 99(12), 1542-1547.

Ussher, M.H., Taylor, A., & Faulkner, G. (2012). Exercise interventions for smoking cessation. *Cochrane Database of Systematic Reviews*, 1, CD002295.

Ussher, M., West, W., McEwen, A., Taylor, A.H., & Steptoe, A. (2003). Efficacy of exercise counselling as an aid for smoking cessation: A randomized controlled trial. *Addiction*, 98(4), 523-532.

Ussher, M., West, W., McEwen, A., Taylor, A.H., & Steptoe, A. (2007). Randomized controlled trial of physical activity counseling as an aid to smoking cessation: 12 month follow-up. *Addictive Behaviors*, 32(12), 3060-3064.

Van Rensburg, K.J., Taylor, A., & Hodgson, T. (2009). The effects of acute exercise on attentional bias towards smoking-related stimuli during temporary abstinence from smoking. *Addiction*, 104(11), 1910-1917.

Verkooijen, K.T., Nielsen, G.A., & Kremers, S.P. (2008). The association between leisure time physical activity and smoking in adolescence: An examination of potential mediating and moderating factors. *International Journal of Behavioural Medicine*, 15(2), 157-163.

Vickers, K.S., Patten, C.A., Bronars, C., Lane, K., Stevens, S.R., Croghan, I.T., et al. (2004). Binge drinking in female college students: The association of physical activity, weight concern, and depressive symptoms. *Journal of American College Health*, 53(3), 133-140.

Vickers, K.S., Patten, C.A., Lane, K., Clark, M.M., Croghan, I.T., Schroeder, D.R., & et al. (2003). Depressed versus nondepressed young adult tobacco users: Differences in coping style, weight concerns and exercise level. *Health Psychology*, 22(5), 498-503.

Werch, C.C., Moore, M.J., DiClemente, C.C., Bledsoe, R., & Jobli, E. (2005). A multihealth behavior intervention integrating physical activity and substance use prevention for adolescents. *Prevention Science*, 6(3), 213-226.

Werch, C., Moore, M., DiClemente, C.C., Owen, D.M., Jobli, E., & Bledsoe, R. (2003). A sport-based intervention for preventing alcohol use and promoting physical activity among adolescents. *Journal of School Health*, 73(10), 380-388.

West, R., Hajek, P., & Belcher, M. (1989). Severity of withdrawal symptoms as a predictor of outcome of an attempt to quit smoking. *Psychological Medicine*, 19(4), 981-985.

Winnail, S.D., Valois, R.F., McKeown, R.E., Saunders, R.P., & Pate, R.R. (1995). Relationship between physical activity level and cigarette, smokeless tobacco, and marijuana use among public high school adolescents. *Journal of School Health*, 65(10), 438-442.

Youngstedt, S.D. (2005). Effects of exercise on sleep. *Clinics in Sports Medicine*, 24(2), 355-365.

Exercise Dependence, Eating Disorders and Body Dysmorphia

Brian Cook, PhD

Neuropsychiatric Research Institute, Fargo, North Dakota, United States

Heather Hausenblas, PhD

University of Florida, Jacksonville, Florida, United States

Chapter Outline

Editors' Introduction

For the vast majority of people, exercise has a positive effect on mental health; many of these beneficial effects are described in the previous chapters of this text. However, a minority of individuals experience exercise dependence and exercise excessively to the detriment of their mental and physical health. This chapter explains how to define and assess exercise dependence and describes researchers' current understanding of the relationship between exercise and eating disorders. The role of exercise in muscle dysmorphia is also explained. This chapter provides a greater awareness and understanding of exercise dependence and offers practical advice about how to identify it and strategies for minimising the risk of occurrence.

Any amount of participation in health behaviours is expected to produce measureable gains in health status. Thus, recommendations to engage in behaviours that either are ordinarily avoided or are not inherently part of daily routines seem to imply that the simple act of doing something will produce a desired health effect and that better health outcomes will occur the more often one engages in such behaviours. Therefore, the relationship between behaviour and health status is commonly conceptualised as linear. However, many volitional behaviours that are considered healthy may exhibit curvilinear relationships to physical, psychological and social health status.

For example, epidemiological research shows that cardiovascular disease is lower in countries where red wine is consumed in moderation (i.e., 1-2 glasses/day; Lippi et al., 2010). However, repeatedly consuming 5 or more glasses/day would indicate a pattern of binge drinking or addiction and consequently increase several health risks (Standridge, Zylstra & Adams, 2004). Understanding the motivation for drinking alcohol (e.g., to avoid negative thoughts and feelings, for enjoyment) may help distinguish addiction or dependence from excessive amount. Extending the same conceptualization of dependence to exercise reveals that exercise may also become problematic for some.

Current exercise guidelines identify the minimum amount of exercise needed to experience health benefits. The guidelines also recommend that an increased amount of exercise is associated with additional benefits (U.S. Department of Health and Human Services, 2008). Although increases above the minimum guidelines are encouraged, no cutoff exists for how much is too much. Thus, it is unknown whether a point exists at which increased exercise may become detrimental to one's health.

Exercise dependence occurs when regular exercise becomes excessive and thus detrimental to an individual's physical and psychological health. Simply stated, exercise dependence is a craving for leisure-time physical activity that results in uncontrollably excessive exercise behaviour that manifests in physiological (e.g., tolerance) or psychological (e.g., withdrawal) symptoms (Hausenblas & Symons Downs, 2002a). Characteristics of exercise dependence include exercising despite injury or illness, experiencing withdrawal effects and giving up social, occupational and family obligations in order to exercise (Hausenblas & Symons Downs, 2002a). Exercise dependence may also play a pivotal role in explaining the function of exercise behaviour in the development and maintenance of body-image disturbance and eating disorders.

The continuum model of eating disorders states that the behaviours and attitudes (e.g., body dissatisfaction, overconcern about weight and shape, excessively exercising) observed in individuals with full-threshold eating disorders begin with less severity and progress linearly, culminating in either anorexia or bulimia nervosa (Fairburn & Bohn, 2005; Fairburn, Cooper & Shafran, 2003; Hay & Fairburn, 1998). Furthermore, compensatory behaviours that one engages in to prevent weight gain after binge eating (e.g., self-induced vomiting, misuse of laxatives, fasting or excessive exercise) may cause serious health detriments before the development of eating disorders (Sobel, 2004). The antecedents and causes of eating disorders are myriad and complex. However, excessive exercise has been the focus of much research and clinical attention. Thus, this chapter focusses primarily on excessive exercise behaviour, exercise dependence and the relationship of excessive exercise with body image, body dysmorphia, eating disorders and quality of life.

1   Exercise Dependence

In 1970, Fredrick Baekeland accidentally discovered exercise dependence while attempting to recruit habitual male exercisers (i.e., exercising 5 or 6 days/wk) for a study that would examine the effect of 1 month of exercise deprivation on sleep. Unfortunately for Baekeland (1970), men who exercised at this frequency refused to give up exercising to participate. This was the case even when Baekeland offered monetary compensation. Consequentially, he reduced his definition of habitual exercise to 3 or 4 days/wk. Interestingly, even with this criterion for exercise, Baekeland found that participants reported increased anxiety, nocturnal awakening and sexual tension (i.e., withdrawal symptoms) during the 1 month of exercise deprivation.

Baekeland's (1970) study is important in the discovery of exercise dependence because he identified an obligatory drive for continued exercise and documented that withdrawal effects (i.e., a key component of addiction) may occur once exercise has become routine. Because exercise is a healthy and socially desirable behaviour and increased psychological distress is considered undesirable, subsequent researchers questioned whether exercise addiction may be considered a positive addiction (Glasser, 1976; Hailey & Bailey, 1982; Morgan, 1979); that is, an increased amount of exercise is desired because the beneficial effects of regular exercise will result in improved psychological and physical health. Conversely, the increased amount and intensity of exercise seen in exercise dependence commonly result in varying degrees of injuries, detriments to social life and occupational problems. Thus, the current general consensus is that exercise addiction may be viewed as a negative addiction as well as a positive addiction (Morgan, 1979).

1.1 Defining Exercise Dependence

Research attempting to identify and accurately measure exercise dependence has been hampered by a lack of consensus on terminology. Researchers have used a variety of terms and labels in an attempt to identify a common phenomenon. However, most have focussed on the individual's perception that exercise is a mandatory prerequisite for daily routines (i.e., the obligatory aspects of exercise dependence). Labels indicating pathological attitudes and excessive amounts of exercise have typically been focussed around addiction, commitment, problems related to exercise in general and running-specific factors.

The terms most commonly applied in an attempt to define exercise dependence (Hausenblas & Symons Downs, 2002a) are as follows:

Addiction

- Bodybuilder addiction
- Exercise addiction
- Exercise addiction and commitment
- Negative addiction
- Running addiction
- Running addiction and commitment

KEY CONCEPTS

- Exercise dependence is an intense craving for leisure-time physical activity that results in uncontrollable, excessive exercise and manifests in physiological or psychological symptoms.

- Several terms have been used to describe exercise dependence (e.g. exercise commitment, exercise addiction).

- Current measurement and assessment tools quantify exercise dependence in terms of the seven criteria of substance dependence as applied to excessive exercise behaviour and cognitions.

- Eating disorders and body dysmorphia are severe mental health conditions that include pathological attitudes toward one's body and often include the use of excessive exercise as a compensatory behaviour.

- Exercise dependence may explain why exercise behaviour can become problematic for some individuals with eating disorders yet be a protective factor against the onset of an eating disorder for others.

Commitment

- Attitudinal commitment
- Commitment and addiction
- Commitment to exercise
- Commitment to physical activity
- Commitment to running
- Exercise commitment
- Running commitment
- Obsessive commitment to running

Exercise

- Exercise dependence
- Excessive exercise
- Fitness fanaticism
- Obligatory athlete
- Obligatory exercise

Running Behaviours

- Compulsive runner
- Chronic jogger
- Habitual running
- High-intensity running
- Running dependence
- Obligatory running

Although no standard description of exercise dependence (or any other specific type of dependence) exists, recommendations have been made to frame exercise dependence using definitions of substance dependence (Szabo, 2000; Veale, 1995). However, evidence for using such a framework is equivocal. Exercise, similar to several other potentially harmful behaviours, is beneficial when performed in appropriate amounts, and these amounts are somewhat subjective. For example, public health paradigms suggest using the following four categories to define the extent to which behaviours are beneficial or problematic (Health Officers Council of British Columbia, 2005):

1. Beneficial use: Use has positive health, spiritual or social effects (e.g., exercise results in positive improvements in physi-

cal, psychological and social aspects of health).

2. Casual or nonproblematic use: Use has negligible health or social effects (e.g., exercise results in minor disruptions in daily routine, minor injuries or financial investment).

3. Problematic use: Use begins to have negative consequences for individual, friends, family or society (e.g., exercise results in detriments in social or professional relationships or in overuse injuries such as tendintious and pulled muscles).

4. Chronic dependence: Use becomes habitual and compulsive despite negative health and social effects (e.g., use of steroids or other drugs, development of an eating disorder, chronic physical injuries, intense need and craving for exercise in order to avoid anxiety or depression).

Applying the *Diagnostic and Statistical Manual (DSM-IV)* (American Psychiatric Association, 2000) definition of substance dependence to exercise yields a more comprehensive, reasonable and objective operational definition of exercise dependence. Using the DSM definition as a guide, exercise dependence occurs when an individual engages in a maladaptive pattern of exercise that leads to clinically significant impairment or distress, as manifested by 3 or more of the following constructs occurring at any time in the same 12 mo period: tolerance, withdrawal, intention, loss of control, time, conflict and continuance (see "Exercise-Dependence Criteria").

1.2 Assessment of Exercise Dependence

Because running and weightlifting are the exercise behaviours of choice in many individuals with exercise dependence, exercise-dependence measures are initially related to specific sports and exercises such as running and bodybuilding. However, simply measuring sport-related constructs or exercise amount alone may not be sufficient to

Exercise-Dependence Criteria

Exercise dependence occurs when three or more of the following occur within a 12 mo period:

- Tolerance: The individual either needs significantly increased amounts of exercise in order to achieve the desired effect or feels diminished effect with continued use of the same amount of exercise.

- Withdrawal: The individual experiences withdrawal symptoms (e.g., anxiety, fatigue) when they participate in less than their regular amount of exercise, or the individual engages in their regular (or closely related) amount of exercise to relieve or avoid withdrawal symptoms.

- Intention effects: The individual often exercises in larger amounts or over a longer period than intended.

- Loss of control: The individual has a persistent desire or unsuccessful effort to cut down or control exercise.

- Time: The individual spends a great deal of time in activities that facilitate their engagement in exercise (e.g., vacations are related to exercise).

- Conflict: The individual gives up or reduces important social, occupational or recreational activities because of exercise.

- Continuance: The individual continues exercising despite knowledge of having a persistent or recurrent physical or psychological problem that is likely caused or exacerbated by exercise (e.g., continues running despite severe shin splits).

Based on the *Diagnostic and statistical manual of mental disorders*, 4th ed. 2000.

identify those who may be experiencing a problem. Thus, it may be difficult to determine how much exercise is too much. Therefore, assessments of exercise-dependence status should focus on the psychological aspects of exercise as well as the physical aspects. More recent measurement tools attempt to quantify risk by applying DSM criteria for substance dependence to exercise behaviour. These measures assess exercise amount, physical constructs or psychological constructs that may indicate pathological patterns of exercise behaviour. Table 13.1 lists self-report measures commonly used to assess exercise dependence. Sport-specific measures are listed first, and exercise-specific measures follow.

2 Eating Disorders and Body Dysmorphia

The *Diagnostic and Statistical Manual of Mental Disorders, Fourth Edition, Text Revision* (DSM-IV TR) (American Psychiatric Association, 2000)

defines eating disorders as severe disturbances in eating behaviour and identifies anorexia nervosa and bulimia nervosa as the two main variants. A multisite international study (Shroff et al., 2006) reported that 43.5% of individuals with a lifetime diagnosis of either anorexia or bulimia engage in excessive amounts of exercise. Closer examination of the prevalence rates by eating disorder subtype shows that 37.4% of anorexics who exhibit bingeing and purging, 40.3% of anorexics who exhibit restrictive eating, 54.5% of anorexics who exhibit purging, 20.2% of bulimics who exhibit purging and 24% of bulimics who exhibit bingeing engage in excessive exercise (Shroff et al., 2006). Similarly, clinical interviews with female eating disorder inpatients who failed to respond to outpatient treatment found that rates of compulsive exercise are higher in patients with restrictive-type anorexia (80%) than in those with binge–purge anorexia (43.3%) or purging-type bulimia (39.3%; Dalle Grave, Calugi & Marchesini, 2008).

Table 13.1 Self-Report Measures of Exercise Dependence

Scale	Source	Items (n)	Constructs assessed	Chronbach's alpha	Population used in validation
Bodybuilding Dependence Scale	Smith, Hale & Collins (1998)	9	Social dependenceTraining dependence Mastery dependence	.75-.93	Adult bodybuilders and weight-lifters
Chapman's Running Addiction Scale	Chapman & De Castro (1990)	11	Psychological correlates of running addiction	.82	University student runners
Commitment to Running Scale	Carmack & Martens (1979)	12	Positive addiction	Not reported	Runners of varying ability
Running Addiction Scale	Estok & Rudy (1986)	17	Negative addiction	.66	Marathon runners
Commitment to Exercise Scale	Davis, Brewer & Ratusny (1993)	8	Obligatory exercise Psychological aspects of exercise	.77-.88	University students
Exercise Addiction Inventory	Terry, Szabo & Griffiths (2004)	6	Salience Mood modification Tolerance Withdrawal symptoms Conflict Relapse	.84	Habitual exercisers
Exercise Beliefs Questionnaire	Loumidis & Wells (1998)	21	Social desirability Physical appearance Mental and emotional functioning Vulnerability to disease and aging	.67-.89	University students and adult exercisers
Exercise Dependence Questionnaire	Ogden, Veale & Summers (1997)	29	Withdrawal symptoms Exercise for weight control Positive reward Stereotyped behaviour Exercise for health reasons Interference with social, family, and work obligations Insight into problem Exercise for social reasons	.52-.84	Individuals exercising ≥4 h/wk recruited from sport- and fitness-oriented clubs and facilities
Exercise Dependence Scale	Hausenblas & Symons Downs (2002b)	21	Tolerance Withdrawal Intention Lack of control Time Reduction in other activities Continuance	.78-.92	University students
Exercise Salience Scale	Kline, Franken & Rowland (1994); Morrow & Harvey (1990)	40	Response-omission anxiety Response persistence Four more minor unnamed factors	Not reported	Undergraduate students
Obligatory Exercise Questionnaire	Pasman & Thompson (1988)	20	Psychological characteristics of committed athletes	.66-.96	Obligatory runners, weight-lifters and sedentary individuals

2.1 Defining Eating Disorders and Body Dysmorphia

The criteria for diagnosis with anorexia nervosa and bulimia nervosa are described in more detail as follows as well as diagnostic criteria for body dysmorphic disorder, which has also been associated with excessive exercise.

2.1.1 Anorexia Nervosa

The DSM IV criteria for anorexia (see "Diagnostic Criteria for 307.1 Anorexia Nervosa") include an intense and unrealistic fear of becoming fat, engaging in behaviours intended to produce distinct weight loss and amenorrhea (the absence of three consecutive menstrual cycles in women) that results from the refusal to maintain a healthy weight. The disturbance of self-evaluation and consequential denial of one's low weight are defined as anorexia nervosa if the individual maintains a weight that is less than 85% of what is considered an ideal body weight.

Anorexia nervosa is categorised into two specific types—restricting type and binge-eating–purging type—based on how the individual reaches and maintains the extreme low weight. The restricting type is defined as the absence of bingeing and purging behaviours. In the binge-eating–purging type, the individual engages in binges (i.e., eating inappropriately massive amounts of food in one period of time) or purging behaviour (i.e., self-induced vomiting; misuse of laxatives, diuretics or enemas) during the current episode of anorexia nervosa.

2.1.2 Bulimia Nervosa

The DSM-IV criteria for bulimia (see "Diagnostic Criteria for 307.51 Bulimia Nervosa") are similar to those for anorexia in that bulimia also includes an intense fear of becoming fat. However, they differ in that bulimia includes powerful urges to overeat and subsequent binges that are followed by engaging in some sort of purging

Diagnostic Criteria for 307.1 Anorexia Nervosa

1. Refusal to maintain body weight at or above a minimally normal weight for age and height (e.g., weight loss leading to maintenance of body weight less than 85% of that expected; or failure to make expected weight gain during period of growth, leading to body weight less than 85% of that expected).

2. Intense fear of gaining weight or becoming fat, even though underweight.

3. Disturbance in the way in which one's body weight or shape is experienced, undue influence of body weight or shape on self-evaluation, or denial of the seriousness of the current low body weight.

4. In postmenarcheal females, amenorrhea (the absence of at least three consecutive menstrual cycles). (A woman is considered to have amenorrhea if her periods occur only following hormone [e.g., estrogen] administration.)

Specific Types

- Restricting type: During the current episode of anorexia nervosa the person has not regularly engaged in binge eating or purging behaviour (i.e., self-induced vomiting or the misuse of laxatives, diuretics or enemas).

- Binge-eating–purging type: During the current episode of anorexia nervosa the person has regularly engaged in binge eating or purging behaviour (i.e., self-induced vomiting or the misuse of laxatives, diuretics or enemas).

Reprinted with permission from the Diagnostic and Statistical Manual of Mental Disorders, Fourth Edition, Text Revision. (Copyright © 2000). American Psychiatric Association.

or compensatory behaviour in an attempt to avoid the fattening effects of excessive caloric intake. Similar to anorexia, people with bulimia experience fear regarding self-evaluation, which leads to compensatory behaviours for evading weight gain. The contradiction is the presence of the uncontrollable urges to overeat. These binges occur within a 2 h period and include a sense of lack of control and consumption of an amount of food that is larger than most people would consume in a similar time and setting (American Psychiatric Association, 2000). Similar to anorexia, compensatory behaviours are separated into purging type (i.e., self-induced vomiting; use of laxatives, diuretics or enemas; medication abuse) and nonpurging type (i.e., other compensatory behaviours such as fasting or excessively exercising). Unlike with anorexia, no criteria that define maintenance of body weight or presence of amenorrhea exist.

2.1.3 Body Dysmorphic Disorder

The *DSM-IV* (American Psychiatric Association, 2000) defines body dysmorphic disorder, also commonly referred to as body dysmorphia, as a somatoform disorder in which the individual maintains a preoccupation with an imagined or trivial defect in their appearance that causes marked distress or impairment in social, occupational or other areas of function (see "Diagnostic Criteria for 300.7 Body Dysmorphic Disorder"). Furthermore, this preoccupation with body parts must not occur in conjunction with other disorders, such as anorexia nervosa. Dissatisfaction with musculature is a common specific feature of body dysmorphic disorder (Pope, Phillips & Olivardia, 2000). Because exercise can increase muscle size and appearance, individuals with body dysmorphic disorder may experience an increased drive for muscularity. Dissatisfaction with musculature that results in feeling unacceptably small is the

Diagnostic Criteria for 307.51 Bulimia Nervosa

1. Recurrent episodes of binge eating. An episode of binge eating is characterised by both of the following:
   - Eating, in a discrete period of time (e.g., within any 2 h period), an amount of food that is definitely larger than most people would eat during a similar period of time and under similar circumstances, and
   - A sense of lack of control over eating during the episode (e.g., a feeling that one cannot stop eating or control what or how much one is eating)
2. Recurrent inappropriate compensatory behaviour undertaken in order to prevent weight gain (e.g., self-induced vomiting; misuse of laxatives, diuretics, enemas or other medications; fasting; or excessive exercise).

3. The binge eating and inappropriate compensatory behaviours both occur, on average, at least 2 times/wk for 3 mo.
4. Self-evaluation is unduly influenced by body shape and weight.
5. The disturbance does not occur exclusively during episodes of anorexia nervosa.

Specific Types

- Purging type: During the current episode of bulimia nervosa the person has regularly engaged in self-induced vomiting or the misuse of laxatives, diuretics or enemas.
- Nonpurging type: During the current episode of bulimia nervosa the person has used other inappropriate compensatory behaviours such as fasting or excessive exercise but has not regularly engaged in self-induced vomiting or the misuse of laxatives, diuretics or enemas.

Diagnostic Criteria for 300.7 Body Dysmorphic Disorder

- Preoccupation with an imagined defect in appearance. If a slight physical anomaly is present, the person's concern is markedly excessive.

- The preoccupation causes clinically significant distress or impairment in social,

occupational or other important areas of functioning.

- The preoccupation is not better accounted for by another mental disorder (e.g., dissatisfaction with body shape and size in anorexia nervosa).

Reprinted with permission from the Diagnostic and Statistical Manual of Mental Disorders, Fourth Edition, Text Revision. (Copyright © 2000). American Psychiatric Association.

main source of body-image disturbance in men. When the individual's preoccupation is focussed on musculature, the dysmorphic disorder is often called muscle dysmorphic disorder or muscle dsymorphia (Pope, Phillips & Olivardia, 2000).

2.2 Assessment of Eating Disorders

Semistructured clinical interviews, self-monitoring and self-report measure are the methods most commonly used to assess eating disorder status. Clinical interviews remain the gold standard for assessment (Garner, 2002). Each method of assessment has unique advantages and disadvantages, and one should think out the aims of the assessment and logistical considerations when choosing an assessment tool. For example, interviews are the most accurate and in-depth method for assessing the type and severity of an eating disorder, but they are typically lengthy and expensive and rely on the expertise of a well-trained clinician. For these reasons, they may not be practical for anonymously assessing large groups of individuals. Similarly, self-monitoring has the potential to elicit valuable insights into the individual's affect, motivation, food intake and energy expenditure but relies heavily on the awareness and honesty of the individual. Because individuals with eating disorders are notoriously secretive about their behaviours and cognitions and because admission of a problem may be socially undesirable (American Psychiatric Association, 2000), self-monitoring may

not be as reliable as either clinical interviews or self-report methods. Finally, most self-report methods are generally considered reliable and valid but typically are not as accurate as clinical interviews. When selecting a self-report measure, one should pay close attention to the items, constructs assessed and population used during development and validation. Table 13.2 provides a partial list of commonly used measurements of eating disorder. The following sections describe clinical interviews, self-monitoring and self-report measures in more detail.

2.2.1 Clinical Interviews

Several interview techniques have received considerable research attention and are well validated. For example, the Eating Disorder Examination (Cooper & Fairburn, 1987) is a semistructured interview that assesses the psychopathology specific to eating disorders. This interview assesses individuals on four subscales—restraint, eating concern, shape concern and weight concern—and has been validated for use in diagnosis.

2.2.2 Self-Monitoring

Self-monitoring techniques gather information about eating-disordered behaviours and cognitions through diary-type recording of food intake, exercise, extreme weight control behaviours and cognitions (see Fairburn, 1985).

2.2.3 Self-Reporting

Generally, self-reports are economical, brief, easily administered and objectively scored. Most self-report measures assess the frequency and

Table 13.2   Measures of Eating Disorder

Scale	Source	Items (n)	Constructs	Chronbach's alpha	Populations used in validation
Binge Eating Questionnaire	Halmi, Falk & Schwartz (1981)	23	Weight Bingeing Vomiting Sex differences Weight change Diuretics	Not reported	Undergraduates
Binge Eating Scale	Gormally et al. (1982)	16	Cognitions Behavioural manifestations	.85-.89	Overweight individuals
Bulimia Test Revised	Thelen & Farmer (1991); Vincent, McCabe & Ricciardelli (1999)	28 scored, 8 nonscored	Bulimia nervosa diagnostic criteria	.88-.98	Adolescents and adults
Children's Eating Attitudes Test	Maloney, McGuire & Daniels (1988)	26	Dieting Bulimia Food preoccupation Oral control	.71-.87	Children
Compulsive Eating Scale	Dunn & Ondercin (1981)	16	Emotional states related to food and eating Body type Medical information Weight gain or loss Binge eating	.72	University students
Dutch Eating Behavior Questionnaire	Van Strien et al. (1986)	33	Restrained eating Emotional eating External eating	.80-.95	Children and adults, dieters, patients with eating disorders, individuals without eating disorders
Eating Attitudes Test	Garner et al. (1982)	26	Dieting Bulimia and food preoccupation Oral control	.90	Females with and without anorexia
Eating Behaviors and Body Image Test for Preadolescent Girls	Candy & Fee (1998)	38	Body image dissatisfaction and restrictive eating Binge eating behaviours	.75-.91	Girls in fourth through sixth grade
Eating Disorder Diagnostic Scale	Stice, Telch & Rizvi (2000)	22	Anorexia Bulimia Binge eating disorder	.89	Females aged 13-65 yr
Eating Disorder Inventory-2	Garner (1991)	91	Drive for thinness Bulimia Body dissatisfaction Ineffectiveness Perfectionism Interpersonal distrust Interceptive awareness Maturity fears Asceticism Impulse regulation Social insecurity	.56-.91	Clinical and community samples

Scale	Source	Items (n)	Constructs	Chronbach's alpha	Populations used in validation
Eating Disorders Examination Questionnaire	Cooper & Fairburn (1987)	36	Dietary restraint Eating concern Shape concern Weight concern	Not reported	Adolescents and adults
Eating Question-naire—Revised	Williamson et al. (1989)	15	Follows DSM-III criteria for bulimia	.87	Female undergradu-ates with and without bulimia
Interview for Diagnosis of Eating Disorders	Kutlesic et al. (1998)	21	Anorexia Bulimia Compulsive overeating	.75-.96	Clinical and community samples
Minnesota Eating Behavior Survey	von Ranson et al. (2005)	30	Body dissatisfaction Compensatory behaviour Binge eating Weight preoccupation	.80-.91	Twins and university students
Questionnaire of Eating and Weight Patterns	Spitzer et al. (1992)	8	Binge eating Binge eating disorder Binge eating syndrome Binge eating syndrome and distress Episodic overeating Possible bulimia No diagnosis	Not reported	Binge eaters and comparison group; adults and children
Setting Condi-tions for Anorexia Nervosa Scale	Slade & Dewey (1986)	40	Life dissatisfaction and loss of control Perfectionism Social and personal anxiety Adolescent problems Need for weight control	Not reported	Adults
Structured Clinical Interview for DSM-IV	Spitzer et al. (1992)	Not reported	Not reported	Not reported	Not reported
Structured Inter-view for Anorexia and Bulimia Nervosa for expert rating	Fichter et al. (1998)	87	Body image and slimness ideal General psychopathology Sexuality and social integration Bulimic symptoms Measures to counteract weight gain Fasting Substance abuse Atypical binges	.43-.91	Anorexia patients and community controls
Survey for Eating Disorders	Ghaderi & Scott (2002); Gotestam & Agras (1995)	36	Bulimia nervosa Anorexia nervosa Binge eating disorder Eating disorders not otherwise speci-fied	Not reported	Binge eating disorder patients and university students
Three-Factor Eating Scale	Stunkard & Messick (1985)	51	Dietary restraint Disinhibition Hunger	.85-.93	Community sample
Yale-Brown-Cornell Eating Disorder Scale	Gearhardt, Corbin & Brownell (2009); Mazure et al. (1994)	65	Interview checklist Features of eating disorders	Not reported	Inpatients and outpa-tients

severity of cardinal features of eating disorders. More recent measures, such as the Eating Disorder Diagnostic Scale (Stice, Telch & Rizvi, 2000), are validated to provide a tentative diagnosis. Although several self-report measures currently exist, the Eating Attitudes Test (available online at www.eat-26.com/index.php; Garner et al., 1982) and the Eating Disorder Inventory (Garner, 1991) are the measures most commonly used (Garner, 2002).

3 Impact of Exercise Dependence on Well-Being and Health

The relationship between exercise amount and health is fairly linear: Increased amounts of exercise result in additional health benefits (U.S. Department of Health and Human Services, 2008). Although public health recommendations such as this accurately reflect the behavioural aspects of health, they fail to account for pathological motivations for behaviour. Thus, pathological motivations may supersede engagement in normal amounts of a behaviour and result in detrimental health effects due to excessive amounts of a behaviour. Exercise dependence is such a case where the psychological side of behaviour can overshadow the anticipated health effects. For example, research examining symptoms of exercise dependence and quality of life (i.e., physical, psychological and social aspects of health) found that the relationship between these two constructs is in fact curvilinear (Cook & Hausenblas, 2010). That is, as exercise amount increases, so do some symptoms of exercise dependence (e.g., tolerance) and overall health. However, this linear relationship ends once exercise becomes excessive and results in increased symptoms of exercise dependence that are also accompanied by decreases in health-related quality of life. Findings such as these should not be surprising considering that the diagnostic criteria of exercise dependence include continuing exercise routines despite injuries or illness (i.e., physical health), exercising to avoid withdrawal effects such as anxiety

and depression (i.e., psychological health) and reduction of time spent in other areas of life such as social, family and work commitments (i.e., social health).

A growing body of equivocal research has begun to quantify the exact aspects of health that are affected by exercise dependence. Specifically, compared with nondependent controls, individuals with exercise dependence often experience an increased number of overuse injuries (e.g., tendinitis, sprains and strains, muscle injuries, iliotibial band syndrome; Hausenbas & Symons Downs, 2002a), negative affect—particularly during exercise cessation (Szabo, 1995), eating pathology and body image disturbances (De Coverley Veale, 1987), anxiety about the shape of one's body (McCabe & Ricciardelli, 2004), hypochondria (Currie et al., 1999) and compulsive shopping or buying (Lejoyeaux et al., 2008).

Despite these health detriments, some researchers have argued that exercise dependence can be considered beneficial or a positive form of addiction (Glasser, 1976). For example, exercise-dependent individuals self-report less smoking or tobacco use (Lejoyeaux et al., 2008) and increased vigilance about monitoring and reacting to one's health (Currie et al., 1999; Hadjistravropoulos & Lawrence, 2007). Lejoyeaux and colleagues (2008) proposed two hypotheses that may explain the potential health benefits of exercise dependence. First, exercise dependence is a socially acceptable or socially tolerated addiction that appears to be a reasonable form of dependence. Second, exercise dependence generates anxiety about physical aspects of the self, thus increasing the likelihood that individuals will address minor health concerns before they become problematic.

Finally, research has indicated that sex differences may occur in the health detriments experienced by exercise-dependent individuals. For example, in a sample of college students with exercise dependence, women reported greater craving for exercise and feelings of being tense when unable to exercise more often than did men (Zmijewski & Howard, 2003). A more in-depth study of sex differences in symptoms of exercise dependence found that men report significantly greater detriments in general health and physical functioning, whereas women report more bodily pain and problems with work or other daily activities (Cook & Hausenblas, 2010). Simply stated, these results show, by sex, where health is affected when exercise motivations and behaviours become pathological. The pathological and psychological motivations associated with exercise dependence may limit the health improvements that one expects to gain with increased levels of exercise. Future research should continue to examine pathological motivations for exercise behaviour and health differences in symptoms of exercise dependence.

4   Relationship Between Exercise Dependence and Eating Disorders

The relationship between exercise and eating pathology is complex and controversial. Diagnostic criteria, correlational research and clinical observation show a higher prevalence of exercise in all forms of eating disorders compared with the general population (American Psychiatric Association, 2000). This is in part due to the ability of exercise to offset caloric balance, resulting in weight loss. Simply stated, for many individuals beginning to experience an eating pathology, diet and compensatory behaviours such as picky eating, skipping meals and fasting may only reduce the number of calories consumed. Consequently, weight loss is slowed and the individual may seek complementary methods in order to accelerate weight loss. If weight-loss progress seems slow, the individual may add compulsive exercise in an attempt to increase weight loss. Although this explanation seems reasonable and sufficient for explaining the role of exercise in eating disorders, simply examining the amount of exercise does not explain either why or for whom excessive exercise may become problematic. Thus, more recent investigations reveal that psychological factors such as exercise dependence may better explain the role of exercise in eating disorders (Cook & Hausenblas,

2008, 2011; Cook et al., 2011). Therefore, a closer examination of prevalence rates and psychological factors indicates that a much more complicated relationship exists between exercise and eating disorders.

Exercise-dependent individuals typically exhibit perfectionistic personality characteristics (Hagan & Hausenblas, 2003) and psychological distress; these features are similar to those of anorexia. Furthermore, a higher prevalence of excessive exercise is observed in all variants of anorexia (Shroff et al., 2006). Thus, studies initially examined exercise dependence as a possible variant of anorexia (i.e., anorexia analogue hypothesis; Yates, Leehey & Shisslak, 1983). However, Yates, Leehey and Shisslak's (1983) anorexia analogue hypothesis was based on a lack of pertinent data, poor methodology, lack of relevance to most exercisers, overreliance on extreme examples and overstating similarities between exercisers and people with anorexia (Hausenblas & Symons Downs, 2002a). Subsequently, better research designs have failed to find similarities between exercise dependence and anorexia (Blumenthal, O'Toole & Chang, 1984; Coen & Ogles, 1993; Dishman & Buckworth, 1997; Kreslestein, 1983; Larsen, 1983; Powers, Schocken & Boyd, 1998).

The notion that behaviour (i.e., exercise amount) alone may somehow be responsible for the development of eating pathologies is based on overstated similarities between individuals who engage in high amounts of exercise (e.g., athletes, distance runners) and those with eating disorders, increased amounts of exercise seen in some subtypes of eating disorders (Shroff et al., 2006) and the inclusion of excessive exercise as a potential diagnostic criterion for bulimia (American Psychiatric Association, 2000). However, psychological variables that may mediate the potential relationship between exercise behaviour and eating disorders have historically been overlooked. Recent research examined the role of psychological variables—in particular, symptoms of exercise dependence—that may mediate the relationship between exercise behaviour and eating disorder. Understanding the end that an individual is attempting to accomplish through exercising may distinguish primary versus secondary dependence. (See "Primary Versus Secondary Dependence" for further elaboration.) Simply stated, it is important to distinguish whether the individual is exercising excessively to satisfy the need to exercise (i.e., primary dependence) or whether they are engaging in increased amounts of exercise as a compensatory behaviour that is secondary to some other pathology, such as an eating disorder (i.e., secondary dependence). For example, Adkins and Keel (2005) found that obligatory attitudes and behaviours, not exercise amount, positively predicted negative eating attitudes and behaviours. Zmijewski and Howard (2003) found that exercise dependence, but not exercise behaviour, positively correlated with bulimia symptoms. Similarly, Cook and Hausenblas (2008) found that exercise-dependence symptoms, not exercise behaviour, mediated the relationship between exercise and eating pathology. Thus, psychological factors, not the amount of exercise, better explained why the relationship between exercise dependence and eating disorders exists.

4.1 Definition of Excessive Exercise

The belief that exercise is associated with the development and maintenance of eating disorders is based largely on cross-sectional, retrospective and case study designs that fail to adequately assess and quantify the term *excessive exercise*. For example, a long-standing clinical observation is that most hospitalised inpatients receiving treatment for anorexia engage in excessive amounts of exercise during the development or maintenance of their eating disorder (Katz, 1996). However, no definition exists for what is considered excessive exercise. Similarly, recent studies have correlated participation in athletics (i.e., populations that engage in large amounts of physical activity) with deleterious eating attitudes that are related to eating disorders (Holm-Denoma et al., 2009; Levitt, 2008). Thus, researchers have focussed on exercise amount

as contributing to the development and maintenance of eating disorders. However, focussing on exercise amount may be misleading because much of the research examining excessive exercise has relied on biased sampling methods and used nonvalidated self-report measures of exercise that lack a clear, concise and consistent definition of how much exercise is excessive (American College of Sports Medicine, 2000; Adkins & Keel, 2005; Hausenblas, Cook & Chittester, 2008; Peñas-Lledó, Leal & Waller, 2002; Solenberger, 2001). Furthermore, many of the operational definitions of excessive exercise list exercise amounts that are less than the minimum amount needed to achieve the health-related benefits of physical activity (American College of Sports Medicine, 2000; U.S. Department of Health and Human Services, 2008).

4.2 Inconsistencies in Diagnostic Criteria

The higher prevalence of excessive exercise in people with anorexia (Shroff et al., 2006) further adds to the confusion of why excessive exercise is explicitly used as a criterion for bulimia but not anorexia. Furthermore, defining exercise as excessive when "it significantly interferes with important activities, when it occurs at inappropriate times or in inappropriate settings or when the individual continues to exercise despite injury or other medical complications" (American Psychiatric Association, 2000, pp. 590-591) fails to quantify the amount needed to determine whether exercise is excessive. Because researchers have studied excessive exercise and its negative health outcomes far less than the other diagnostic symptoms, more research is needed to better understand excessive exercise and eating disorders (Lewisohn et al., 2002). In an attempt to clarify the construct of excessive exercise, researchers advocate for either revising the diagnostic criteria with regard to excessive exercise or eliminating excessive exercise as a diagnostic criterion because of lack of empirical support for it (Hebebrand et al., 2004; Mond et al., 2004). In short, considerable debate exists regarding classification of eating disorders in general (Mitchell, Cook-Myers & Wonderlich, 2005; Sloan, Mizes & Epstein, 2005; Williamson, Gleaves & Steward, 2005) and, in particular, how best to define excessive exercise (Walsh, 2004) or whether to even include excessive exercise as a compensatory behaviour for bulimia nervosa (Herzog & Delinsky, 2001; Mond et al., 2006). Currently, the DSM-V Eating Disorder Work Group is assessing the clinical utility of, and possible alterations to, existing diagnostic criteria (e.g., excessive exercise) of all variants of eating disorders (Walsh, 2009).

4.3 Primary Versus Secondary Dependence

Much of the research examining the relationship between excessive exercise and eating disorders has focussed on the contribution of exercise amount to the development of eating disorders but has overlooked psychological variables that may mediate such a relationship. Understanding the psychological antecedents of exercise may offer insight into the distinction of primary versus secondary exercise dependence and help clarify the relationship between eating disorders and excessive exercise. Primary exercise dependence occurs when the individual meets criteria for exercise dependence and continually exercises solely for the psychological gratification that results from the exercise behaviour. Secondary exercise dependence occurs when an exercise-dependent individual uses exercise to accomplish some other end. Because exercise can be used as a compensatory behaviour to prevent or reverse weight gain, secondary exercise dependence in the context of eating disorders occurs when an individual meets criteria for exercise dependence and continually exercises in order to manipulate and control their own body (Hausenblas & Fallon, 2006; Hausenblas & Symons Downs, 2002a). In this case, exercise dependence is secondary to an eating disorder.

Adkins and Keel (2005) found that obligatory exercise attitudes and behaviours (i.e., exercise-dependence symptoms), not time spent exercis-

ing (i.e., amount), was a positive predictor of negative eating attitudes and behaviours. Zmijewski and Howard (2003) found that exercise-dependence scores, but not exercise behaviour, in female undergraduate students were positively correlated with bulimia symptoms. These results indicate that many college women may be exercising in association with either formal or subclinical eating disorders (Zmijewski & Howard, 2003). Similarly, Cook and Hausenblas (2008) and found that exercise-dependence symptoms, not exercise behaviour, mediated the relationship between exercise and eating pathology. Thus, psychological factors such as exercise dependence and not exercise behaviour or amount may explain how or why the relationship exists.

5 Models of Exercise Dependence and Eating Disorders

The limitations of biased clinical observations (Katz, 1996), retrospective research designs (Davis, Katzman & Kirsh, 1999), vague operational definitions of excessive exercise (American Psychiatric Association, 2000), inconclusive animal research (Cai et al., 2008) and overlooking potential mediating psychological variables (Adkins & Keel, 2005; Cook & Hausenblas, 2008; Zmijewski & Howard, 2003) supports the need for theoretically driven models that explain the relationship between eating disorders and the psychological motivation as well as the physical effect of exercise (Jansen, 2001; Thome & Espelage, 2007). Few models have empirically tested the relationship between exercise dependence and eating disorders. Davis, Katzman and Kirsh (1999) presented a model based on Eisler and le Grange's (1990) theory stating that personality characteristics, obligatory exercising (i.e., psychological characteristics similar to those of exercise dependence) and eating disorders are related. This theory extends the anorexia analogue hypothesis by postulating that obsessive–compulsive disorder or other affective disorders may explain obligatory exercise. Specifically, Davis and colleagues (1999) hypothesised and found initial support for the following: that attitudes and exercise behaviour are reinforcing and reciprocal; that obsessive–compulsive personality influences the development of pathological attitudes toward exercise; that these personality traits indirectly influence behaviour through exercise attitudes; and that excessive exercise was more likely to develop among individuals who were physically active before the onset of anorexia nervosa.

Expanding on Davis' model, Thome and Espelage (2007) confirmed that obligatory exercise attitudes are related to eating pathology in nonclinical, college-age samples. Models resulting from these studies show the need to further explore the relationship between exercise and eating disorders and to carefully examine potential psychological components of this behavioural relationship.

Although the development of models that postulate how and why obligatory attitudes toward exercise may influence the development and maintenance of eating pathology has advanced the understanding of such relationships, these models are retrospective in nature and offer limited insight into why the benefits typically experienced as a result of regular exercise do not occur in individuals with eating disorders. For example, exercise may impart positive improvements on the eating disorder risk factors of anxiety (Landers & Arent, 2001; Taylor, 2003), body image (Hausenblas & Fallon, 2006), depression (Landers & Arent, 2001), stress reactivity (Taylor, 2003) and self-esteem in populations without eating disorders (but not in populations with eating disorders) (Landers & Arent, 2001; Taylor, 2003). Similarly, cardiovascular benefits such as increased cardiac mass, increased stroke volume and cardiac output at rest and during exercise, lower resting heart rate and blood pressure and a decreased tendency for blood clotting are pertinent to research on eating disorders because cardiac damage can occur early during the development of eating disorders (Klump et al., 2009; Mehler & Krantz, 2003; Pearson, Goldklang & Streigel-Moore, 2002). Exercise also has the ability to reduce adiposity, thus contributing to a leaner, fit and culturally ideal body type (Thompson et al., 1999). More-

over, sociocultural pressures to be thin and social comparison are risk factors for the development of eating disorders (Jacobi et al., 2004; Levine & Smolak, 2006; Stice, 2002; Streigel-Moore & Bulik, 2007). Furthermore, the metabolic benefits of exercise include decreased triglycerides and increased high-density cholesterol, increased insulin-mediated glucose uptake and a possible increase in resting metabolism (Haskell, 1994). Finally, exercise increases skeletal muscle mass and bone density in youths and is related to the retention of bone mineral density in older adults. This has implications in the development of osteoporosis, a common consequence of prolonged eating-disordered behaviours (Klump et al., 2009; Sobel, 2004). Exercise is an effective intervention for many physical and psychological health issues, yet recent recommendations for research to re-examine the role of exercise in eating disorders (Meyer, Taranis & Touyz, 2008) have largely been overlooked.

Hausenblas, Cook and Chitttester (2008) presented a conceptual model that examines relationships between exercise and eating disorders (see figure 13.1). Their exercise and eating disorders model states that regular exercise is associated with improvements in several physical (i.e., cardiovascular and metabolic benefits, decreased adiposity and increased bone density; Haskell, 1994; Mehler & Krantz, 2003), psychological (i.e., body image, depression, anxiety, stress reactivity and self-esteem; Fox, 1999; Hausenblas & Fallon, 2006; Paluska & Schwenk, 2000; Taylor, 2003) and social benefits that are risk factors, maintenance factors, outcomes or diagnostic criteria for eating disorders. Hence, the exercise and eating disorders model has consolidated and supported several narrative and meta-analytic reviews that have shown the ability of exercise to impart positive improvements on eating disorder risk, development and maintenance factors. The model also extends current understanding of the relationship between exercise and health status by including exercise dependence. That is, exercise dependence may explain why the development of eating disorders may supersede the expected benefits of exercise. Simply stated, this model posits that the benefits conveyed by regular exercise (e.g., improvements in depression, anxiety, stress reactivity, self-esteem and body composition) may counteract the risk factors for eating disorders (e.g., body dissatisfaction, depression, anxiety, increased body mass) in the absence of pathological or psychological factors such as exercise dependence.

Two recent studies have found initial support for the exercise and eating disorder model. First, university students completed self-report measures of physical and psychological quality of life, exercise behaviour, eating disorder risk and exercise-dependence symptoms. Structural equation modelling analysis found support for the mediation effect of exercise dependence on eating disorders as well as the effect of psychological well-being on eating disorders. Together, exercise behaviour, psychological well-being and exercise-dependence symptoms predicted 22.9%

of the variation in eating disorders. These results indicate that the psychological health benefits conveyed by exercise reduced eating disorder risk (Cook et al., 2011). These results were replicated in a more diverse sample of college students (Cook & Hausenblas, 2011). Thus, initial tests of the exercise and eating disorders model suggest that the model may synthesise two divergent lines of research. That is, exercise may play a role in the development of eating disorders when exercise dependence is simultaneously present. Similarly, the psychological health benefits of exercise may also reduce risk of eating disorders for individuals without exercise dependence.

6 Exercise in Body Dysmorphia

An individual's subjective sense of dissatisfaction with their own body commonly results in

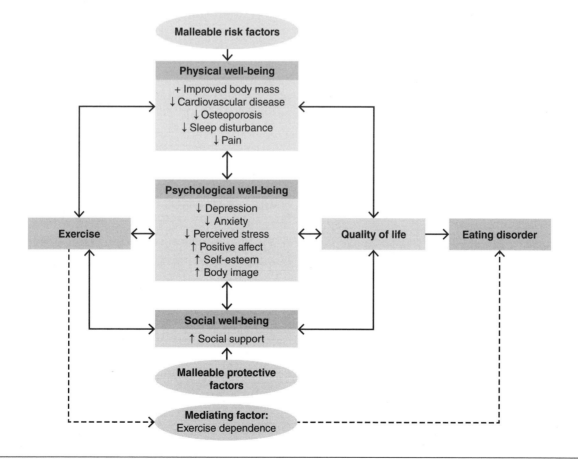

Figure 13.1 The exercise and eating disorder model.

Reprinted, by permission, from H.A. Hausenblas, B.J. Cook, and N.I. Chittester, 2008, "Can exercise treat eating disorders?," *Exercise and Sport Sciences Reviews* 36: 43-47.

efforts to reduce body mass and lose weight, as described previously. However, cultural ideals for men emphasise a larger, more muscular body ideal (Pope, Phillip & Olivardia, 2000). For some, this cultural ideal seems unattainable and may result in body dysmorphia. More specifically, the excessive preoccupation with aspects of their physique and musculature arises from a feeling of being unacceptably small or puny, an under-estimation of muscle mass and an overestimation of fat mass. The individual may then undertake exercise in an attempt to gain muscle mass. Simply stated, the relationship between body mass and body-image disturbance is twofold (Kostanski, Fisher & Gullone, 2004; Kostanski & Gullone, 1998; Presnell, Bearman & Stice, 2004):

1. The individual possesses a self-perception that they are too heavy, which results in a drive to simultaneously lose body fat and add muscle, or

2. the individual possesses a self-perception they are too thin, which results in a drive for muscularity.

Drive for muscularity and preoccupation with perceptions of body fat are the main sources of body-image disturbance in men (Pope, Phillips & Olivardia, 2000). Engaging in exercise in an attempt to gain muscle mass and conform to cultural male body ideals may result in muscle dysmorphia. Thus, muscle dysmorphia is a specific type of body dysmorphia (Pope et al., 1997) in which individuals perceive themselves as unacceptably small (Pope, Katz & Hudson, 1993). Individuals with muscle dysmorphia are

- pathologically preoccupied with the appearance of their whole body,
- concerned that they are not sufficiently large or muscular, and
- consumed by weightlifting, dieting or use of steroids or other supplements.

Because this pursuit of a physical ideal seems to be the opposite of anorexia, various terms such as *reverse anorexia*, *bigorexia*, *bodybuilder anorexia*, *inverse anorexia* and *megorexia* have

been used to describe muscle dysmorphia (Pope et al., 1997). Also similar to anorexia (Pope, Katz & Hudson, 1993), a positive predictive relationship exists between muscle dysmorphia and social physique anxiety (Ebbeck et al., 2009; Grieve et al., 2008), depression (Ebbeck et al., 2009) and perfectionism (Kuennen & Waldren, 2007), and a negative predictive relationship exists between muscle dysmorphia and perceived body attractiveness (Ebbeck et al., 2009).

Exercise is a main focus for individuals with muscle dysmorphia because it has an anabolic affect. Therefore, individuals subsequently initiate resistance exercise (i.e., weightlifting, bodybuilding) in order to increase muscle mass and decrease fat mass. Ironically, individuals with muscle dysmorphia increase exercise amounts and intensities despite possessing a large, muscular physique that actually meets or exceeds the male cultural ideal. That is, because the preoccupation with one's body is pathological, individuals with muscle dysmorphia do not attain satisfaction with their body despite appearing muscular to the casual observer. Moreover, Chittester and Hausenblas (2008) found that weightlifting, supplement use and exercise dependence predict the drive for muscularity. Thus, the pathological role of exercise may lead to exercise dependence (Hausenblas & Symons Downs, 2002a,b; Smith & Hale, 2004; Smith, Hale & Collins, 1998) and the associated physical and psychological difficulties (e.g., withdrawal symptoms, decreased time spent with family or friends, overuse injuries) (Andersen, Cohn & Holbrook, 2000; Pope, Phillips & Olivardia, 2000).

The resulting increases in musculature from increased amounts of exercise often plateau, further contributing to body dissatisfaction. Consequently, individuals often use dietary supplements and anabolic steroids in an attempt to increase muscle mass, decrease fat mass and satisfy their subjective sense of becoming sufficiently big (Kanayama, Pope & Hudson, 2001; Varnado-Sullivan, Horton & Savoy, 2006). However, supplements are generally expensive, typically show little impact on muscle mass (Kreider, 1999) and may promote dependence

(Kanayama, Pope & Hudson, 2001). Steroids are efficacious in producing gains in muscle mass (Cox, 2012; Olrich & Ewing, 1999) but also are associated with significant health risks such as hypertension, disturbed lipid profiles, increased irritability, increased aggression, body-image disturbance and mood disturbances (Hartgens & Kuipers, 2004).

In summary, muscle dysmorphia is a specific type of body-image disturbance that is associated with exercise, exercise dependence and use of dietary supplements and steroids. See "Muscle Dysmorphia Case Studies" for two recent case studies that illustrate the nature of muscle dysmorphia.

7 Strategies for Minimizing the Risk of Exercise Dependence

Identifying individuals who are at risk for exercise dependence is a major challenge because exercise is considered a positive health behaviour. Thus, excessive exercise often goes unnoticed as a negative health behaviour until it has reached an extreme. A key warning sign for distinguishing between healthy and dependent exercise is that healthy exercisers organise exercise around their lives, whereas dependents organise their lives round exercise. The following are other key warning signs of exercise dependence:

- Always working out alone, isolated from others
- Always following the same rigid exercise pattern
- Fixation on weight loss or calories burned
- Exercising when sick or injured
- Exercising to the point of pain and beyond
- Skipping work, class or social plans in order to work out

In individuals with exercise dependence, the psychological torment of not exercising is greater than the negative consequences that affect their physical and social well-being. When exercise is withheld, these individuals often experience irritability and depression. Exercising relieves these symptoms and thus the cycle is continued.

Muscle Dysmorphia Case Studies

CASE STUDY 1

Murray and colleagues (2012) reported on a 20-yr-old male diagnosed with muscle dysmorphia. The male is described as engaging in weightlifting exercise 6 days/wk for 2 h at a time in an effort to obtain a desired musculature and an additional 30 min of cardiovascular exercise in an attempt to reduce fat mass. He is also described as eating high-protein, low-fat and low-carbohydrate foods that are "more for functionality than for taste" and is preoccupied with his perceived lack of muscularity, which affects his capacity to concentrate.

CASE STUDY 2

Leone's (2009) case study describes a 23-yr-old female bodybuilder who presented with questions about use of androgenic anabolic steroids. She reported engaging in 2.5 h/day of weight training during the midafternoon followed by 30 to 45 min of cardiovascular exercise in an attempt to burn fat and 20 min of abdominal exercises before bedtime. Furthermore, she reported ingesting 250 to 300 g of protein supplements as well as various undisclosed "fat burners." She outwardly acknowledged that her exercise is obsessive and her lifestyle is distressing because of the inordinate amount of time spent in the gymnasium. Interestingly, she also reported weightlifting hours after receiving several stitches in her wrist. Such compulsion to exercise despite a clear medical contraindication illustrates aspects of exercise dependence in muscle dysmorphia.

EVIDENCE TO PRACTICE

Exercise dependence may result in serious physical, psychological or social problems. Table 13.1 lists tools for identifying and assessing the severity of exercise dependence. Practitioners are also encouraged to do the following:

- Make a distinction between primary dependence (i.e., excessive exercise is an end in itself) and secondary dependence (i.e., excessive exercise occurs in conjunction with some other pathology, such as an eating disorder or dysmorphia, and is used to manipulate the individual's body).

- Educate the client about specific health affects resulting from their exercise dependence or associated pathology.

- Help the client reframe their exercise goals, expectations and intentions to reflect realistic possibilities and focus on overall health.

- Create a plan for the client that includes healthy amounts of—and attitudes toward—exercise routines, social support, progress monitoring and appropriate rewards for successfully adhering to a recommended exercise programme or routine.

- Refer the client to appropriate and qualified psychological health professionals.

Regardless of the reason behind the excessive exercise and whether or not it is caused by an eating disorder, the effects are harmful to the individuals on psychological, physiological and psychosocial levels.

Although debate exists about the relationship between exercise dependence and eating disorders, it is important to realise that exercise dependence is a real addiction that affects real people and families. Regardless of the cause, more research on effectively minimizing the risk of exercise dependence is needed. Ultimately, the goal is to help these individuals overcome this harmful dependence.

The following self-help strategies can be incorporated into the exercise routine of an individual who may be at risk for dependence:

- Use cross-training to avoid overuse injuries. Remember that aerobic fitness, strength and flexibility are all important aspects of fitness.

- Schedule a reasonable rest between two exercise bouts in order to prevent physical and psychological fatigue.

- Schedule 1 day/wk of complete rest and note how energetic you are the next day.

- Exercise your mind by getting involved in mental and social activities that can reduce anxiety and increase self-esteem.

- Try to learn stress-management techniques such as relaxation, yoga and meditation.

8   Summary

Pathological motivations can result in excessive and detrimental exercise patterns. Exercise dependence is defined as an intense craving for leisure-time physical activity that results in excessive amounts of exercise and physiological or psychological symptoms. Because exercise dependence is associated with several disorders (e.g., body-image disturbance, eating disorders and dysmorphia), distinction should be made between primary exercise dependence (i.e., exercise is the sole desired outcome) and secondary exercise dependence (i.e., exercise is secondary to some other pathology). Interest in exercise dependence is relatively recent and provides context for why the relationship exists between exercise and other pathologies (e.g., body-image disturbance, eating disorders). Finally, exercise dependence may result in serious and sometimes severe detriments to health and well-being. Recent research has begun to uncover sex differences in these effects. Future research and clinical practice are encouraged to further refine the measurement and treatment of exercise dependence.

9   References

Adkins, C.E., & Keel, P.K. (2005). Does "excessive" or "compulsive" best describe exercise as a symptom of bulimia nervosa? *International Journal of Eating Disorders, 38*, 24-29.

American College of Sports Medicine. (2000). *ACSM's guidelines for exercise testing and prescription* (6th ed.). Baltimore: Lippincott Williams & Wilkins.

American Psychiatric Association. (2000). *Diagnostic and statistical manual of mental disorders* (4th ed. Text revision). Washington, D.C.: American Psychiatric Association.

Andersen, A., Cohn, L., & Holbrook, T. (2000). *Making weight: Men's conflicts with food, weight, shape and appearance*. Carlsbad, CA: Gurze Books.

Baekland, F. (1970). Exercise deprivation: Sleep and psychological reactions. *Archives of General Psychiatry, 22*, 365-369.

Blumenthal, J.A., O'Toole, L.C., & Chang, J.L. (1984). Is running an analogue of anorexia nervosa? An empirical study of obligatory running and anorexia nervosa. *Journal of the American Medical Association, 27*, 520-523.

Cai, W., Bocarsly, M.E., Arner, C.N., Walsh, B.T., Foltin, R.W., Hoebel, B.G., & Barbarich-Marsteller, N.C. (2008). Activity-based anorexia during adolescence does not promote binge eating during adulthood in female rats. *International Journal of Eating Disorders, 41*, 681-685.

Candy, C.M., & Fee, V.E. (1998). Underlying dimensions and psychometric properties of the Eating Behaviors and Body Image Test for preadolescent girls. *Journal of Clinical Child Psychology, 27*, 117-127.

Carmack, M.A., & Martens, R. (1979). Measuring commitment to running: A survey of runners' attitudes and mental states. *Journal of Sports Psychology, 1*, 25-42.

Chapman, C.L., & De Castro, J.M. (1990). Running addiction: Measurement and associated psychological characteristics. *The Journal of Sports Medicine and Physical Fitness, 30*, 283-290.

Chittester, N.I., & Hausenblas, H.A. (2009). Correlates of drive for muscularity: The role of anthropometric measures and psychological factors. *Journal of Health Psychology, 14*, 872-877.

Coen, S.P., & Ogles, B.M. (1993). Psychological characteristics of the obligatory runner: A critical examination of the anorexia analogue hypothesis. *Journal of Sport and Exercise Psychology, 15*, 338-354.

Cook, B.J., & Hausenblas, H.A. (2008). The role of exercise dependence for the relationship between exercise behavior and eating pathology: Mediator or moderator? *Journal of Health Psychology, 13*, 495-502.

Cook, B.J., & Hausenblas, H.A. (2010). Gender differences in exercise dependence's effect on quality of life. *Annals of Behavioral Medicine, 39*, S101.

Cook, B.J., & Hausenblas, H.A. (2011). Eating disorder specific health-related quality of life and exercise in college females. *Quality of Life Research, 20*(9), 1385-1390.

Cook, B.J., Hausenblas, H.A., Tuccitto, D., & Giacobbi, P. (2011). Eating disorders and exercise: A structural equation modeling analysis of a conceptual model. *European Eating Disorders Review, 19*, 216-225.

Cooper, Z., & Fairburn, C. (1987). The eating disorder examination: A semi-structured interview for the assessment of the specific psychopathology of eating disorders. *International Journal of Eating Disorders, 6*, 1-8.

Cox, R.H. (2012). *Sports psychology* (7th ed.). New York: McGraw-Hill.

Currie, A., Potts, S.G., Donovan, W., & Blackwood, D. (1999) Illness behaviour in elite middle and long distance runners. *British Journal of Sports Medicine, 33*, 19-21.

Dalle Grave, R., Calugi, S., & Marchesini, G. (2008). Compulsive exercise to control shape or weight in eating disorders: Prevalence, associated features, and treatment outcome. *Comprehensive Psychiatry, 49*, 346-352.

Davis, C., Brewer, H., & Ratusny, D. (1993). Behavioral frequency and psychological commitment: Necessary concepts in the study of excessive exercising. *Journal of Behavioral Medicine, 16*, 611-628.

Davis, C., Katzman, D., & Kirsh, C. (1999). Compulsive physical activity in adolescents with anorexia nervosa. A psychobehavioral spiral of pathology. *Journal of Nervous and Mental Disorders*, 187, 336-342.

De Coverley Veale, D.M.E. (1987). Exercise dependence. *British Journal of Addiction*, 82, 735-740.

Dishman, R.K., & Buckworth, J. (1997). Adherence to physical activity. In W.P. Morgan (Ed.), *Physical activity and mental health* (pp. 63-80). Washington, D.C.: Taylor & Francis.

Dunn, P.K., & Ondercin, P. (1981). Personality variables related to compulsive eating in college women. *Journal of Clinical Psychology*, 37, 43-49.

Ebbeck, E., Watkins, P.L., Concepcion, R.Y., Cardinal, B.J., & Hammermeister, J. (2009). Muscle dysmorphia symptoms and their relationship to self-concept and negative affect among college recreational exercisers. *Journal of Applied Sport Psychology*, 21, 262-275.

Eisler, I., & le Grange, D. (1990). Excessive exercise and anorexia nervosa. *International Journal of Eating Disorders*, 9, 377-386.

Estok, P., & Rudy, E. (1986). Physical, psychosocial, menstrual changes/risks and addiction in female marathon and nonmarathon runners. *Health Care for Women International*, 7, 187-202.

Fairburn, C.G. (1985). Cognitive-behavioral treatment for bulimia. In D.M. Garner & P.E. Garfinkel (Eds.), *Handbook of psychotherapy for anorexia nervosa and bulimia* (pp. 160-192). New York: Guilford Press.

Fairburn, C.G., & Bohn, K. (2005). Eating disorders NOS (EDNOS): An example of troublesome "not otherwise specified" (NOS) category in DSM-IV. *Behaviour Research and Therapy*, 43, 691-701.

Fairburn, C.G., Cooper, Z., & Shafran, R. (2003). Cognitive behavior therapy for eating disorders: A transdiagnostic theory and treatment. *Behavior Research and Treatment*, 41, 509-528.

Fichter, M.M., Herpertz, S., Quadflieg, N., & Herpertz-Dahlmann, B. (1998). Structured interview for anorexia and bulimic disorders for DSM-IV and ICD-10: Updated (third) revision. *International Journal of Eating Disorders*, 24, 227-249.

Fox, K.R. (1999). The influence of physical activity on mental well-being. *Public Health Nutrition*, 2, 411-418.

Garner, D.M. (1991). *The Eating Disorder Inventory-2 professional manual*. Odesa, FL: Psychological Assessment Resources.

Garner, D.M. (2002). Measurement of eating disorder psychopathology. In C.G. Fairburn & K.D. Brownell (Eds.), *Eating disorders and obesity: A comprehensive handbook* (2nd ed.) (pp. 141-150). New York: Guilford.

Garner, D.M., Olmsted, M.P., Bohr, Y., & Garfinkle, P.E. (1982). The eating attitudes test: Psychometric features and clinical correlates. *Psychological Medicine*, 12, 184-187.

Gearhardt, A.N., Corbin, W.R., & Brownell, K.D. (2009). Preliminary validation of the Yale food addiction scale. *Appetite*, 52, 430-436.

Ghaderi, A., & Scott, B. (2002). The preliminary reliability and validity of the Survey for Eating Disorders (SEDs): A self-report questionnaire for diagnosing eating disorders. *European Eating Disorders Review*, 10, 61-76.

Glasser, W. (1976). *Positive addiction.* New York: Harper & Row.

Gormally, J., Black, S., Daston, S., & Rardin, D. (1982). The assessment of binge eating severity among obese persons. *Addictive Behaviors*, 7, 47-55.

Gotestam, K.G., & Agras, W.S. (1995). General population-based epidemiological study of eating disorders in Norway. *International Journal of Eating Disorders*, 18, 119-126.

Grieve, F.G., Jackson, L., Reece, T., Marklin, L., & Delaney, A. (2008). Correlates of social physique anxiety in men. *Journal of Sport Behavior*, 31, 329-337.

Hadjistavropoulos, H.D., & Lawrence, B. (2007). Does anxiety about health influence eating patterns and shape-related body checking among females? *Personality and Individual Differences*, 43, 319-328.

Hagan, A., & Hausenblas, H. (2003). The relationship between exercise dependence symptoms and perfectionism. *American Journal of Health Studies*, 18, 133-137.

Hailey, B.J., & Bailey, L.A. (1982). Negative addiction in runners: A quantitative approach. *Journal of Sport Behavior*, 5, 150-154.

Halmi, K.A., Falk, J.R., & Schwartz, E. (1981). Binge-eating and vomiting: A survey of a college population. *Psychological Medicine*, 11(4), 697-706.

Hartgens, F., & Kuipers, H. (2004). Effects of androgenic-anabolic steroids in athletes. *Sports Medicine*, 34, 513-554.

Haskell, W.L. (1994). Physical/physiological/biological outcomes of physical activity. In H.A. Quinney,

L. Gauvin, & A.E.T. Wall (Eds.), *Toward active living: Proceedings of the International Conference on Physical Activity, Fitness, and Health* (pp. 17-24). Champaign, IL: Human Kinetics.

Hausenblas, H.A., Cook, B.J., & Chittester, N.I. (2008). Can exercise treat eating disorders?, *Exercise and Sport Sciences Reviews*, 36, 43-47.

Hausenblas, H.A., & Fallon, E.A. (2006). Exercise and body image: A meta-analysis. *Psychology and Health*, 21, 33-47.

Hausenblas, H.A., & Symons Downs, D. (2002a). Exercise dependence: A systematic review. *Psychology of Sport and Exercise*, 3, 89-123.

Hausenblas, H.A., & Symons Downs, D. (2002b). How much is too much? The development and validation of the exercise dependence scale. *Psychology and Health*, 17, 387-404.

Hay, P.J., & Fairburn, C.G. (1998). The validity of the DSM-IV scheme for classifying bulimic eating disorders. *International Journal of Eating Disorders*, 23, 7-15.

Health Officers Council of British Columbia. (2005). *A public health approach to drug control in Canada*. Victoria, British Columbia: Public Health Association of British Columbia.

Hebebrand, J., Casper, R., Treasure, J., & Schweiger, U. (2004). The need to revise the diagnostic criteria for anorexia nervosa. *Journal of Neural Transmission*, 111, 827-840.

Herzog, D.B., & Delinsky, S. (2001). Classification of eating disorders. In R.H. Striegel-Moore & L. Smolak (Eds.), *Eating disorders: Innovations in research, treatment, and prevention* (pp. 31-50). Washington, D.C.: American Psychological Association.

Holm-Denoma, J.M., Scaringi, V., Gordon, K.H., Van Orden, K.A., & Joiner, T.E. (2009). Eating disorder symptoms among undergraduate varsity athletes, club athletes, independent exercisers, and non-exercisers. *International Journal of Eating Disorders*, 42, 47-53.

Jacobi, C., Hayward, C., de Zwaan, M., Kraemer, H.C., & Agras, W.S. (2004). Coming to terms with risk factors for eating disorders: Application of risk terminology and suggestions for a general taxonomy. *Psychological Bulletin*, 130, 19-65.

Jansen, A. (2001). Toward effective treatment of eating disorders: Nothing is as practical as a good theory. *Behavior Research and Therapy*, 39, 1007-1022.

Kanayama, G., Pope, H.G. Jr., & Hudson, J.I. (2001). "Body image" drugs: A growing psychosomatic problem. *Psychotherapy and Psychosomatics*, 70, 61-65.

Katz, J.L. (1996). Clinical observations on the physical activity of anorexia nervosa. In W.F. Epling & W.D. Pierce (Eds.), *Activity anorexia: Theory, research, and treatment.* Mahwah, NJ: Lawrence Erlbaum Associates.

Kline, T.J.B., Franken, R.E., & Rowland, G.L. (1994). A psychometric evaluation of the Exercise Salience Scale. *Personality and Individual Differences*, 16, 509-511.

Klump, K.L., Bulik, C.M., Kaye, W.H., & Treasure, J. (2009). Academy for eating disorders position paper: Eating disorders are serious mental illnesses. *International Journal of Eating Disorders*, 42, 97-103.

Kostanski, M., Fisher, A., & Gullone, E. (2004). Current conceptualization of body image dissatisfaction: Have we got it wrong? *Journal of Child Psychology and Psychiatry*, 45, 1317-1325.

Kostanski, M., & Gullone, E. (1998). Adolescent body image dissatisfaction: Relationships with self-esteem, anxiety, and depression controlling for body mass. *Journal of Child Psychology and Psychiatry*, 39, 255-262.

Kreider, R.B. (1999). Dietary supplements and the promotion of muscle growth with resistance exercise. *Sports Medicine*, 27, 97-110.

Kreslestein, M. (1983). Is running an analogue of anorexia nervosa? *New England Journal of Medicine*, 309, 48.

Kuennen, M.R., & Waldren, J.J. (2007). Relationships between specific personality traits, fat free mass indices, and the Muscle Dysmorphia Inventory. *Journal of Sports Behavior*, 30, 453-470.

Kutlesic, V., Williamson, D.A., Gleaves, D.H., & Barbin, J.M. (1998). The interview for the diagnosis of eating disorders-IV: Application to DSM-IV diagnostic criteria. *Psychological Assessment*, 10, 41-48.

Landers, D.M., & Arent, S.M. (2001). Physical activity and mental health. In R.N. Singer, H.A. Hausenblas, & C.M. Janelle (Ed.), *Handbook of sport psychology* (2nd ed.) (pp. 740-765). New York: Wiley.

Larsen, K.D. (1983). Is running an analogue of anorexia nervosa? *New England Journal of Medicine*, 309, 47.

Lejoyeaux, M., Avril, M., Richoux, C., Embouazza, H., & Nivoli, F. (2008). Prevalence of exercise dependence and other behavioral addictions among clients of a Parisian fitness room. *Comprehensive Psychiatry*, 49, 353-358.

Leone, J. (2009). MUSCLE dysmorphia symptomatology and extreme drive for muscularity in a 23-year-old woman: A case study. *Journal of Strength and Conditioning*, 23, 988-995.

Levine, M.P., & Smolak, L. (2006). *The prevention of eating disorders: Theory, research, and practice.* Mahwah, NJ: Erlbaum.

Levitt, D.H. (2008). Participation in athletic activities and eating disordered behavior. *Eating Disorders*, 16, 393-404.

Lewinsohn, P.M., Seeley, J.R., Moerk, K.C., & Striegel-Moore, R.H. (2002). Gender differences in eating disorder symptoms in young adults. *International Journal of Eating Disorders*, 32, 426-440.

Lippi, G., Franchini, M., Favaloro, E.J., & Targher, G. (2010). Moderate red wine consumption and cardiovascular disease risk: Beyond the "French paradox." *Seminars in Thrombosis and Hemostasis*, 36, 59-70.

Loumidis, K., & Wells, A. (1998). Assessment of beliefs in exercise dependence: The development and preliminary validation of the exercise beliefs questionnaire. *Personality and Individual Differences*, 25, 553-567.

Maloney, M.J., McGuire, J.B., & Daniels, S.R. (1988). Reliability testing of a children's version of the eating attitudes test. *Journal of the American Academy of Child and Adolescent Psychiatry*, 27, 541-543.

Mazure, C.M., Halmi, K.A., Sunday, S.R., Romano, S.J., & Einhorn, A.M. (1994). The Yale-Brown-Cornell eating disorder scale: Development, use, reliability, and validity. *Journal of Psychiatric Research*, 28, 425-445.

McCabe, M.P., & Ricciardelli, L.A. (2004a). A longitudinal study of pubertal timing and extreme body change behaviors among adolescent boys and girls. *Adolescence*, 39, 145-166.

Mehler, P.S., & Krantz, M. (2003). Anorexia nervosa medical issues. *Journal of Women's Health*, 12, 331-340.

Meyer, C., Taranis, L., & Touyz, S. (2008). Excessive exercise in the eating disorders: A need for less activity from patients and more from researchers. *European Eating Disorders Review*, 16, 81-83.

Mitchell, J.E., Cook-Myers, T., & Wonderlich, S.A. (2005). Diagnostic criteria for anorexia nervosa: Looking ahead to DSM-V. *International Journal of Eating Disorders*, 37, S95-S97.

Mond, J.M., Hay, P.J., Rodgers, B., & Owen, C. (2006). An update on the definition of "excessive exercise" in eating disorders research. *International Journal of Eating Disorders*, 39, 147-153.

Mond, J.M., Rodgers, B., Hay, P.J., Owens, C., & Beaumont, P.J.V. (2004). Relationship between exercise behaviour, eating disordered behaviour and quality of life in a community sample of women: When is exercise "excessive"? *European Eating Disorders Review*, 12, 265-272.

Morgan, W.P. (1979). *Physical activity and mental health.* Washington D.C.: Taylor & Francis.

Morrow, J., & Harvey, P. (1990). Exermania! *American Health*, 9, 31-32.

Murray, S.B., Maguire, S., Russell, J., & Touyz, S. (2012). The emotional regulatory features of bulimic episodes and compulsive exercise in muscle dysmorphia: A case report. *European Eating Disorders Review*, 20(1), 68-73.

Ogden, J., Veale, D., & Summers, Z. (1997). The development and validation of the exercise dependence questionnaire. *Addiction Research*, 5(4), 343-356.

Olrich, T.W., & Ewing, M.E. (1999). Life on steroids: Bodybuilders describe their perceptions of the anabolic-androgenic steroid use period. *The Sports Psychologist*, 13, 299-312.

Paluska, S.A., & Schwenk, T.L. (2000). Physical activity and mental health. *Sports Medicine*, 29, 167-180.

Pasman, L., & Thompson, J. K. (1988). Body image and eating disturbance in obligatory runners, obligatory weightlifters, and sedentary individuals. *International Journal of Eating Disorders, 7,* 759-769.

Pearson, J., Goldklang, D., & Streigel-Moore, R. (2002). Prevention of eating disorders: Challenges and opportunities. *International Journal of Eating Disorders*, 31, 233-239.

Peñas-Lledó, E.F., Leal, V., & Waller, G. (2002). Excessive exercise in anorexia nervosa and bulimia nervosa: Relation to eating characteristics and general psychopathology. *International Journal of Eating Disorders*, 31, 370-375.

Pope, H.G., Gruber, A.J., Choi, P., Olivardia, R., & Phillips, K.A. (1997). Muscle dysmorphia. An underrecognised form of body dysmorphia disorder. *Psychosomatics*, 38, 548-557.

Pope, H.G. Jr., Katz, D.L., & Hudson, J.I. (1993). Anorexia nervosa and "reverse anorexia" among 108 male bodybuilders. *Comprehensive Psychiatry*, 34, 406-409.

Pope, H.G. Jr., Phillips, K.A., & Olivardia, R. (2000). *The Adonis complex: The secret crisis of male body obsession.* New York: The Free Press.

Powers, P.S., Schocken, D.D., & Boyd, F.R. (1998). Comparison of habitual runners and anorexia nervosa patients. *International Journal of Eating Disorders*, 23, 133-143.

Presnell, K., Bearman, S.K., & Stice, E. (2004). Risk factors for body dissatisfaction in adolescent boys and girls: A prospective study. *International Journal of Eating Disorders*, 36, 389-401.

Shroff, H., Reba, L., Thornton, L.M., Tozzi, F., Klump, K., Berrettini, W.H., et al. (2006). Features associated with excessive exercise in women with eating disorders. *International Journal of Eating Disorders*, 39, 454-461.

Slade, P.D., & Dewey, M. (1986). Development and preliminary validation of SCANS: A screening instrument for identifying individuals at risk of developing anorexia and bulimia nervosa. *International Journal of Eating Disorders*, 5, 517-538.

Sloan, D.M., Mizes, J.S., & Epstein, E.M. (2005). Empirical classification of eating disorders. *Eating Behaviors*, 6, 53-62.

Smith, D., & Hale, B. (2004). Validity and factor structure of the bodybuilding dependence scale. *British Journal of Sports Medicine*, 38, 177-181.

Smith, D.K., Hale, B.D., & Collins, D. (1998). Measurement of exercise dependence in bodybuilders. *Journal of Sports Medicine and Physical Activity*, 38, 66-74.

Sobel, S.V. (2004). Eating disorders. *Continuing Medical Education Resource*, 118, 69-114.

Solenberger, S. (2001). Exercise and eating disorders: A 3-year inpatient hospital record analysis. *Eating Behavior*, 2, 151-168.

Spitzer, R.L., Devlin, M., Walsh, B.T., Hasin, D., Wing, R., Marcus, M., et al. (1992a). Binge eating disorder: A multi-site field trial of the diagnostic criteria. *International Journal of Eating Disorders*, 11, 191-203.

Spitzer, R.L., Williams, J.B., Gibbon, M., & First, M.B. (1992b). The Structured Clinical Interview for DSM-III-R (SCID). I: History, rationale, and description. *Archives of General Psychiatry, 49,* 624-629.

Standridge, J.B., Zylstra, G., & Adams, S.M. (2004). Alcohol consumption: An overview of benefits and risks. *Southern Medical Journal*, 97, 664-672.

Stice, E. (2002). Risk and maintenance factors for eating pathology: A meta-analytic review. *Psychological Bulletin*, 128, 825-848.

Stice, E., Telch, C.F., & Rizvi, S.L. (2000). Development and validation of the eating disorder di-agnostic scale: A brief self-report measure of anorexia, bulimia, and binge-eating disorder. *Psychological Assessment*, 12, 123-131.

Streigel-Moore, R., & Bulik, C. (2007). Risk factors for eating disorders. *American Psychologist, 62*, 181-198.

Stunkard, A.J., & Messick, S. (1985). The three factor eating questionnaire to measure dietary restraint, disinhibition, and hunger. *Journal of Psychosomatic Research*, 29, 71-83.

Szabo, A. (1995). The impact of exercise deprivation on well-being of habitual exercisers. *The Australian Journal of Science and Medicine in Sport*, 27, 68-75.

Szabo, A. (2000). Physical activity and psychological dysfunction. In S. Biddle, K. Fox, & S. Boutcher (Eds.), *Physical activity and psychological well-being* (pp. 130-153). London: Routledge.

Taylor, A.H. (2003). Physical activity, anxiety, and stress. In S.J.H. Biddle, K.R. Fox, & S.H. Boutcher (Eds.), *Physical activity, mental health, and psychological well-being* (pp. 10-45). London: Routledge & Kegan Paul.

Terry, A., Szabo, A., & Griffiths, M.D. (2004). The exercise addiction inventory: A new brief screening tool. *Addiction Research and Theory*, 12, 489-499.

Thelen, M.H., & Farmer, J. (1991). A revision of the bulimia test: The BULIT-R. Psychological Assessment: A Journal of Consulting and Clinical Psychology, *3*, 119-124.

Thome, J.L., & Espelage, D.L. (2007). Obligatory exercise and eating pathology in college females: Replication and development of a structural model. *Eating Behaviors*, 8, 334-349.

Thompson, J.K., Heinberg, L.J., Altabe, M., & Tantleff-Dunn, S. (1999). *Exacting beauty. Theory, assessment, and treatment of body image disturbance.* Washington, D.C.: American Psychological Association.

U.S. Department of Health and Human Services. (2008). 2008 physical activity guidelines for Americans. Available: www.health.gov/paguidelines/guidelines/default.aspx.

van Strien, T., Frijters, J.E.R., Bergers, G.P.A., & Defares, P.B. (1986). The Dutch eating behaviour questionnaire (DEBQ) for assessment of restrained, emotional, and external eating behaviour. *International Journal of Eating Disorders*, 5, 295-315.

Varnado-Sullivan, P.J., Horton, R., & Savoy, S. (2006). Differences for gender, weight and exercise in body image disturbance and eating disorder symptoms. *Eating and Weight Disorders*, 11, 118-125.

Veale, D. (1995). Does primary exercise dependence really exist? In J. Annett, B. Cripps, & H. Steinberg (Eds.), *Exercise addiction: Motivation for participation in sport and exercise* (pp. 1-5). Leicester: British Psychological Society.

Vincent, M.A., McCabe, M.P., & Ricciardelli, L.A. (1999). Factorial validity of the Bulimia Test-revised in adolescent boys and girls. *Behaviour Research and Therapy*, 37, 1129-1140.

von Ranson, K.M., Klump, K.L., Iacono, W.G., & McGue, M. (2005). The Minnesota Eating Behavior Survey: A brief measure of disordered eating attitudes and behaviors. *Eating Behaviors*, 6, 373-392.

Walsh, B.T. (2004). The future of research on eating disorders. *Appetite*, 42, 5-10.

Walsh, B.T. (2009). Eating disorders in DSM-V: Review of existing literature (Part 1). *International Journal of Eating Disorders*, 42, 579-580.

Williamson, D.A., Davis, C.J., Goreczmy, A.J., Bennett, S.M., & Watkins, P.C. (1989). The Eating Questionnaire-Revised: A new symptom checklist for bulimia. In P.A. Keller & L.G. Ritt (Eds.), *Innovations in clinical practice: A sourcebook* (pp. 321-326). Sarasota, FL: Professional Resource Exchange.

Williamson, D.A., Gleaves, D.H., & Steward, T.M. (2005). Categorical versus dimensional models of eating disorders: An examination of the evidence. *International Journal of Eating Disorders*, 37, 1-10.

Yates, A., Leehey, K., & Shisslak, C.M. (1983). Running—An analogue of anorexia? *New England Journal of Medicine*, 308, 251-255.

Zmijewski, C.F., & Howard, M.O. (2003). Exercise dependence and attitudes toward eating among young adults. *Eating Behaviors*, 4, 181-195.

Recommendations for Research, Policy and Practice

Angela Clow, PhD
University of Westminster, London, United Kingdom

Sarah Edmunds, PhD
University of Westminster, London, United Kingdom

The evidence discussed in this text demonstrates strong relationships between physical activity, well-being and mental health. These relationships have impact at both the population and clinical levels. For example, at the population level, social gradients in physical activity are associated with health inequalities, and decreased physical activity with age is associated with accelerated aging. In addition, physical activity can help buffer the negative effects of stress and has been shown to benefit those with conditions such as schizophrenia, addiction, depression or dementia. Physical activity has broad applications and few negative side effects and should be available to all in one form or another. Despite this awareness, physical activity remains a largely untapped resource.

This text makes the case that population-level increases in physical activity promote well-being and have the potential to shift more people away from clinically diagnosed mental health conditions toward the flourishing end of the mental health continuum. At the same time, physical activity can be used to manage clinical conditions. In other words, physical activity can be used in the prevention, treatment and management of ill mental health.

Accordingly, this book reviews in detail the evidence of a relationship between physical activity and mental health in the general population as well as in older adults and those with mental health conditions, addictions and long-term physical health conditions. Evidence-based guidelines provide recommendations for the type and amount of physical activity that are necessary to promote physical health and well-being in the general population. However, debate still exists about the optimal type and amount of physical activity for people with mental health conditions and other psychologically vulnerable individuals, such as older people and those with long-term conditions. As a result, the benefits of physical activity for mental health are often neglected in national physical activity guidelines and by mental health practitioners. Intensity, duration, frequency and type of physical activity all potentially influence the relationship between physical activity and mental health. Research is beginning to explore how these factors affect well-being in people with those mental health conditions as well as in the general population. Some emerging evidence suggests that higher-intensity and resistance exercise are particularly beneficial. However, there is still much more to learn in this area.

Physical limitations and poor motivation are significant barriers to physical activity for many groups. Motivation for physical activity is not the focus of this text. However, we need to better understand how to help as many people as possible tap into physical activity as a resource for well-being. Those with low mental health have the most to gain but may be the hardest to motivate. One thing that emerges from the evidence presented in this text is that doing any physical activity is better than doing none in terms of quality of life and mental health. Getting started is the most important thing. Even small increases in levels of activity and the associated factors (e.g., increased social interaction) can generate a chain of events that improve well-being and reinforce the motivation to continue and gain the maximum benefits that physical activity can confer (see figure 1.4 in chapter 1).

Longitudinal studies show that maintaining high levels of physical activity over several years has a positive impact on mental health and well-being. However, the majority of exercise-intervention programmes described in the research literature run over a set period of weeks or months and have a fixed end point. Some studies include long-term follow-up measures, typically 6 months or 1 year after the intervention ended. However, due to practical limitations and funding issues, little if any research using a randomised controlled design explores the impact of supervised exercise programmes over a period of several years on mental health outcomes. Understanding the impact of longer-term physical activity interventions would be useful, and these studies might be more relevant to practitioners who work with patients over a period of years than the type of short-term intervention frequently described in research papers.

The physiological underpinnings of the relationship between physical activity and mental health are becoming better understood. However, there is still a long way to go in understanding the complex physiological systems that are affected by physical activity and the interaction of these systems with social and environmental factors. Research should further investigate the role of stress as a mediator between physical activity and mental health problems.

1 Recommendations for Priorities in Future Research

Accurately measuring physical activity is challenging. Chapter 3 describes in detail the issues of this area. Advances in technology are leading to the development of objective physical activity monitors that provide accurate and valid data yet are small enough that participants accept wearing them for several days. Furthermore, the cost of these devices is decreasing to a level where research groups can purchase a sufficient number and conduct relatively large-scale studies using objective physical activity measurement. Future research should focus on accurately assessing physical activity and should use this assessment to understand the relationship between mental health and well-being in more detail in both the general and mental health populations. People with dementia, depression or schizophrenia may find it particularly difficult to accurately recall their physical activity. It will be particularly important to gather data from these groups using objective measurement devices.

More longitudinal studies need to investigate the direction of causality between physical activity and mental health. These should be carefully controlled, use objective measures and have long-term follow-up and be conducted separately for each mental health condition. Future research should also explore the experience of physical activity at an individual level. Research into the effect of short bursts of physical activity on mood has shown that emotional responses to physical activity differ from individual to individual. Exploring these varied individual responses qualitatively, and perhaps using biological markers, would be a useful alternative approach to understanding interacting mechanisms and may inform optimal physical activity recommendations for different subpopulations. This approach would also provide an alternative means of exploring the interacting systems that underpin the relationship between physical activity and mental health (e.g., the contribution of genotype, social factors or being in a green environment).

Better methodologies are needed to evaluate physical activity programmes that are ongoing in the community. Practitioners are doing a lot of good work to develop long-term programmes that go unevaluated, and researchers put a lot of effort into developing short-term programmes that are often effective but are not maintained or replicated due to funding constraints. All this work must be captured to build the evidence base and provide a resource for practitioners so that they can replicate good practice and produce maximum benefit.

2 Recommendations for Policy Development

Physical activity guidelines for physical health and well-being exist in many developed countries and some developing ones. However, implementing these guidelines remains a challenge in many places. The guidelines are often not publicised as widely as they could be and are not accompanied by strategies that help translate policy into practice and help people become physically active. At present, the evidence is not strong enough to enable the development of physical activity guidelines for people with specific mental health conditions, but this may change as this evidence base develops.

Policy makers should target health practitioners who care for people with mental health problems. All health practitioners should be fully informed about the benefits of physical activity for mental health. Targeting the physical activity behaviour of practitioners may be a time- and cost-effective way of getting the message out there because practitioners who personally experience the benefits of physical activity and believe in its positive effect are likely to be more motivated to promote it to their patients and be more persuasive in doing so.

3 Recommendations for Daily Practice

Practitioners are on the front line and should be active themselves. In addition, practitioners should keep abreast of the developments in understanding how the intensity, frequency, duration and type of physical activity affect mental health and well-being outcomes and adapt exercise-intervention programmes accordingly. In addition, they should encourage patients to become physically active and make lifestyle choices that are practical and feasible to maintain in the long term.

In a small number of individuals exercise becomes problematic. Exercise dependence and overtraining are examples of problems that can occur. Exercise practitioners should be aware of these conditions and look out for any signs or symptoms of them in the people they work with. However, the existence of these conditions should not sway practitioners to ignore the overwhelming evidence that physical activity is a force for good.

Index

Note: The italicized *f* and *t* following page numbers refer to figures and tables, respectively.

About the Editors

Angela Clow, PhD, is a professor of psychophysiology in the department of psychology at the University of Westminster (London, United Kingdom). She also serves as the head of the department of psychology and leader of the psychophysiology and stress research group. Clow has garnered international acclaim for her research in the biological foundations of mental health. In 2002 she received the National Teaching Fellowship Award.

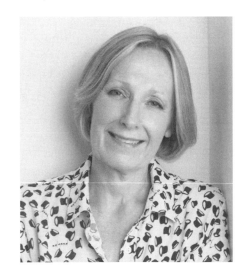

Sarah Edmunds, PhD, is a research fellow in the department of psychology at the University of Westminster. Edmunds is a BPS-chartered psychologist and HCPC-registered sport and exercise psychologist. She is well regarded as both a researcher and teacher in sport and exercise psychology.

As research partners, Clow and Edmunds combine their expertise in the areas of mental health and sport and exercise psychology to bring unique insight to the exploration of the connections between physical activity and mental health.

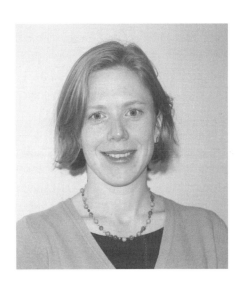

About the Contributors

F. Hülya Aşçı, PhD, is director of the sport sciences department of Başkent University in Ankara, Turkey, where she studies physical self-perception and psychological effects of physical activity on psychological well-being. She earned her bachelor's degree in physical education and sport from Middle East Technical University in 1991. Dr. Aşçı received her MS degree in sport psychology and PhD in guidance and counseling in 1993 and 1998, respectively. She has presented papers at international and national congresses and published articles in refereed international journals such as *Journal of Sport and Exercise Psychology*, *International Journal of Sport Psychology*, and *Psychology of Sport and Exercise*, the latter of which she is an associate editor. She received the Best Educator Award for the 1998-1999 academic year while working in the physical education and sports department of Middle East Technical University. Recently she received the Developing Scholar Award from the International Society of Sport Psychology.

Adrian Bauman, PhD, is the sesquicentenary professor of public health and director of the Prevention Research Collaboration at the University of Sydney, Australia. Dr. Bauman has research interests in prevention of chronic disease, with a longstanding focus on physical activity epidemiology and interventions to promote physical activity. He directs the WHO Collaborating Centre on Physical Activity, Nutrition and Obesity and has assisted in the development of national physical activity policies and strategies in many countries. He is extensively published in the peer-reviewed literature (H index 57) and has secured several millions of dollars in research funds since 2004. Recent interests include the epidemiology and public health aspects of inactivity and sitting time, and translation and upscaling of physical activity programs to the population level.

Fiona Bull, PhD, is codirector of the Loughborough University and University of Western Australia British Heart Foundation National Centre for Physical Activity and Health and is professor of physical activity and public health. She earned a PhD in physical activity and public health from the University of Western Australia (1997), MSc in sport science from Loughborough University (1990) and a BEd with honors from Exeter University (1988). Before joining Loughborough in 2004, Dr. Bull worked at the U.S. Departments of Health and Social Security in the Centers for Disease Control and Prevention, the World Health Organization in Geneva and the school of public health and the school of human movement and exercise science at the University of Western Australia. Dr. Bull continues to play an active role in international work, specifically in the comparison and measurement of physical activity, the development of national policy on physical activity and the establishment of the Global Alliance on Physical Activity in 2005.

Brian Cook, PhD, teaches courses in sport and exercise psychology, history of sport and physical education and nutrition and fitness at the Neuropsychiatric Research Institute. He received his PhD in exercise physiology in relation to eating disorders from the University of Florida in 2010. Before that, he earned a BA in psychology and an MS in exercise psychology. His research interests are quality of life, body image and eating disorders, and exercise during pregnancy and the postpartum period. He, along with coauthor Heather Hausenblas, has authored a number of research articles, chapters and manuscripts in this area.

Amanda Daley, PhD, is a senior lecturer in health psychology at the University of Birmingham and holds a National Institute for Health Research Senior Research Fellowship award. Her PhD focussed on the mental health benefits of regular physical activity. She has completed a number of trials in this area in both healthy and clinical populations. Dr. Daley has a particular research interest in depression and postnatal depression. She has published widely in this field and has served on the editorial boards of several related journals.

Guy Faulkner, PhD, is an assistant professor of physical education and health at the University of Toronto and coordinates the activities of the exercise psychology unit. After completing a PhD in exercise psychology in 2001 at Loughborough University, Dr. Faulkner worked for 3 years as director of the exercise and sport psychology unit at the University of Exeter in England. He has a cross-appointment with the Institute for Human Development, Life Course and Aging and is a mentor with the Canadian Institutes of Health Research Strategic Training Program in Tobacco Research, an investigator with the Ontario Tobacco Research Unit, and a research affiliate of the Alberta Centre for Active Living. He is also a member of the editorial board of *Psychology of Sport and Exercise*. His current research concerns the physical health needs of users of mental health services in relation to antipsychotic medication, weight gain, diabetes and medication compliance; mediated health messages; and the role of physical activity in harm reduction and smoking cessation.

Paul Gorczynski is pursuing his doctoral studies at the University of Toronto under the supervision of Guy Faulkner. He plans to examine the effects of motivational interviewing, a behaviour modification intervention, on increasing physical activity and improving dietary habits in order to decrease adiposity of obese individuals with schizophrenia who are taking antipsychotic medication.

Mark Hamer, PhD, is a senior research fellow based in the epidemiology and public health division of population health at University College London. He studied sport and exercise at undergraduate and graduate levels and has a PhD in physical activity and health from De Montfort University. Since 2007 at University College London he has carried out seminal research, sponsored by the British Heart Foundation, using the Health Surveys for England and Scotland and the English Longitudinal Study of Ageing. His work involved innovative analyses relating to psychosocial stress, physical activity and health. Since 2008 he has served as first author of more than 60 papers and has authored a total of more than 90 papers. Dr. Hamer was awarded a grant by the National Prevention Research Initiative for studying physical activity and mortality risk in South Asians in the United Kingdom.

Heather Hausenblas, PhD, is director of the exercise psychology laboratory at the University of Florida. She has taught courses in exercise psychology and has conducted research on the psychological effects of physical activity in a variety of special populations. Dr. Hausenblas has extensive research experience and has published more than 70 peer-reviewed journal articles. In 2006 she received the University of Florida Research Foundation Professorship. Dr. Hausenblas' key research area is the cognitive, behavioral and affective components of body image and eating and their relationship to exercise in special populations (e.g., eating-disordered patients, overweight women, pregnant women and exercise-dependent people).

Goran Kenttä, PhD, has a passion for building bridges between the domains of sport psychology research, education and applied work in elite sports. He earned his doctorate in psychology at Stockholm University in 2001. The majority of his research and publications have focussed on elite-level athletes and the training process with a stress–recovery perspective. He has an extensive coaching background with various national and club teams in flatwater sprint kayaking. Over the years Dr. Kenttä has been involved with both the Swedish Olympic Committees and the Swedish National Sport Federation and several Olympic sports in order to develop strategies for psychological support for elite athletes and coaches. Dr. Kenttä holds a research position at the Swedish School of Sport and Health Sciences in Stockholm and is a director of the coach education program at the university; he is also the past president of the Swedish Sport Psychological Association.

Magnus Lindwall, PhD, is a research fellow at the University of Gothenburg in Sweden, where his primary research interest is the relationship between physical activity, exercise, and training and mental health (exercise psychology). He has also conducted research into psychometrics, focussing on using advanced statistical models (e.g., structural equation modelling) to evaluate self-assessment instruments in sport and health psychology. In recent years he has focussed on the relationship between physical activity and psychological health (including depression and cognition) in the elderly and has worked with data from both large, longitudinal, epidemiological studies and intervention studies. The focus for his postdoctoral research is the relationship between lifestyle, physical activity and psychological health in the elderly.

Juan Tortosa Martinez, PhD, works at the Clínica Mediterranea de Neurociencias in Alicante, Spain, where he is responsible for implementing physical activity programmes for patients with various mental and physical health problems. Dr. Martinez is an assistant professor in physical activity and sport sciences at the University of Alicante and teaches public employees in psychiatric institutions about the benefits of physical activity and recreation programmes for mental health. His current research projects include conducting physical activity programmes for people with mild cognitive impairment, dementia and severe mental health problems such as schizophrenia and bipolar disorder.

Juan M. Murias, PhD, is a postdoctoral fellow in the exercise biochemistry laboratory at the University of Western Ontario, researching vascular adaptations to exercise training in healthy and clinical populations. After completing studies in physical education and exercise physiology in Buenos Aires, Argentina, Dr. Murias moved to Canada where he completed a PhD in the Cardiovascular Exercise Laboratory in the Canadian Centre for Activity and Aging at the University of Western Ontario. This work focussed on central and peripheral cardiovascular adaptations to exercise training interventions in older and young individuals.

Donald H. Paterson, PhD, is a professor in the school of kinesiology (faculty of health sciences) and is research director of the Canadian Centre for Activity and Aging. Over the years his research has focussed on cardiorespiratory responses to exercise, initially with emphasis on the cardiovascular system and respiratory function and more recently on muscle metabolism. At the same time his research has focussed on population groups and, since 1988, on understanding the exercise responses and limitations of older adults and the relationships of fitness to health and overall well-being of older adults. His recently published papers extensively review the evidence regarding the best guidelines and recommendations for physical activities (exercise programmes) for maintaining health and independence in older adults. Dr. Paterson has been an invited speaker at exercise physiology conferences and international gerontology meetings in Canada, the United States, Japan, Australia and Brazil. He also has served as president and treasurer of the Canadian Association of Sport Sciences (now Canadian Society for Exercise Physiology), performs reviews for granting agencies and journals and has participated in government and agency task groups.

John S. Raglin, PhD, is a professor in the department of kinesiology at the Indiana University School of Public Health in Bloomington. His work addresses the interaction between psychological and biological processes as they apply to various phenomena in exercise and sport. Dr. Raglin's research interests include the influence of physical activity on mental health in recreational exercisers and athletes, emotions in sport and the influence of perceptual factors on pacing in endurance sport tasks. He is a fellow of the American College of Sports Medicine, American Psychological Association and American Academy of Kinesiology.

Natalie Taylor, PhD, has been working as a project manager and senior research fellow at Bradford Institute for Health Research since March 2011. She completed her PhD at the Institute of Psychological Sciences at the University of Leeds in 2010. Dr. Taylor has expertise in physical activity and its measurement; she developed the online measure of physical activity (OSWEQ). Dr. Taylor develops and tests theoretically informed interventions for the improvement of a range of health behaviours and works with NHS services to promote physical activity using behaviour change strategies. As part of her role as a fellow in honorary research in the Institute of Psychological Sciences at the University of Leeds, she coordinates and delivers a CPD course for health care professionals that aids in developing knowledge and skills for using evidence of behaviour change in practice.

Michael Ussher, PhD, is a senior lecturer in psychology at St. George's University of London, where he specialises in health psychology, physical activity promotion and smoking cessation. He is the chief investigator on a National Institute for Health Research–funded multisite randomised control trial assessing whether a physical activity intervention helps women quit smoking during pregnancy and postpartum.

Gregory Wilson, PED, FACSM, is a professor and chair of the department of exercise science at the University of Evansville in Indiana. He received his doctorate and master's degrees from Indiana University. Dr. Wilson has numerous publications in exercise and sport psychology, covering topics such as health behaviors of college students and overtraining and staleness in athletes. He has edited two textbooks, *Exploring Exercise Science* and *Applying Sport Psychology: Four Perspectives*. He is a fellow of the American College of Sports Medicine and a member of the Psychobiological Interest Group of ACSM.

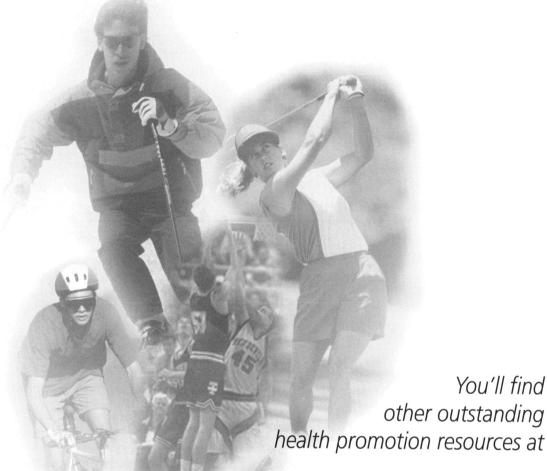

*You'll find
other outstanding
health promotion resources at*

www.HumanKinetics.com

In the U.S. call

1-800-747-4457

Australia...08 8372 0999
Canada 1-800-465-7301
Europe..+44 (0) 113 255 5665
New Zealand...0800 222 062

HUMAN KINETICS
The Information Leader in Physical Activity & Health
P.O. Box 5076 • Champaign, IL 61825-5076 USA